Anthropometric Standards for the Assessment of Growth and Nutritional Status

Anthropometric Standards for the Assessment of Growth and Nutritional Status

A. Roberto Frisancho

A. Roberto Frisancho is a research scientist at the Center for Human Growth and Development and professor of biological anthropology at the University of Michigan.

Ann Arbor

The University of Michigan Press

1993   1992   1991   1990   4   3   2   1

Library of Congress Cataloging-in-Publication Data

Frisancho, A. Roberto, 1939–
    Anthropometric standards for the assessment of growth and
nutritional status / A. Roberto Frisancho.
        p.   cm.
    Includes bibliographical references.
    ISBN 0-472-10146-3
    1. Nutrition.   2. Malnutrition.   3. Anthropometry.   I. Title.
    [DNLM: 1. Anthropometry—methods.   2. Growth—tables.
3. Nutritional Status—tables.   QU 16 F917a]
TX345.F66   1989
612.6′ 00287—dc20
DNLM/DLC
for Library of Congress   89-20695
                                                                    CIP

Preface

Anthropometric techniques have become indispensable instruments for the evaluation of the nutritional and health status of children and adults. It is a general truism that the reference point determines the extent to which a given measurement can be considered to be within the normal range. An anthropometric reference that is derived from a restricted sample will provide a narrower range of variability than one that is based upon samples that include a wide spectrum of the population. Therefore, when evaluating an individual's anthropometric status, depending on the reference used, different conclusions can be reached. In general, the larger the sample size and the more representative the sample, the better the reference. For this reason, in previous publications I have published several sets of norms of anthropometric dimensions which were based on large and representative samples from the U.S.A. Continuing this endeavor I have written this book, which is based on a sample of 43,774 subjects aged 1 to 74 years and derived from the combined samples of the first and second National Health Examination Surveys of the U.S.A. conducted during 1971–74 and 1976–80.

This book presents: (1) the theoretical rationale for the use of anthropometric dimensions in the evaluation of nutritional status; (2) a unified set of anthropometric techniques of data collection; (3) the statistical basis for the anthropometric classification of individuals or populations; (4) the anthropometric standards in tabular form giving means, standard deviations, and percentile ranges of anthropometric dimensions used in the evaluation of growth and nutritional status; (5) anthropometric reference data for blacks and whites; and (6) and anthropometric graphs that facilitate the interpretation of anthropometric data. In addition, it provides interpretation of anthropometric dimensions illustrated with practical examples.

Acknowledgments

I thank Drs. Stanley M. Garn, Victor Katch, and William Leonard for their constructive criticisms. I also thank Ms. Shelley Smith, Mr. Tom TenHave, my son Roberto Javier Frisancho, and Ms. Teryl Lynn who have assisted in the process of preparing this manuscript for publication.

Research Support

The research and preparation of this monograph was supported in part by Grant MCJ-2600560-01-0 awarded by the Division of Maternal and Child Health, Bureau of Health Care Delivery and Assistance of the U.S. Department of Health and Human Services.

Contents

I
Necessity for New
Anthropometric Standards

Assessment of anthropometric dimensions has become an indispensable approach for the assessment of nutritional status of clinical and nonclinical populations. Recently, a great deal of attention has been given to the development of standards of anthropometric dimensions. Uniform anthropometric standards are necessary, because any inferences regarding individual or population nutritional status are dependent on the standards used for comparison. For example, the same individual may be classified as obese using one set of reference values and as normal according to another set of standards. This section will discuss the anthropometric approaches currently used and the necessity for incorporating measurements of body composition in the evaluation of nutritional status of children and adults.

Children

Evaluations of growth and nutritional status are usually done with reference to height and weight. The standards used include (1) the Stuart and Stevenson's growth curves, which is based upon studies conducted during the 1950s of children from Boston and Iowa City; (2) the National Center for Health Statistics (NCHS) growth curves, which were compiled from a combined sample of data derived from the NCHS's Health Examination Surveys (HES), conducted during 1963–65 and 1970–74, and data from the Fels Research Institute; (3) the British standards of height and weight velocity published by Tanner and Davies (3).

Using these standards as a reference, investigators have determined the extent to which children are growing either normally, advanced, or delayed for their age. Furthermore, these standards are used to infer whether children are either obese or undernourished for their height. In 1977 Waterlow et al. (4) suggested that by using height and weight standards malnourished children can be classified as either stunted if they have low height-for-age, or wasted if they have low weight-for-height. While this approach has the advantage of being based upon easily obtainable measurements, it is ineffective for accurately distinguishing the truly malnourished child from the simply underweight. Protein-energy malnutrition (PEM) is characterized by a decrease in both fat and muscle tissue. Usually a child suffering from PEM will have a low weight-for-height, but a tall and normally lean child can also have a low weight-for-height. Even under conditions of chronic malnutrition a child could develop low weight-for-height without losing weight at all when gain in weight stops while gain in height continues. As indicated by Rivers (5), in Costa Rica with the introduction of situation development projects the prevalence of wasting rose because children started to gain height faster than weight. Similarly, even under conditions of famine, classifications based only on measurements of weight and height are inadequate for detecting interpopulation differences in nutritional status (5). The use of indices of weight-for-height are also inadequate for predicting mortality risk in a community. This is because the mortality associated with wasting depends on the extent of stunting: wasted and stunted children have higher risk than children who are wasted but not stunted. Therefore, *paradoxically*, low levels of wasting in a community where wasting is prevalent could indicate a higher prospective mortality than high levels of wasting in previously nonstunted children (5). Probably because of the same inaccuracy of the weight-for-height indices, the prevalence of wasting reported for the third world countries (6) was higher than that observed in regions affected by famine (5).

The ineffectiveness of the weight-for-height indices is also evident under conditions of affluence. Because obesity is characterized by excess fat, an obese child usually has a high weight-for-height; but a muscular and large-framed child can also have a high weight-for-height. In other words, excess weight does not necessarily imply excess fat, and underweight is not necessarily associated with protein-energy malnutrition. For this reason, assessment of nutritional status based only on weight and height, especially when the degree of underweight or overweight is moderate, is bound to be ineffective in distinguishing the truly wasted (i.e., low fat and muscle) from the normally low-weight child, and the truly obese from the normally heavy child. It is evident then that because of the lack of an appropriate anthropometric standard, and/or because of artifacts of sampling and statistics, evaluations of malnutrition are either grossly overestimated or underestimated (5, 7–10).

At present, there are two references that can be used for the evaluations of body composition. These include (1) the anthropometric standards for British children published by Tanner and associates (11–12) and (2) the National Center for Health Statistics (NCHS) anthropometric charts (13). The British reference provides graphs for growth in height, weight, sitting height, biacromial breadth, and skinfold thicknesses derived from investigations of British children studied before 1960 (11). These standards do not provide the age- and sex-specific sample size, means, and standard deviations of the anthropometric dimensions, which are necessary for statistical comparisons of individuals or population anthropometric nutritional status. Furthermore, because of the natural distortion of figures or graphs, determining the percentile position of an individual or population is subject to inaccuracies, especially in borderline cases. Moreover, as pointed out by Buckler (11) these "charts are only appropriate for the population from which they were derived (British children)," and the "values may not apply to populations from different regions, countries or races." On the other hand, the NCHS reference (13) does provide adequate information on skinfold thicknesses, body circumference, and body proportions of U.S. children and adults. However, because this reference is based only upon data derived from the NCHS's First Health Examination Surveys (NHANES I) conducted during 1971–1975 the sample size is small, especially when considered by one year intervals. Furthermore, this reference does not provide information on muscle size, which is important for an adequate of children's growth and nutritional data. Similarly, several studies have documented the fact that non-Western populations have different body proportions than those of Western nations (14–17).

Thus, there is a critical need for a more timely and nonpopulation-specific anthropometric standard that can permit the evaluation of growth, body proportions, and the components of overweight and underweight and hence determine the nutritional status of children.

Adults

The so-called desirable weight tables published by the Metropolitan Life Insurance Company (18–19) are often used for the evaluation of nutritional status of adults. These tables, despite their wide use, are not adequate for assessing nutritional status. It is generally assumed that a value greater than the desirable weight is synonymous with obesity. This assumption is invalid because the *desirable* weight tables do not give information on body composition, which is essential for an assessment of fatness. Indeed, lack of measurements of body composition can lead to erroneous conclusions (see fig. I.1). For example, as demonstrated by Welham and Behnke (20), a group of football players who were rejected by the armed forces for being obese actually had a low percentage of fat; the elevated weight was due to a high percentage of muscle. Similarly, recent studies (21) have compared estimates of obesity based on skinfold thickness with those estimated using weight/height indices. These studies have shown that among individuals whose weight is below the 85th percentile, overweight is not associated with a high level of subcutaneous fat. Fat and overweight are synonymous *only* among individuals whose weight exceeds the 95th percentile (21). In other words, an overweight measure cannot be equated with an obesity measure. Moreover, excess weight per se is a poor indicator of risk of heart disease. A recent study by Hubert et al. (22) reports that in Framingham men subscapular skinfold thickness was significantly associated with myocardial infarction, while Metropolitan relative weight (i.e., weight greater than

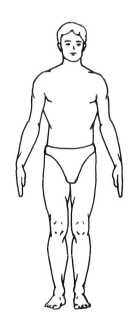

Fig. I.1. Heavy weight does not necessarily mean fat. This individual's weight is above the 50th percentile of the weight by height standard but in terms of fatness he is below the 50th percentile.

20% of ideal weight) was not. In other words, excess *weight* per se is not the causative factor in heart disease; *excess fat*, which is associated with excess weight, is the causative factor.

Weight represents the sum of fat, protein, water, and bone mineral, and any of these components may change in an unpredictable manner. Edema and ascites increase water retention, resulting in maintenance of weight even though fat and protein may have been lost. Similarly, measurements of weight in patients that are stressed by trauma, burns, infection, or sepsis are not useful for assessment of nutritional status. For example, the early postadmission weight of a thermally injured patient may be elevated by 12% to 15% above his/her preinjury weight due to fluid resuscitation. Under these circumstances initial weight is useless unless it is considered with preinjury reported weight (23). Measurement of weight is also a poor guide when energy intake is adequate but protein intake is inadequate. In this case, fat can be preserved while protein mass declines. This situation can occur in both the juvenile and adult forms of kwashiorkor. Typical cases are patients receiving nutritional support during the catabolic phase of a severe injury, and patients on simultaneous hyperalimentation and elevated doses of corticosteroid therapy. Similarly, in wasting malnutrition as it occurs in elderly patients or those suffering from surgical intervention, better information about nutritional status is obtained from measurements of upper arm muscle area than from measurements of weight or skinfold thickness. This is because weight can vary deceptively as a result of differences in hydration, occurrence of edema, ascites, or tumor, while wasting malnutrition involves the depletion of body protein stores and is indicated by a very low upper arm muscle area.

Third, weight and body composition are also directly related to frame size, so that the bigger the frame the greater the weight. To take into account the role of frame size, the Metropolitan Life Insurance Company gave weights by height and frame size categories in both the 1959 and 1983 tables (18–19). However, the Metropolitan Life Insurance Company had no data on the frame sizes of their policyholders. The categories of frame size in the 1959 tables were not based on anthropometric measurements of the policy holders, but rather represent an arbitrary division of the population into the lowest (small frame), middle two (medium frame), and highest (large frame) quartiles for weight (24). Thus, the frame size categories used bear no relationship to skeletal size. Similarly, the frame size categories given in the 1983 Metropolitan Height and Weight Tables (19) are arbitrary because no measurements of elbow breadth were included in the insurance examination data. In an attempt to overcome this difficulty, the Metropolitan Life Insurance Company used the elbow breadths derived from the NHANES I data sets, while the weights associated with these frame size categories were derived from the Metropolitan Insurance policyholder population. In other words, to establish frame size categories, they combined measurements derived from two different populations. This approach is arbitrary, and consequently the weights associated with such categories of frame size are also arbitrary. It is evident that the Metropolitan weight tables, despite their widespread use, have limited value for assessing nutritional status of contemporary populations.

Body Fat and Body Muscle

A basic principle of living organisms is that they require a continuous supply of energy and nutrients to maintain their normal metabolic activities, to continue tissue replacement, and to grow. The organism is in equilibrium when the energy intake equals the energy expenditure. When the energy intake exceeds the needs, all three major dietary components—carbohydrates, fats, and proteins—are converted into fatty acids and stored as a reserve of energy in cellular adipose tissue. Then when the energy intake is low, the organism reconverts the fatty acids into glucose through a series of biochemical processes and uses the glucose as a source of energy. Therefore, whatever the cause, variability in the thickness of adipose tissue as indicated by skinfold thickness indicates variability in the amount of stored energy.

In the same manner that variability in skinfold thickness implies variability in energy storage, differences in the amount of skeletal muscle indirectly imply variability in protein and energy intake. Since most body tissues consist of protein, which can be formed only from amino acids, tissue growth and maintenance can be achieved only when the diet provides sufficient protein and calories. If the calorie intake is insufficient to meet energy needs, or if the essential amino acids are not all present simultaneously, body tissues are broken down and used as energy. As has been learned from surgical patients, when dietary intake of protein and energy is low, the blood concentration of the amino acids valine, isoleucine, and leucine is reduced (25–28). If chronic, such dietary deficiency leads to reduction of muscle tissue as this tissue is broken down to provide essential amino acids (27–28). As shown in figure I.2, among postoperative patients or those suffering from cancer or other debilitating diseases, the reduction in upper arm muscle area is directly related to the severity of the disease. In other words, the muscle tissues of the body are in a dynamic equilibrium with dietary protein availability, and hence variability in the amount of body muscle tissue implies variability in the availability of nutrients. This is why nutritional restriction is characterized by reduction of both body fat and muscle tissue.

Fig. I.2. Changes in upper arm muscle area with various degrees of malnutrition among patients suffering from diverse debilitating diseases. (Adapted from Heymsfield et al. 1982. Anthropometric measurements of muscle mass. Am. J. Clin. Nutr. 36:680–90.)

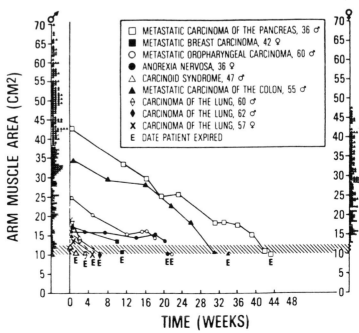

As evaluated by 24-hour creatinine excretion (among subjects ingesting a creatinine-free diet), measurements of upper arm muscle tissue in healthy and chronically undernourished subjects provide a practical guide to body muscle mass (29–30) (see fig. I.3). Hence, variability in upper arm muscle area implies variability in the availability and utilization of nutrients.

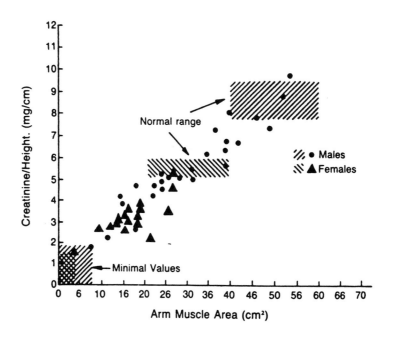

Fig. I.3. Relationship of mid upper arm muscle area to creatinine-height index in healthy and chronically undernourished subjects. Each point represents the average of three consecutive study days on metabolic ward. During the study period the subjects ingested a meat-free diet. The minimal values represent boundaries below which adults show limited survival. The close relation between upper arm muscle area and urinary creatinine indicates that the arm muscle area does measure body protein. (Adapted from Heymsfield et al. 1982. Anthropometric measurements of muscle mass. Am. J. Clin. Nutr. 36:680–90.)

In summary, high amounts of body fat and muscle do imply high energy reserves, while low amounts of body fat and muscle imply low energy reserves.

Objectives

In view of the lack of an adequate anthropometric reference this book has the following objectives:

1. To describe the general protocol for obtaining anthropometric measurements compatible with the present standards and with the recommendations of the Anthropometric Standardization Committee. As such this information can be used across disciplines.

2. To present descriptive information (means, standard deviations, and percentiles) by age, sex, and frame size, of anthropometric dimensions of body size and body composition used in the evaluation of growth and nutritional status of children and adults.

3. To illustrate the use of statistical criteria for classifying the anthropometric dimensions of children and adults into five categories of growth and nutritional status.

4. To illustrate with practical examples the use of anthropometric dimensions in diagnosing the nutritional status of clinical and nonclinical populations.

II
Methods and Materials

This chapter gives a description of the total NHANES sample. Thereafter, the general procedures for obtaining measurements of anthropometric dimensions and indices of body size, body proportion, and body composition are described. The chapter concludes with a discussion of concerns regarding reliability in the collection of anthropometric data.

Sample

This study is based on a cross-sectional sample of 43,774 subjects aged 1 to 74 years derived from the first and second National Health and Nutrition Examination Surveys (the NHANES I and II) of 1971–74 and 1976–80. The NHANES I was conducted by the National Center for Health Statistics (NCHS) according to a multistage, stratified sampling approach which included the selection of 28,043 persons who represented the 194 million noninstitutionalized civilians, aged 1 to 74 years, of the United States. Of the 28,043 individuals who made up the sampling universe of NHANES I, 23,808 (84.9%) were included in the present study.

The NHANES II was conducted by the NCHS following the same sampling and data collection methods as NHANES I. The stratified probability sample included the selection of 27,801 persons aged 6 months to 74 years who represented the population of 196 million noninstitutionalized civilians in the United States. Of the 27,801 individuals who made up the sampling universe of NHANES II, 20,322 (73.1%) were interviewed and examined. Hence, the present study includes a total sample of 44,130 (23,808 for NHANES I and 20,322 for NHANES II).

The distribution of the height and weight of the NHANES I subsample, when appropriately weighted for sampling variability, was indistinguishable from that of the NHANES II subsample. Similar results were found by Abraham (1). For this reason, and in view of the critical need for a large sample size, we decided to merge the data of NHANES I with NHANES II, treating them as a single sample. To do so, we calculated a new sampling weight by dividing each subject's sampling weight by two, as recommended by the NCHS. The mathematical derivation for this approach has already been given (2).

The total combined sample of NHANES I and II surveys consisted of a sample of 7,125 blacks, 35,931 whites, and 718 of other ethnic groups. The ages ranged from 1 to 74 years. It should be noted, however, as shown in table II.1, that the number of cases was not the same for all the anthropometric dimensions.

The anthropometric data for the combined NHANES I and II samples are given in chapter IV. In addition, in Appendix A and Appendix B the anthropometric data for blacks and whites are given separately. It should be noted that these percentiles are not weighted for sampling size as was the case for the combined samples that are given in chapter IV. Furthermore, due to small sample size for blacks anthropometric data by frame size are not given.

Table II.1.
Sample size distribution by ethnic group in the combined samples
derived from NHANES I and II surveys

Variables	Blacks	Whites	Other	Total
Age	7,125	35,931	718	43,774
Weight	7,122	35,904	718	43,744
Height	6,954	35,436	708	43,098
Sitting Height	6,736	34,637	681	42,054
Elbow Breadth	7,119	35,881	718	43,714
Arm Circumference	7,116	35,864	718	43,698
Triceps Skinfold	7,080	35,801	716	43,597
Subscapular Skinfold	7,052	35,694	714	43,460

Measurements

Although the data included in the present study were collected before the publication of the Anthropometric Standardization Reference Manual (3), the general protocol for obtaining the measurement did follow the recommended technique given in the above-mentioned manual. For this reason, the general procedures for obtaining measurements have been worded so as to follow the recommended technique. This section describes the guidelines for the anthropometric variables used in the present standard. These include measurements of: (1) weight, (2) height, (3) sitting height, (4) elbow breadth, (5) mid upper arm circumference, (6) triceps skinfold thickness, (7) subscapular skinfold thickness, (8) computation of mid upper arm muscle and fat area and arm fat index, and (9) calculation of sitting height index, body mass index, and frame size.

Weight

Weight of children under 2 years of age is measured on a leveled pan scale with a beam and movable weight. A quilt is left on the scale at all times and the scale is calibrated to zero. The scale should be calibrated every month using objects with known weight. When the scale is not in use, the beam should be locked in place to reduce wear. The infant, with or without a diaper, is placed on the scale making sure the weight is distributed equally on each side of the center of the pan (see fig. II.1). Weight is recorded to the nearest 10 grams. (In cases where infants cannot be weighed alone on the pan scale, they can be weighed with their mother on the platform weight scale. But such a measurement is less accurate because the mother's weight is recorded to the nearest 100 grams.) If a diaper is worn, to obtain a nude weight, the diaper's weight is subtracted from the observed weight of the infant.

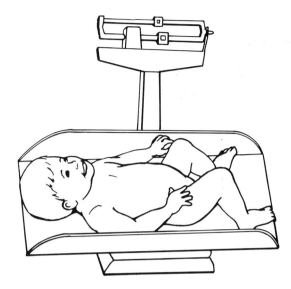

Fig II.1. Measuring weight. Infants less than 2 years of age are weighed while lying down naked on a pan pediatric scale. (Adapted from Lohman, T. G., Roche, A. F., and Martorell, R. [eds]. 1988. Anthropometric Standardization Reference Manual. Champaign, Ill.: Human Kinetics Books.)

For subjects older than 2 years, the body weight should be measured using a platform–beam scale with movable weights or an instrument of equivalent accuracy (see fig. II.2). The beam of the platform scale must be graduated so that it can be read from both sides. The calibration of the scale should also be done every month using objects with known weight. The subjects stand still over the center of the platform with body weight evenly distributed between both feet. Light indoor clothing such as hospital gowns or shorts can be worn. Do not subtract the weight of the clothing when comparing to the weights given in the present monograph because the weights are given with light clothing but without shoes. Weight is recorded to the nearest 100 grams.

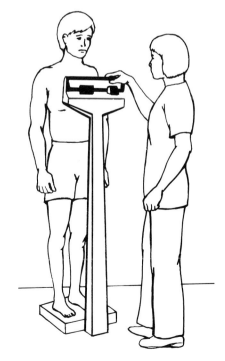

Fig. II.2. Measuring weight. Subjects older than 2 years of age are measured with shorts or standard gown on a platform-beam scale. (Adapted from Chumlea, W. C., Roche, A. F., and Mukherjee, D. 1987. Nutritional Assessment of the Elderly through Anthropometry. Columbus, Ohio: Ross Laboratories.)

Height

Recumbent Length. In children under 3 years of age, length should be obtained in the recumbent position using an infantometer. An infantometer is a device which consists of a flat board with a fixed headboard and a movable footboard which are perpendicular to the table surface. The device has a fixed measuring tape marked off in millimeters or inches with its zero end at the edge of the headboard. Infant length is recorded as the distance between the headboard and footboard. To obtain accurate measurements two people are required (see fig. II.3). The assistant stands at the head of the table and holds the infant's head so the infant looks vertically upward with the crown of the head against the headboard. The examiner straightens the infant's legs holding the feet with toes pointed directly up, and moves the footboard against the feet. The measurement is indicated by the position of the footboard and is recorded to the nearest 0.1 cm.

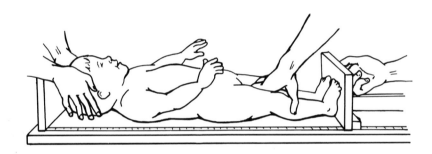

Fig. II.3. Measurements of recumbent length in infants (aged less than 3 years) with an infantometer. (Adapted from Moore, W. M., and Roche, A. F. 1982. Pediatric Anthropometry. Columbus, Ohio: Ross Laboratories.)

Stature. The length of subjects older than 3 years of age is measured, without shoes, with a standiometer (see fig. II.4). A standiometer consists of a metric tape affixed to a vertical surface, such as a wall or a rigid free-standing measuring device, and a movable block, attached to the vertical surface at a right angle, that can be brought down to the crown of the head. In the absence of a standiometer, height can be measured on a platform scale, but this device is less accurate than the standiometer. In either case, the subject should stand with heels together and back as straight as possible; the heels, buttocks, shoulders, and head should touch the wall or the vertical surface of the measuring device as shown in fig. II.4. The weight of the subject is distributed evenly on both feet and the head is positioned in the Frankfort horizontal plane. The arms hang freely by the sides with the palms facing the thighs. The subject should be asked to inhale deeply and maintain a fully erect position. The movable block is brought down until it touches the head; make sure to put sufficient pressure to compress the hair. The measurement is recorded to the nearest 0.1 cm. Two measurements are taken and if the difference between both readings is less than 1 cm, the mean measurement is recorded.

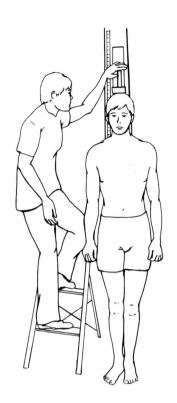

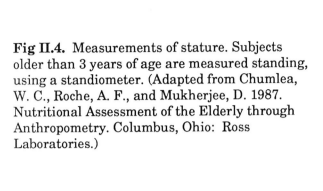

Fig II.4. Measurements of stature. Subjects older than 3 years of age are measured standing, using a standiometer. (Adapted from Chumlea, W. C., Roche, A. F., and Mukherjee, D. 1987. Nutritional Assessment of the Elderly through Anthropometry. Columbus, Ohio: Ross Laboratories.)

Knee Height in the Handicapped. When stature cannot be measured due either to inability to stand or to excessive spinal curvature, it can be estimated from measurements of knee height.

The knee height is measured with a sliding broad-blade caliper known as a Mediform Caliper (Mediform Printers and Publishers, 5150 S.W. Griffith Drive, Beaverton, OR 97005). As shown in figure II.5, while lying supine the subject being measured bends the knee and ankle to a 90-degree angle. The fixed blade of the caliper is placed under the heel of the foot, and the other blade is placed over the anterior surface of the thigh over the condyle of the femur. The shaft of the caliper is held parallel to the shaft of the tibia, and pressure is applied to compress the tissue. Measurements are recorded to the nearest 0.1 cm. The average of two measurements is then converted to stature using the following equation (4):

Males = 64.19 - (0.04 x age) + (0.02 x knee height)

Females = 84.88 - (0.24 x age) + (1.83 x knee height)

Sitting Height

Sitting height is measured with an anthropometer. The subject sits erect on a measuring table or bench, with the legs hanging unsupported over the edge of the table and with the hands resting on the thighs (see fig. II.6). The subject sits as erect as possible, with the head in the Frankfort horizontal plane and the eyes also in a horizontal plane looking straight ahead. The head, shoulders, and buttocks should touch the vertical surface of the measuring device. The subject should be asked to

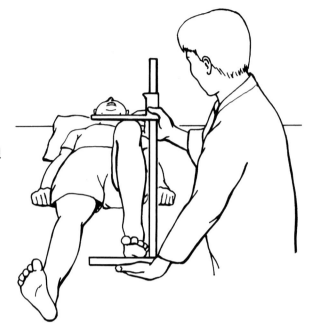

Fig II.5. Measurements of knee height in the handicapped with a broad-blade caliper. (Adapted from Chumlea, W. C., Roche, A. F., and Mukherjee, D. 1987.   Nutritional Assessment of the Elderly through Anthropometry. Columbus, Ohio: Ross Laboratories.)

inhale deeply and maintain a fully erect position, and the measurement is made just before the subject exhales. The movable block is brought down until it touches the head. Sufficient pressure is applied to compress the hair. The measurement is recorded to the nearest 0.1 cm. Two measurements are taken and if the difference between both readings is less than 1 cm, the mean is then recorded.

Fig. II.6. Measurements of sitting height. Sitting height is measured with an anthropometer while the subject sits on a bench. (Adapted from Martin, D. A., Carter, J. E. L., Hendy, K. C., and Malina, R. M. Segment Lengths. In: Lohman, T. G., Roche, A. F., and Martorell, R. [eds]. 1988. Anthropometric Standardization Reference Manual. Champaign, Ill.: Human Kinetics Books.)

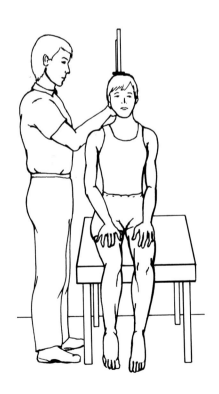

Sitting Height Index

The sitting height index (%), also known as the Cormic index, is derived by computation as the ratio of sitting height to stature (or recumbent length) times 100:

Sitting Height Index (%) = [sitting height (cm) / stature (cm)] x 100

Body Mass Index

The body mass index (kg/sq. m), also known as the weight-height index or Quetelet index, is derived by computation as the quotient of weight (kg) divided by height (in meters) squared (5):

Body Mass Index (BMI) = weight (kg) / height (m²)

Bitrochanteric Breadth

The measurement of bitrochanteric breadth, although some investigators have used it as component of frame size index (5–7), is not much used in the evaluation of nutritional status. To measure the bitrochanteric breadth the subject stands with the heels together and the arms folded over the chest. An anthropometer with straight blades is used. The examiner stands behind the subject (see fig. II.7). The maximum distance between the trochanters is measured and is recorded to the nearest 0.1 cm. Considerable pressure must be applied with the anthropometer blades to compress the soft tissues.

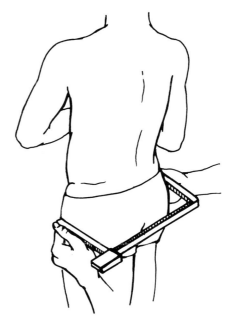

Fig. II.7. Measurements of bitrochanteric breadth with an anthropometer. Applying pressure, the maximum distance between the trochanters is measured.

Elbow Breadth

To measure elbow breadth, two instruments are available: (1) an anthropometric sliding caliper, and (2) the Frameter.

Sliding Caliper. A broad-faced sliding caliper is recommended for measuring elbow breadth. The subject's right arm is raised forward to the horizontal and the forearm is flexed to a right (90-degree) angle at the elbow, with the dorsum of the hand facing the examiner. The examiner stands in front facing the subject, palpates the lateral and medial epicondyles of the humerus, and then places the caliper jaws parallel or slightly at a slant to these two sites and measures the greatest bony width across the elbow joint (see fig. II.8). Obtaining accurate measurements of elbow breadth with the sliding caliper requires expertise in measurement techniques. Erroneous information can be obtained because of difficulties in locating the anatomical landmarks and positioning the caliper jaws on the subject's arms. When this occurs, use the Frameter instead.

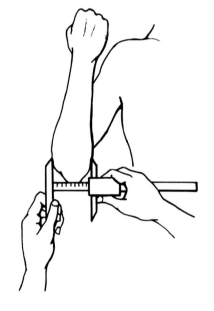

Fig. II.8. Measurements of elbow breadth with the sliding caliper. Elbow breadth is measured at the epicondyles of the humerus.

Frameter. The Frameter (distributed by Health Products, 2126 Ridge, Ann Arbor, MI 48104) includes components that accurately measure the distance between the bony landmarks that demarcate elbow breadth, the medial and lateral epicondyles of the humerus. The procedure for measuring elbow breadth and frame size using the Frameter is as follows: Direct the subject to extend his or her right arm and bend the forearm towards the shoulder at a 90-degree angle, turning the palm of the hand toward his or her body (see fig. II.9). Place the subject's elbow on the baseboard against the fixed endboard, making sure that the fixed endboard is to the subject's left and the mobile board is to his or her right. Then slide the mobile board against the right side of the subject's elbow as firmly as possible, and read the actual elbow breadth measurement and the corresponding frame size for his or her sex. Record both the elbow breadth and the frame size category.

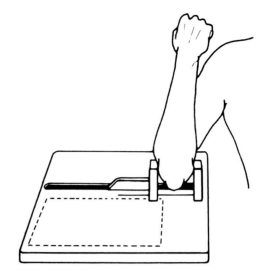

Fig. II.9. Measurements of elbow breadth with the Frameter. Elbow breadth is measured while the arm rests on a fixed baseboard.

Mid Upper Arm Circumference

To obtain the mid upper arm circumference, the subject's right arm is bent at the elbow at a 90-degree angle, with the upper arm held parallel to the side of the body. Then, using either a metallic tape or an insert tape, measure the distance between the acromion (the bony protrusion on the posterior of the upper shoulder) and the olecranon process of the elbow (tip of the elbow) (see fig. II.10a). Mark the midpoint between these two landmarks with indelible ink. (If an insert tape is used, the same number should appear at the top of the shoulder and the elbow, and the midpoint is given by the mark on the tape.) The subject's right arm should then be relaxed and hanging loosely at his or her side (see fig. II.10b). Position the metric tape around the upper arm at the previously marked midpoint. Make sure the tape is snug, but not so tight as to cause skin indentation or pinching. The circumference is recorded to the nearest 0.1 cm.

Fig. II.10a. Measurement of midpoint of the upper arm. The midpoint is located with a metric measuring tape with the subject's elbow flexed at 90 degrees.

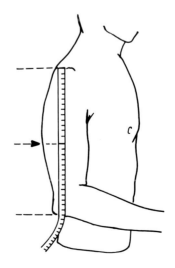

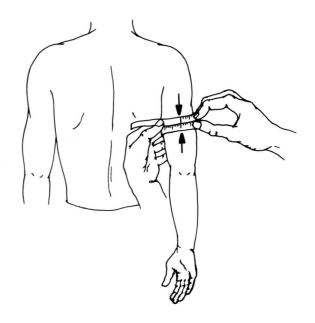

Fig. II.10b. Measurement of upper arm circumference. The upper arm circumference is measured with the metric measuring tape at the midpoint of the upper arm with the subject's arm relaxed and the elbow extended.

Triceps Skinfold Thickness

Triceps skinfold thickness is measured with a skinfold caliper (see fig. II.11). Skinfold thickness is measured at the previously marked midpoint of the right upper arm (posterior or back side). The subject should stand with right arm hanging loosely by his or her side. The examiner should palpate the subject's measuring site to become familiar with soft tissues. Then the examiner should grasp a vertical pinch of skin and subcutaneous fat between thumb and forefinger about 1 cm above the previously marked midpoint. The skinfold should be gently pulled away from underlying muscle.

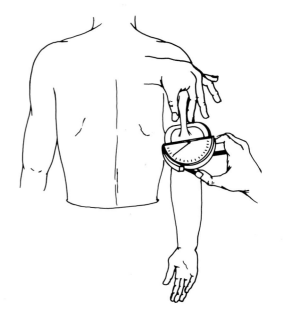

Fig. II.11. Measurement of triceps skinfold thickness with a Lange skinfold caliper. The triceps skinfold is measured with the subject's arms hanging loosely and comfortably at his/her side. The triceps skinfold is picked up with the left thumb and index finger of the examiner, approximately 1 cm proximal to the midpoint marked in figure II.10a.

The skinfold caliper should be placed on the skinfold at the midpoint marked, while maintaining a grasp of the skinfold. Three readings should be taken in quick succession, and the average of the three recorded in mm. Each reading should be taken as soon as the jaws of the caliper come into contact with the skin and the dial reading stabilizes.

Subscapular Skinfold Thickness

The subscapular skinfold is picked up on a diagonal, inclined infero-laterally approximately 45 degrees to the horizontal plane in the natural cleavage lines of the skin. The site is just below the inferior angle of the scapula (see fig. II.12). The subject stands comfortably erect with the hands relaxed at the sides of the body. The examiner palpates the subject's scapula to locate the inferior border of the scapula. The examiner should grasp a horizontal pinch of skinfold at about 1 cm below the inferior angle of the right scapula (shoulder blade). The jaws of the caliper are applied 1 cm infero-lateral to the thumb and finger raising the skinfold, and three readings are taken rapidly. The average of the three readings is recorded in mm.

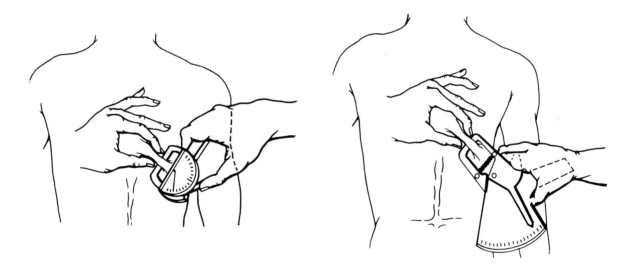

Fig II.12. Measurement of subscapular skinfold thickness with (a) a Lange skinfold caliper and (b) a Slim Guide caliper. Subscapular skinfold thickness is measured with the subject standing with arm and shoulder relaxed. The examiner should grasp a horizontal pinch of skinfold at about 1 cm below the tip of the right scapula (shoulder blade). The jaws of the caliper are applied 1 cm infero-lateral to the thumb and finger raising the fold, and three readings are taken rapidly.

Note. In both triceps and subscapular skinfolds the amount of tissue elevated must be sufficient to form a fold with sides that are approximately parallel to each other. The amount of skin and subcutaneous fat to be elevated depends on the thickness of the subcutaneous fat at the site. The thicker the fat layer, the larger should be the separation between thumb and index finger when the anthropometrist begins to elevate the skinfold. Furthermore, the fold should be kept elevated until the measurement has been completed. It is recommended that all sample measurements be practiced until good measurement reliability is obtained (see section on reliability and interpretation of measurements).

Upper Arm Muscle, Fat Area, and Arm Fat Index

Upper Arm Muscle Area. Calculations of upper arm muscle and fat areas are based on measurements of the upper arm circumference and triceps skinfolds (see fig. II.13). The technique of computing upper arm areas using brachium radiographic shadow was originally used by Best and Kuhl (8) and Baker and associates (9–10), who assumed that the upper arm and its constituents are cylindrical. Since then this approach has been applied to determine upper arm muscle and fat areas and circumferences from measurements of upper arm circumference and skinfold thickness (2, 11–19). Since this technique assumes that the upper arm and its constituents are cylindrical, the corresponding areas of cross section are computed from the formula that yields the areas of a circle from its circumference. Letting C equal the circumference of the upper arm,

$$\text{Total Upper Arm Area (TUA)} = C^2 / (4 \times \pi)$$

Similarly, letting Ts equal the triceps skinfold thickness,

$$\text{Upper Arm Muscle Area (UMA)} = [C - (Ts \times \pi)]^2 / (4 \times \pi)$$

Then the upper arm fat area is calculated by subtraction:

$$\text{Upper Arm Fat Area (UFA)} = \text{Total Upper Arm Area} - \text{Upper Arm Muscle Area}$$

The arm fat index (or percentage of fat in the upper arm) is derived by this equation:

$$\text{Arm Fat Index (AFI)} = (\text{Upper Arm Fat Area} / \text{Total Arm Area}) \times 100$$

Example:

If the upper arm circumference (C) is 30.0 cm, and the triceps skinfold is 25 mm (or 2.5 cm):

$$\text{Total Upper Arm Area (TUA)} = C^2 / (4 \times \pi)$$

$$\text{TUA} = 30^2 / 12.57 = 71.6 \text{ cm}^2$$

$$\text{Upper Arm Muscle Area (UMA) (cm}^2) = [C - (3.1416 \times Ts)]^2 / 12.57$$

$$\text{UMA} = [30.0 - (3.1416 \times 2.5)]^2 / 12.57 = 39.0 \text{ cm}^2$$

To adjust for the area of the bone (20) and obtain the bone-free arm muscle area (UBMA), for males subtract 10.0 cm² (UBMA = 39.0 - 10.0 = 29.0 cm²); for females subtract 6.5 cm² (UBMA = 39.0 - 6.5 = 32.5 cm²).

The upper arm fat area (UFA) is calculated as follows:

Upper Arm Fat Area (UFA) (cm²) = Total Upper Arm Area (TUA) - Uncorrected Upper Arm Muscle Area (UMA)

UFA = 71.6 - 39.0 = 32.6 cm²

Arm Fat Index (AFI) (% fat area) = (32.6 / 71.6) x 100 = 45.53%

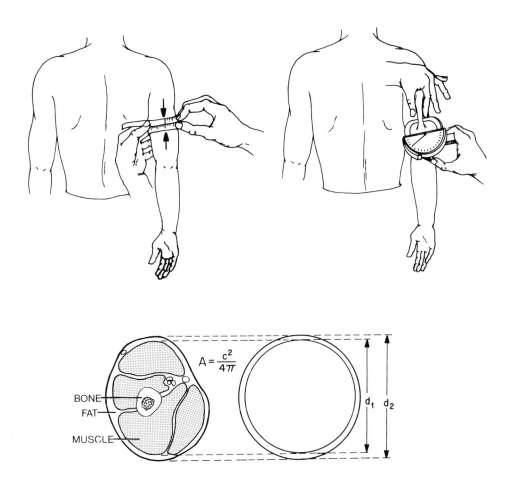

Fig. II.13. Cross-sectional view of the upper arm tissue areas derived from measurements of upper arm circumference and triceps skinfold thickness.

A rapid estimate of arm muscle area and arm fat index (or percent fat in the upper arm area) may be obtained using the nomogram given in figure II.14. Note that for adults muscle area values obtained using this nomogram must be corrected for bone area by subtracting 10.0 cm² for males and 6.5 cm² for females.

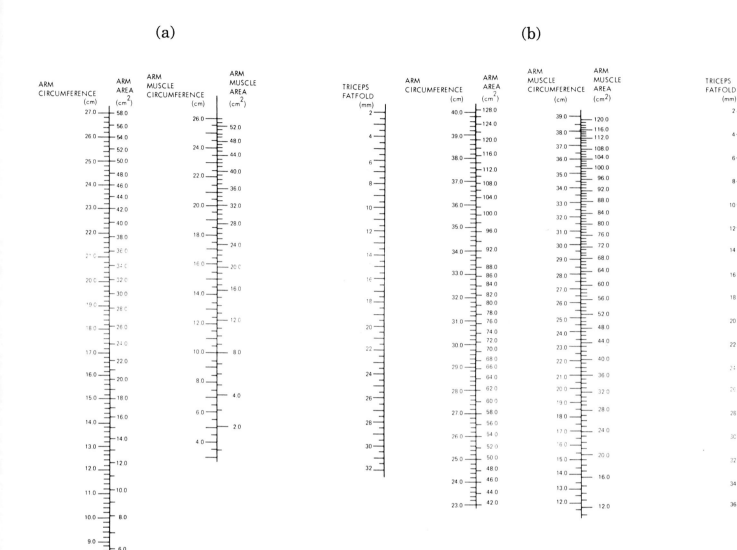

Fig. II.14. Nomogram to calculate upper arm muscle area for (a) children and for (b) adults. Locate the measurement of upper arm circumference (cm) on the left scale and the triceps skinfold thickness (mm) on the right scale. Then, with a ruler, connect these two points and read the total arm area (cm²), and the muscle area (cm²) where this line intercepts the respective areas. To obtain the fat area (cm²) subtract from the total arm area the muscle area. Note: For adults the muscle area should be corrected by subtracting 10 cm² from males and 6.5 cm² from females. (Adapted from Gurney and Jelliffe, 1973. Arm anthropometry in nutritional assessment: Nomogragram for rapid calculation of muscle circumference and cross-sectional muscle areas. Am. J. Clin. Nutr. 26:12–15).

Limitation of Muscle Area among the Obese. As indicated by Forbes et al. (21), arm muscle area estimated by anthropometry overestimates the arm muscle area determined by CAT (computerized axial tomography) scan, and the degree of overestimation varies directly with the degree of adiposity. As a result an anthropometric estimate of muscle area especially among the obese or those whose triceps skinfold thickness exceeds the 85th age and sex percentiles can give an excessive estimate of body muscle. For this reason, evaluation of nutritional status based upon anthropometric estimates of muscle area among the obese should be done with great caution.

Percent Fat Estimated from Skinfolds

Although at present there is no generally applicable equation which converts skinfolds or other anthropometric variables into estimates of density and percent of fat (22–31), estimates of percent fat weight, albeit crude, do provide an additional indication of body fatness. For this reason, we decided to derive estimates of percent fat from the regression equations of the logarithm of skinfold thickness on density given by Durnin and Womersley (31) (see table II.2). The range of variability in skinfold thickness, height, weight, and age upon which these equations were based was comparable to the data included in the present standards, and was also derived from a large sample size.

Table II.2.
Regression equations for the estimation of body density (D)
from the logarithm of skinfold thickness

Age Groups	Males	Females
D = a - (b x log of Triceps)		
17–19	D = 1.1252 - (0.0625 x log Ts	D = 1.1159 - (0.0648 x log Ts)
20–29	D = 1.1131 - (0.0530 x log Ts)	D = 1.1319 - (0.0776 x log Ts)
30–39	D = 1.0834 - (0.0361 x log Ts)	D = 1.1176 - (0.0686 x log Ts)
40–49	D = 1.1041 - (0.0609 x log Ts)	D = 1.1121 - (0.0691 x log Ts)
50–72	D = 1.1041 - (0.0662 x log Ts)	D = 1.1160 - (0.0762 x log Ts)
D = a - (b x log of Subscapular)		
17–19	D = 1.1312 - (0.0670 x log Subs)	D = 1.1081 - (0.0621 x log Subs)
20–29	D = 1.1360 - (0.0700 x log Subs)	D = 1.1184 - (0.0716 x log Subs)
30–39	D = 1.0978 - (0.0416 x log Subs)	D = 1.0979 - (0.0567 x log Subs)
40–49	D = 1.1246 - (0.0686 x log Subs)	D = 1.0860 - (0.0505 x log Subs)
50–72	D = 1.1334 - (0.0760 x log Subs)	D = 1.0899 - (0.0590 x log Subs)
D = a - (b x log of Triceps + Subscapular)		
17–19	D = 1.1561 - (0.0711 x log Ts + Subs)	D = 1.1468 - (0.0740 x log Ts + Subs)
20–29	D = 1.1525 - (0.0687 x log Ts + Subs)	D = 1.1582 - (0.0813 x log Ts + Subs)
30–39	D = 1.1165 - (0.0484 x log Ts + Subs)	D = 1.1356 - (0.0680 x log Ts + Subs)
40–49	D = 1.1519 - (0.0771 x log Ts + Subs)	D = 1.1230 - (0.0635 x log Ts + Subs)
50–72	D = 1.1527 - (0.0793 x log Ts + Subs)	D = 1.1347 - (0.0742 x log Ts + Subs)

Source: Adapted from Durnin, J., and Womersley, J. 1974. Body fat assessed from total body density and its estimation from skinfold thickness: measurements on 481 men and women aged from 16 to 72 years. Br. J. Nutr. 32:77–97.

The estimation of percent body fat was made as follows: First, for each group and sex, three densities (i.e., density based on triceps skinfold, density based on subscapular skinfold, and density based on sum of both triceps and subscapular skinfold thicknesses) were predicted using the corresponding regression equation relating the $\log_{10}$ of triceps, the $\log_{10}$ of subscapular skinfold thicknesses, and the $\log_{10}$ of the sum of triceps and subscapular skinfold thicknesses. Second, the percent fat weight associated with each density was calculated using Siri's equation (32) {% fat = [(4.95 / Density) - 4.50] x 100}. Third, the three estimates of percent fat weight were then averaged.

Frame Size Classification

Elbow Breadth as a Marker of Skeletal Frame

It is generally recognized that weight not only varies with height and age, but is also influenced by factors such as body width, bone thickness, muscularity, and length of trunk relative to total height. Therefore, an appropriate evaluation of individual variability in weight should include some measurements that reflect these factors. Frame size is one such measurement. However, few systematic studies have been made to assess this variable as a factor affecting body weight independently of height and percent body fat.

Frame is a skeletal concept, and therefore measurements to quantify frame size should be based on skeletal dimensions. Several approaches have been used for quantifying frame size. Some, like the Metropolitan Life Insurance Tables (33–34), rely almost totally on self-appraisal. Katch et al. (6–7) classified frame size based on measurements of biacromial and bitrochanteric breadths. Although the mathematical basis for this approach is good, it cannot fully represent skeletal variability because the measurements of shoulder and hip width are more significantly affected by adiposity than ankle and elbow breadth (35). Similarly, Grant (36) developed an index of frame size based on the wrist circumference of 100 adults. Since this index is based on wrist circumference, which is affected by variability in soft tissue, it is not indicative only of skeletal frame. Garn et al. (37) also established frame size categories based on bony chest breadths derived from lateral radiographs. While this approach is indeed excellent for assessing actual skeletal dimensions it cannot be applied to the population at large, because of the problems associated with exposure to radiation. For these reasons, in the present work we have used measurements of elbow breadth as a marker of skeletal frame (38).

The effectiveness of elbow breadth as a marker of skeletal width can be evaluated through correlation analysis. For this purpose, we have calculated the coefficients of $\log_{10}$ subscapular skinfold thickness to elbow breadth, frame index, and bitrochanteric breadth, using the merged samples. Since body fat and fat fold mass are not independent, especially in obese individuals, and both fatness and lean body mass change with age, the association between the above measurements and fatness needs to be partialled out for the effects of lean body mass and age. Because in the NHANES data sets there are no measurements of lean body mass, we have used the upper arm muscle area (39) instead. Furthermore, we used only the subscapular skinfold thickness rather than the sum of triceps and subscapular skinfolds, because the upper arm muscle area is computed from both the triceps skinfolds and upper arm circumference, and partialling out the effect of muscle area from that of fat in the upper arm would be redundant. As is demonstrated in table II.3, after accounting for the associations of upper arm muscle area and age in males, neither elbow breadth nor frame index is correlated with subscapular skinfold thickness, while bitrochanteric breadth and weight continue to be related to fatness. Although in females elbow breadth and frame index showed some association with fatness, this relationship is not as strong as that shown by bitrochanteric breadth and weight. Thus, given the availability of good national data, and until better anthropometric dimensions are available, elbow breadth is a good index of frame size.

Table II.3.
Partial correlations (r) of frame size variables with $\log_{10}$ subscapular skinfold
thickness controlling for age and arm muscle area

Measurement	Males (yrs)			Females (yrs)		
	10–17	18–54	55–74	10–17	18–54	55–74
Elbow Breadth	0.15	0.06	0.03	0.19	0.17	0.15
Bitrochanteric Breadth	0.36	0.26	0.11	0.39	0.33	0.17
Weight	0.69	0.65	0.59	0.67	0.63	0.59

Note: Excludes individuals who were either excessively lean or excessively fat.

$r > 0.20$ significance at 0.01 level

If frame measures are not associated with body fat, classification by frame size should not be associated with significant differences in the relative amount of fat. As a measure of relative amount of fat we have used the arm fat index [arm fat index = (upper arm fat area / total arm area) x 100]. Table II.4 gives the median values of weight, upper arm muscle area, and arm fat index (or percent fat in the upper arm) of males and females classified by frame size. From these data it is evident that while there are significant differences in weight and upper arm muscle area between frame sizes, there are no differences in the arm fat index. Furthermore, these data also suggest that frame size contributes to fat free mass, as is shown by the significant differences in upper arm muscle area. Conceptually, this relationship indicates that skeletal robustness is associated with relative muscularity (35). These findings together suggest that evaluations of weight and upper arm muscle area should be performed with reference to height and frame size. Other investigators have indicated that because the inclusion of body diameters such as elbow breadth do not improve statistical predictions of weight/height indices and percent body fat, they may not be useful for the construction of frame size categories of weight by height (40). It may be noted, however, that this conclusion is not correct, because weight/height indices do not distinguish the components of body weight such as fat and muscle; and, as indicated previously, elbow breadth is a good indicator of skeletal dimensions precisely because it is not affected by percent fat weight.

The importance of an accurate assessment of frame size has been illustrated by Katch et al. (7). In their study, self-appraisal either overestimated or underestimated frame size, and thus desirable weight, 42% of the time. For example, an individual who considers himself to be small framed but is actually medium framed can underestimate his desirable weight by as much as 10 kg (22 lb.). According to Katch et al. (6), it would be nearly impossible for this individual to achieve this lower body weight, as it would involve reducing percent body fat to below 5%. Since an appropriate evaluation of frame size requires a reliable measurement of elbow-breadth, it should be measured accurately, not by simple manual touch as suggested by the Metropolitan Life Insurance Company (34), but with broad-faced calipers or other appropriate measuring devices. Otherwise, estimations of desirable weight based on inappropriate frame size estimation may be unrealistic and subject to large errors.

In summary, elbow breadth is a good indicator of skeletal dimensions and

Table II.4.

Median weight (Wt.), upper arm muscle area (A.M.A.), and arm fat index (Fat I.) of males and females of small, medium, and large frame size, by age

Age (yrs)	Small			Medium			Large		
	Wt. (kg)	A.M.A. (cm²)	Fat I. (%)	Wt. (kg)	A.M.A. (cm²)	Fat I. (%)	Wt. (kg)	A.M.A. (cm²)	Fat I. (%)
Males									
18–24	68	45	16	72	50	18	75	55	17
25–29	72	48	19	76	53	20	82	60	19
30–34	75	49	19	78	54	20	85	63	19
35–39	76	51	20	80	56	20	84	60	20
40–44	76	52	20	79	56	20	85	60	20
45–49	76	49	20	80	56	20	84	60	19
50–54	75	48	20	78	54	20	83	59	19
55–59	75	48	20	78	55	20	85	60	20
60–64	73	48	20	77	52	20	80	58	20
65–69	70	45	20	75	49	20	79	54	20
70–74	70	44	20	73	48	20	77	51	20
Females									
18–24	55	26	36	58	28	37	63	32	39
25–29	55	27	40	59	29	40	69	34	42
30–34	58	28	40	61	31	40	73	37	42
35–39	60	29	41	62	31	42	77	39	45
40–44	59	29	41	63	32	42	77	41	45
45–49	60	28	43	63	32	44	77	40	46
50–54	60	29	43	64	34	44	78	40	46
55–59	60	30	42	66	34	44	78	42	45
60–64	61	31	42	65	34	44	77	41	45
65–69	60	30	41	65	34	42	75	41	44
70–74	60	30	41	63	34	42	75	40	44

hence of frame size. It is less affected by adiposity than other anthropometric dimensions and highly associated with lean body mass and muscle size. Finally, it is easily accessible for measurement and the values of elbow breadth are normally distributed. For these reasons, evaluations of weight and muscle area should be done with reference to height and frame size.

Categories of Frame Size

The reader should note that the frame size categories (small, medium, and large) given in previous publications (2, 38,) were made with reference to measurements of elbow breadth only. The present classification is based upon a new index hereafter referred to as *Frame Index 2,* which is derived from measurements of *elbow breadth, height,* and *age.* The formula for calculating Frame Index 2 is as follows:

Frame Index 2 = [elbow breadth (mm) / stature (cm)] x 100

To determine these three frame size categories, age- and sex-specific percentiles of Frame Index 2 were determined. Thereafter, three categories of frame size were established—small, medium, and large—corresponding respectively to values below the 25th, from the 25th to the 75th, and above the 75th sex- and age-specific percentiles of Frame Index 2 (table II.5). With these percentile cutoffs, 25%, 50%, and 75% of the sample of both males and females were classified as either small, medium, or large frame respectively.

The reason why we decided to base the frame size classification on Frame Index 2 rather than elbow breadth alone is that weight increases until about the fifth decade in males and sixth decade in females, while height starts declining by the fourth decade (see figure II.15). Therefore, any classificatory approach of frame

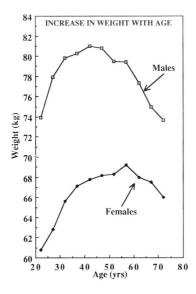 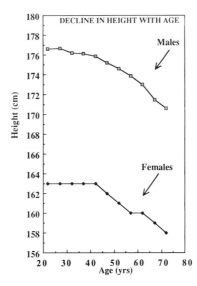

Fig. II.15. Relationship of weight and height to age among adults. Note that weight increases until about the fifth decade in males and sixth decade in females, while height begins to decline after the age of 40 years in both males and females.

size must take into account these age-associated changes. Hence, values of weight for height even when given by frame size are misleading because they do not reflect the naturally occurring changes in weight and height. For this reason, the frame-specific values of weight and upper arm muscle area given in tables IV.22 to IV.25 are presented *by age rather than by height*. The corresponding graphs are presented in figures IV.49 to IV.54.

Table II.5.

Categories of frame size derived with reference to Frame Index 2 {[elbow breadth (mm) / stature (cm)] x 100}, by age and by height

Frame Index 2 = [elbow breadth (mm) / stature (cm)] x 100						
	Male			Female		
	Small	Medium	Large	Small	Medium	Large
Age (yrs.)	Frame Index 1: elbow breadth (mm)					
18.0–24.9	<38.4	38.4 to 41.6	>41.6	<35.2	35.2 to 38.6	>38.6
25.0–29.9	<38.6	38.6 to 41.8	>41.8	<35.7	35.7 to 38.7	>38.7
30.0–34.9	<38.6	38.6 to 42.1	>42.1	<35.7	35.7 to 39.0	>39.0
35.0–39.9	<39.1	39.1 to 42.4	>42.4	<36.2	36.2 to 39.8	>39.8
40.0–44.9	<39.3	39.3 to 42.5	>42.5	<36.7	36.7 to 40.2	>40.2
45.0–45.9	<39.6	39.6 to 43.0	>43.0	<36.7	37.2 to 40.7	>40.7
50.0–54.9	<39.9	39.9 to 43.3	>43.3	<37.2	37.2 to 41.6	>41.6
55.0–59.9	<40.2	40.2 to 43.8	>43.8	<37.8	37.8 to 41.9	>41.9
60.0–64.9	<40.2	40.2 to 43.6	>43.6	<38.2	38.2 to 41.8	>41.8
65.0–69.9	<40.2	40.2 to 43.6	>43.6	<38.2	38.2 to 41.8	>41.8
70.0–74.9	<40.2	40.2 to 43.6	>43.6	<38.2	38.2 to 41.8	>41.8
Frame Index 2: Elbow breadth by height						
	Male			Female		
	Small	Medium	Large	Small	Medium	Large
Height (cm)	Elbow breadth (mm)					
141–146	—	—	—	<56	56 to 61	>61
147–152	—	—	—	<57	57 to 62	>62
153–158	<66	66 to 70	>70	<60	60 to 63	>63
159–164	<66	66 to 71	>71	<61	61 to 65	>65
165–170	<68	68 to 72	>72	<61	61 to 65	>65
171–176	<70	70 to 73	>73	<62	62 to 65	>65
177–182	<71	71 to 75	>75	<62	62 to 66	>66
183–188	<71	71 to 76	>76	—	—	—
189–194	<73	73 to 76	>76	—	—	—

Statistical Notes

Reliability of Anthropometric Measurements

Anthropometric evaluation, like other techniques, is subject to error in both data collection and interpretation. Therefore, researchers need to assess whether the degree of reliability of a given measurement is large or small. There are several statistical approaches at determining the reliability of obtaining information about anthropometric dimensions (41). A widely employed measure of replicability is the *technical error of measurement (tem)*. The technical error of measurement is defined as the squared root of the sum of the squared differences (Σd^2) of replicates (the same measurements are taken on the same subject) divided by twice the number of pairs $(2N)$. The mathematical expression is as follows:

$$\text{Tem} = \sqrt{(\Sigma d^2) / 2N} \quad (1)$$

To evaluate adequately the validity of a given measurement one needs to know both the inter- and intraexaminer technical measurement error. One way of assessing the accuracy of a given measurement is to compare the values of *tem* with values obtained by a well-trained anthropometrist (table II.6). If the examiner's *tem* comes close to the reference value (table II.6) in a series of repeated measurements and if there are no biases in measurement then the measurements can be considered accurate. Reliability of a measurement can also be evaluated with reference to a coefficient calculated as:

$$R = 1 - (tem^2/s^2)$$

Where R is the coefficient of reliability that ranges from 0 to 1, tem^2 is the square of the technical error of measurement, and s^2 is the square of the intersubject variance. The coefficient indicates the degree to which a given measurement is error free. For example, a measurement reliability $R = 0.80$ indicates that the measurement is 80% error free (41). With both the *tem* and the R value the investigator can determine the permissible limits of accepting and interpreting inter- and intrapopulation differences in a given anthropometric dimension. Of course such interpretation depends not only on the *tem* but also on the scale of a given measurement. For example, when measuring upper arm tissues, it is best to evaluate them in terms of areas rather than actual circumferences. This point can be illustrated by the study of Hill et al. (42) who report that the difference in measurement of upper arm circumference of patients before major surgery and patients still in the hospital one week after equaled only 1.1 cm (before = 23.3 cm and after = 22.2 cm). However, when the same values are expressed as areas, there is a difference of nearly 4 cm² (before = 43.19 cm² and after = 39.21 cm²). For a comprehensive evaluation of interobserver error in measurements of upper arm areas, the procedure of Hall et al. (43) should be used.

Since measuring techniques are usually learned via instruction of an expert or supervisor, there is a need to determine when a trainee or anthropometrist is ready to perform the measurement accurately. With this purpose in mind, Zerfas

(44) has developed a versatile method that monitors the measuring ability of trainees as well as other sources of error. A basic principle of this method is to compare the measurements obtained by the trainee to the measurements obtained by the expert or supervisor. Based on more than 50 tests during large-scale nutrition tests on young children in developing countries and from various sources in the literature, four categories have been established for stature (or length), arm circumference, weight, and triceps skinfold thickness. These categories are given in table II.7. From these data, it is evident that a difference of more than 20 mm (2 cm) between the expert's and the trainee's measurements indicates a gross error related to reading or recording imprecision. An error in the range of 10 to 19 mm indicates that the trainee is not yet ready to take accurate measurements. A difference between the expert's and trainee's measurements of 0 to 5 mm indicates that the trainee has reached an acceptable level of proficiency in measuring.

Table II.6.

Reliability of anthropometric dimensions given by mean intra- and interexaminer technical error of measurement

Measurement	Technical Error of Measurement	
	Intraexaminer Mean	Interexaminer Mean
Height, cervical (cm)	0.692	0.953
Sitting Height (cm)	0.535	0.705
Biacromial Breadth (cm)	0.544	0.915
Bitrochanteric Breadth (cm)	0.523	0.836
Elbow Breadth (cm)	0.117	0.154
Wrist Breadth (cm)	0.115	0.139
Upper Arm Circumference (cm)	0.347	0.425
Triceps Skinfold Thickness (mm)	0.800[a]	1.890[a]
Subscapular Skinfold Thickness (mm)	1.830[a]	1.530[a]
Midaxillary Skinfold Thickness (mm)	2.080[a]	1.470[a]

Source: Adapted from Malina, R. M., Hamill, P. V. V., and Lemeshow, S. 1973. Selected body measurements of children 6–11 years. U.S. Vital and Health Statistics, series 11, no. 123, USDHHS, Washington, D.C.

[a] From Johnston, F. E., Hamill, P. V. V., and Lemeshow, S. 1972. Skinfold thicknesses of children 6–11 years. U.S. Vital and Health Statistics, series 11, no. 120, USDHHS, Washington, D.C.

Table II.7.

Evaluation of measurement error among trainees

Measurement	Difference between Trainee and Supervisor			
	Good	Fair	Poor	Gross Error
Height (mm)	0 to 5	6 to 9	10 to 19	20 or >
Arm Circum. (mm)	0 to 5	6 to 9	10 to 19	20 or >
Weight (kg)	0 to 0.1	> 0.2	0.3 to 0.4	0.5 or >
Skinfold (mm)	0 to 0.9	1 to 1.9	2 to 4.9	5 or >

Source: Adapted from Zerfas, A. J. 1985. Checking Continuous Measurements: Manual for Anthropometry. Division of Epidemiology, School of Public Health, University of California, Los Angeles.

III
Anthropometric Classification

Statistical Basis of Anthropometric Classification

A productive way for determining the individual's or population's nutritional status is to classify the measurements into anthropometric categories, using as reference the percentage of median of a given standard (1). A general assumption of this classificatory method is that anthropometric information is normally distributed, but not all anthropometric dimensions are normally distributed. For example, observations of the sex-specific distribution of the anthropometric data utilized in the present standard indicate that stature, elbow breadth, sitting height, and upper arm muscle area are normally distributed. On the other hand, weight, triceps skinfold thickness, subscapular skinfold thickness, sum of skinfold thicknesses, arm fat area, arm fat index, and percent fat weight are skewed to the right. Furthermore, even in the same measurement, the meaning of a cutoff point is not the same because the range of variability is different across ages. For example, a value of less than 60% of the median weight-for-age indicates a much more severe state of malnutrition in infants than in school-age children. Therefore, to maximize the diagnostic effectiveness of anthropometric information any classificatory approach should be based upon statistical techniques applicable to normally and nonnormally distributed variables. For this reason, we propose that anthropometric classification be based on both Z-score (2) and percentile cutoffs. The formula for calculating the Z-score is:

$$\text{Z-score} = (\text{Standard's mean value - value of subject})\,/\,\text{standard deviation of standard}$$

For example, an 8-year-old boy who is 119.0 cm tall when compared to the standard (i.e., in table IV.1, for the 8.0–8.9 age group, the mean = 129.8 cm and the S.D. = 6.3 cm) would have a Z-score of -1.714 [(129.8 - 119.0) / 6.3 = -1.74].

As shown in table III.1 and illustrated in figure III.1, a value that is *less* than 1.65 Z-score from the mean is comparable to a value that is *below* the 5th percentile, and a value that is *less* than 1.04 Z-score from the mean is comparable to a value that is *below* the 15th percentile. Conversely, a value that is *above* the 85th percentile is comparable to a value that is 1.04 Z-score *above* the mean, and a value that is *above* the 95th percentile is comparable to a value that is 1.65 Z-score *above* the mean. Then, based on this information the anthropometric standards can be classified into five statistical categories whose upper limit of normality is the *95th* percentile. Therefore, the corresponding five statistical anthropometric categories are as follows:

Category I   = Below 5th percentile or Z-score is less than -1.650.
Category II = 5.0 to 15th percentile or Z-score is between-1.645 and -1.040.
Category III = 15.1 to 85th percentile or Z-score is between-1.036 and +1.030.
Category IV = 85.1 to 95th percentile or Z-score is between +1.036 and +1.640.
Category V   = 95.1 to 100th percentile or Z-score is equal to or greater than +1.645.

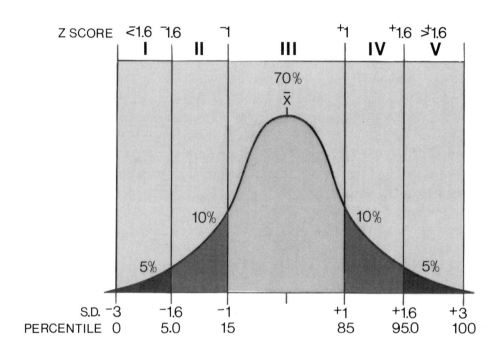

Fig. III.1. Schematization of the statistical relationship of Z-scores, percentile ranges, and standard deviations. Based on this relationship, the five anthropometric categories have been established.

Table III.1.
Equivalents of percentile and Z-scores in a normal distribution

Below Mean		Above Mean	
Percentile	Z-score	Percentile	Z-score
0.0 to 4.9	-3.090 to -1.650	50.0 to 54.9	0.000 to 0.120
5.0 to 9.9	-1.645 to -1.290	55.0 to 59.9	0.126 to 0.250
10.0 to 14.9	-1.282 to -1.040	60.0 to 64.9	0.253 to 0.380
15.0 to 19.9	-1.036 to -0.850	65.0 to 69.9	0.385 to 0.520
20.0 to 24.9	-0.842 to -0.680	70.0 to 74.9	0.524 to 0.670
25.0 to 29.9	-0.675 to -0.530	75.0 to 79.9	0.675 to 0.840
30.0 to 34.9	-0.524 to -0.390	80.0 to 84.9	0.842 to 1.030
35.0 to 39.9	-0.385 to -0.260	85.0 to 89.9	1.036 to 1.280
40.0 to 44.9	-0.253 to -0130	90.0 to 94.9	1.282 to 1.640
45.0 to 50.0	-0.126 to -0.000	95.0 to 99.9	1.645 to 3.090

Classification for Evaluations of Growth and Nutritional Status

As shown in table III.2 these five categories are applied to the evaluation of growth and nutritional status. Based upon measures of linear growth (child's height) children are classified as either short, below average, average, above average, or tall, depending upon whether they fall into one of these five categories. Measurements of upper muscle area provide information about the components of variability in body weight. Thus, a child whose muscle area by height falls in Category I can be classified as wasted, while another whose high muscle area by height falls in Category IV or V certainly indicates good nutritional status, which is also reflected in high stature by age and adequate muscle area by age. On the other hand, if an individual falls in Category I, IV or V of weight status all it can be inferred is that he or she is underweight or overweight, but the components of such variability can not be determined. However, if the underweight or overweight individual also falls in Category I, IV, or V of upper muscle area can indicate an actual risk of undernutrition or reflect a good nutritional status.

Table III.2.

Anthropometric classification for the evaluation of growth
and nutritional status

	Percentile	Z-score	Growth Status[1]	Weight Status[2]	Muscle Status[3]
Category I	0.0 to 5.0	Z < -1.650	Short	Low Weight	Low Muscle Wasted
Category II	5.1 to 15.0	-1.645 < Z < -1.040	Below Average	Below Average	Below Average
Category III	15.1 to 85.0	-1.036 < Z < +1.030	Average	Average	Average
Category IV	85.1 to 95.0	+1.036 < Z < +1.640	Above Average	Above Average	Above Average
Category V	95.1 to 100.0	Z > +1.645	Tall	Heavy Weight	High Muscle: Good Nutrition

Z-score = (standard's mean value - value of subjects / standard deviation of standard).

[1]Growth Status defined with reference to sex-specific standards of height.

[2]Weight Status defined with reference to sex-specific standards of weight by age and/or by frame size.

[3]Muscle Status defined with reference to sex-specific standards of mid arm muscle area by age and/or by frame size.

Classification for the Evaluation of Fat Status

A general assumption in the evaluation of anthropometric nutritional status is that the standard embodies desirable qualities to which the individual or population aims to reach. According to current research, excessive fatness is a negative health risk factor, because it is usually associated with high blood pressures and high lipid levels (3–5), so that age for age, fatter individuals have higher blood pressures and higher lipid levels than leaner ones (5). Therefore, in order to be considered desirable, an anthropometric standard should be based upon individuals who are not excessively fat. Studies of NHANES I data found a direct relationship of weight and skinfold thickness to blood pressure, which was consistent in all ethnic groups, for both sexes, and across the adult age range of 18–74 years (6). In other words, those individuals who were characterized by excessive weight and fatness were also characterized by negative health risk factors.

Since the NHANES I and II data were obtained to derive representative samples of all segments of the U.S. population from the anthropometric point of view, it includes individuals with undesirable traits (high fat) as well as those with desirable traits. For this reason, we decided to determine the association between percentile categories of sum of skinfold thickness and blood pressures, and between percentile categories of sum of skinfold thickness and serum cholesterol levels. Analyses of the data indicated that adults whose skinfold thickness (sum of triceps and subscapular skinfolds) were below the age- and sex-specific percentiles had systolic/diastolic blood pressures that were below 160/90 mmHg. and serum cholesterol levels that were below 270 mg/100 ml. These data suggest that individuals whose fatness is below the *85th* percentile can be considered to have fat levels associated with positive health, since the values for blood pressure and cholesterol are below the hypertensive and hypercholesterimia criteria.

Thus, assuming a normal distribution and using the *85th* percentile of skinfold thickness as the upper limit as shown below, the data on fatness can be classified into five categories:

Category I = Below 5th percentile or Z-score is less than -1.650.
Category II = 5.1 to 15th percentile or Z-score is between -1.645 and -1.040.
Category III = 15.1 to 75th percentile or Z-score is between -1.036 and +0.670.
Category IV = 75.1 to 85th percentile or Z-score is between +0.675 and +1.030.
Category V = 85.1 to 100th percentile or Z-score is equal to or greater than +1.036.

In table III.3, these five categories are applied to measurements of sum of (triceps and subscapular) skinfold thickness, arm fat index, and percent fat weight. The use of these three measurements increases the diagnostic efficiency of determining with certainty the fat status of an examinee. For example, when using all three measurements if an individual falls in Category V one can conclude that the subject has excessive fatness and is at risk of obesity. Conversely, if an individual falls in Category I and if his muscle size is adequate one can ascertain that the individual's low weight is attributable to his leanness.

Table III.3.
Anthropometric classification for the evaluation of fat status

	Percentile	**Z-score**	**Fat Status[1]**
Category I	0.0 to 5.0	$Z < -1.650$	Lean
Category II	5.1 to 15.0	$-1.645 < Z < -1.040$	Below Average
Category III	15.1 to 75.0	$-1.036 < Z < +0.670$	Average
Category IV	75.1 to 85.0	$+0.675 < Z < +1.030$	Above Average
Category V	85.1 to 100.0	$Z > +1.036$	Excess Fat

Z-score = (Standard's mean value - value of subjects + standard deviation of standard).

[1]Fat Status defined with reference to sex- and age-specific standards of sum of triceps and subscapular skinfold thicknesses, mid arm fat area, mid arm fat index, and/or % fat weight.

A basic premise for this classification is that measurements of weight and height are effective for determining variability in body size and linear growth but are less effective for determining the components of variability in body composition. If the goal is ascertaining the sources of variability in body growth and body size a given analytic approach should enable the investigator to differentiate the past and present nutritional status of the examinee. We believe that the present classification, because it incorporates known measures indicative of nutritional status, permits the investigator to determine the magnitude of variability in growth and body size and actually identify the nutritional components of such variability. Furthermore, in this classificatory approach the cutoff points are comparable across anthropometric dimensions and across all ages. For example, a subject whose weight and muscle are in the high category but whose measurements of fat (such as sum of skinfold thicknesses, and arm fat index) approach the average is not at risk of obesity. On the other hand, an individual whose measurements of fat are in the high category (greater than 85th percentile) can be considered to be at risk of obesity, even though the weight may approach the average. Conversely, if the muscle area is below the 5th percentile and is also associated with low fat area and low arm fat index, this indicates that the examinee is at risk of undernutrition. Similarly, if *both* the stature and the mid arm muscle area are below the 5th percentile, or 1.65 Z-scores below the mean, this indicates that the child is short and wasted and thus probably suffering from chronic malnutrition.

As pointed out before, in both clinical and nonclinical populations measures of excess weight or underweight per se are poor indicators of health status. A proper evaluation of nutritional status needs to be based upon measurements of body composition such as those given by measurements of skinfold thickness and estimates of body muscle and skeletal frame. Indeed, clinical studies have shown that for determining protein and calorie depletion anthropometric evaluations are more sensitive than biochemical approaches. For example, the Category I given in the present anthropometric classification does coincide with limits of malnutrition derived from studies of patients suffering from debilitating diseases. According to Heymsfield and associates (7), the lower limit of upper arm (bone-free) muscle area for adults compatible with survival is between 9 to 11 sq cm for muscle, and 2 to 5 sq cm for fat area. In the present standards, these values are found between the 5th percentile and 85th percentile ranges for arm muscle area and fat area, depending on sex, age, and frame size. Similarly, extensive experience in nonclinical populations has shown that better information about the risk of obesity is obtained from measurements of skinfold thickness and estimates of body muscle than from measurements of weight alone. For example, on the basis of information on weight alone a high proportion of Eskimos can be considered to be at risk of obesity, but when evaluated with reference to skinfold thickness they are not.

As shown by the examples presented in chapter V, each anthropometric dimension provides a different set of diagnostic information. Therefore, an appropriate assessment of anthropometric nutritional status requires evaluation of several dimensions. It should also be noted that the diagnostic efficiency of a given measure also depends on the general physiological status of the examinee. For example, small changes in nitrogen balance, especially over short time periods, cannot be measured accurately with anthropometric measurements of muscle area. Similarly, periodic changes in adipose tissue hydration that occur during the menstrual cycle can affect the compressibility of skinfolds. In the same manner, because skinfold compressibility varies with age, sex, and anatomical site, two individuals with the same value of skinfold thickness at a given anatomical location may have different amounts of fat at that location. *Therefore, as a general rule, diagnostic information inferred from anthropometry should be corroborated by data derived from clinical and biochemical observations.*

IV
Anthropometric Standards

Anthropometric Tables by Age, Sex, Height, and Frame Size

Anthropometric Tables

The anthropometric data are presented in two groups: (1) by age, sex, and height, and (2) by height, age, and frame size.

By Age, Sex, and Height. The anthropometric data by age, sex, and height are presented in tables IV.1 to IV.21 as follows:

1. stature by age for adults
2. weight by age for adults
3. weight by height for adults
4. weight by height for adults
5. body mass index by age for adults
6. sitting height by age for adults
7. sitting height index by age for adults
8. bitrochanteric breadth by age for adults
9. elbow breadth by age for adults
10. mid upper arm circumference by age for adults
11. mid upper arm area by age for adults
12. mid upper arm muscle area by age for adults
13. mid upper arm muscle area by height for boys and girls
14. mid upper arm fat area by age for adults
15. mid arm fat index by age for adults
16. triceps skinfold thickness by age for adults
17. subscapular skinfold thickness by age for adults
18. sum of skinfold thickness by age for adults
19. percent fat weight by age for adult adults
20. percent fat weight associated with summed skinfold thicknesses for adult males
21. percent fat weight associated with summed skinfold thicknesses for adult females

By Age, Sex, and Frame Size. The anthropometric data by age, sex, and frame size are presented in tables IV.22 to IV.25 as follows:

22. weight by age and frame size for adult males
23. weight by age and frame size for adult females
24. mid upper arm muscle area by age and frame size for adult males
25. mid upper arm muscle area by age and frame size for adult females

Percentiles. These data are presented in the form of means, standard deviations, and percentile ranges. The 5th, 10th, 15th, 25th, 50th, 75th, 85th, 90th, and 95th percentiles are included.

Age Groups. Following the classificatory approach of the National Center for Health Statistics (NCHS) the sample under18 years of age was classified into one-year age groups (e.g., 1.0 to 1.9, 2.0 to 2.9, etc.). In addition, those aged between 18 and 75 years were grouped into one seven-year age group (e.g., 18.0 to 24.9), and ten five-year age groups (e.g., 25.0 to 29.9, 30.0 to 34.9, 35.0 to 39.9, 40.0 to 44.9, etc.).

Height Groups. The data of weight by height for children and adults were tabulated by 3 cm of height. The children were classified into two age groups: (a) 2 to 11 years and 12 to17 years for boys and (b) 2 to 10 years and 11 to17 years for girls. On the other hand, the data of muscle area by height for children were calculated for every 6 cm of height rather than every 3 cm. This is because there were no major height-associated changes in muscle area when using 3-cm height intervals.

Anthropometric Data for Blacks and Whites. In Appendix A and Appendix B the anthropometric data for blacks and whites are given separately. It should be noted that these percentiles are not weighted for sampling size as was the case for the combined samples given in this chapter. Furthermore, due to small sample size for blacks anthropometric data by frame size are not given.

Table IV. 1.
Means, standard deviations, and percentiles of stature (cm) by age for males and females of 1 to 74 years

Age (yrs)	N	Mean	SD	Percentiles								
				5	10	15	25	50	75	85	90	95
Males												
1.0–1.9	366	82.5	5.1	75.5	76.7	77.8	79.3	82.1	85.6	87.2	88.0	89.8
2.0–2.9	664	91.4	4.3	84.9	86.3	87.2	88.4	91.4	94.4	95.8	96.9	98.0
3.0–3.9	716	99.1	4.7	91.6	93.7	94.7	96.1	98.7	102.0	103.9	104.9	107.0
4.0–4.9	709	106.0	5.1	98.1	99.5	100.5	102.7	106.1	109.3	111.2	112.3	114.1
5.0–5.9	675	112.6	5.3	103.9	105.9	107.4	109.3	112.7	115.7	118.1	119.2	121.2
6.0–6.9	298	119.2	5.4	109.4	112.0	113.3	115.7	119.4	122.8	124.9	126.0	127.7
7.0–7.9	312	125.1	5.7	115.6	118.2	119.6	121.5	125.4	128.5	130.6	131.6	133.5
8.0–8.9	296	129.8	6.3	120.0	122.6	123.9	125.9	130.1	133.7	136.0	137.5	140.0
9.0–9.9	322	135.8	5.8	126.0	128.7	129.7	131.4	135.8	139.9	142.0	143.0	145.0
10.0–10.9	334	140.9	6.9	130.2	132.3	133.8	136.1	140.9	145.8	148.2	150.1	152.7
11.0–11.9	324	146.4	7.4	134.3	136.6	138.8	141.6	146.4	151.5	154.0	155.0	158.1
12.0–12.9	349	152.2	8.1	139.7	141.9	143.6	146.4	151.4	157.9	160.4	162.3	166.0
13.0–13.9	350	159.2	8.8	145.1	147.8	149.6	152.8	159.3	165.6	168.9	170.7	173.2
14.0–14.9	359	167.1	8.2	153.3	156.3	158.6	161.7	166.9	172.8	175.9	178.2	179.9
15.0–15.9	359	170.8	7.3	158.5	161.5	162.9	165.6	171.2	176.2	177.9	179.8	182.5
16.0–16.9	349	174.5	7.1	163.4	165.0	167.3	169.8	174.1	178.7	182.0	183.8	186.7
17.0–17.9	338	175.5	6.9	164.4	166.9	168.6	170.7	175.1	180.5	183.0	184.5	187.3
18.0–24.9	1755	176.6	7.0	165.4	167.8	169.5	171.9	176.6	181.2	183.7	185.5	188.6
25.0–29.9	1255	176.7	7.0	165.1	167.8	169.4	172.0	176.6	181.5	184.0	185.7	188.0
30.0–34.9	947	176.2	6.9	164.8	167.4	169.0	171.5	176.2	180.9	183.3	184.8	187.2
35.0–39.9	839	176.1	7.2	164.0	166.8	168.8	171.9	176.1	181.0	183.5	185.0	187.7
40.0–44.9	829	175.9	6.7	165.0	167.2	168.9	171.4	176.0	180.3	182.7	184.2	186.9
45.0–49.9	871	175.2	7.1	163.8	166.5	168.0	170.6	174.8	180.2	182.9	184.5	186.6
50.0–54.9	882	174.6	6.5	164.2	166.4	167.8	170.1	174.6	178.8	181.4	183.2	185.3
55.0–59.9	807	173.9	6.8	163.2	165.0	166.8	169.3	173.8	178.7	181.0	182.3	184.6
60.0–64.9	1261	173.0	6.6	161.9	165.0	166.4	168.7	173.0	177.4	179.8	181.3	183.7
65.0–69.9	1773	171.5	6.9	159.7	162.9	164.5	166.7	171.6	176.3	178.6	180.1	182.5
70.0–74.9	1257	170.6	6.8	159.5	162.0	163.6	165.8	170.7	175.0	177.4	179.4	182.0
Females												
1.0–1.9	333	80.6	4.8	73.2	74.7	75.6	77.4	80.5	83.6	85.9	86.8	88.6
2.0–2.9	610	90.1	4.5	83.1	84.9	85.6	86.8	90.1	93.0	94.6	95.7	97.4
3.0–3.9	651	97.7	4.5	90.3	92.1	92.9	94.8	97.5	100.6	102.4	103.4	105.0
4.0–4.9	678	105.0	4.9	97.0	98.5	99.6	101.6	104.9	108.3	110.0	111.2	113.6
5.0–5.9	673	112.0	5.4	103.1	105.3	106.7	108.6	111.9	115.4	117.4	119.0	120.6
6.0–6.9	296	118.3	5.6	109.9	111.4	112.4	114.2	118.5	122.2	124.2	125.2	127.6
7.0–7.9	331	124.2	6.0	115.3	117.0	118.3	120.3	124.3	128.4	130.1	131.7	134.5
8.0–8.9	276	129.8	6.0	120.1	122.1	123.7	125.5	129.7	133.5	135.6	137.8	140.1
9.0–9.9	322	135.7	7.2	125.7	127.5	128.4	130.5	135.6	140.4	142.5	143.9	147.2
10.0–10.9	330	141.5	7.4	129.5	132.2	133.9	136.3	141.6	146.0	148.3	150.9	154.4
11.0–11.9	303	148.1	8.2	134.7	138.1	139.8	142.3	148.4	153.4	156.1	158.0	162.1
12.0–12.9	324	154.6	7.2	143.0	145.2	147.0	149.6	154.6	159.3	162.5	164.0	165.5
13.0–13.9	361	158.8	6.2	149.1	151.1	152.8	155.1	158.8	162.8	164.8	165.7	168.3
14.0–14.9	370	160.9	6.2	151.0	153.0	154.5	156.8	160.8	164.9	167.0	168.8	171.7
15.0–15.9	309	163.2	6.5	152.8	155.2	157.1	158.8	162.7	167.2	169.7	172.0	175.4
16.0–16.9	343	162.2	6.6	151.4	153.6	155.5	157.7	162.3	166.4	169.1	171.6	173.2
17.0–17.9	293	162.7	6.0	153.2	155.5	156.9	159.2	162.3	166.4	168.7	169.9	172.8
18.0–24.9	2592	163.0	6.5	152.3	154.8	156.4	158.8	163.1	167.1	169.6	171.0	173.6
25.0–29.9	1935	162.9	6.3	152.6	155.2	156.6	158.6	162.8	167.1	169.5	170.9	173.3
30.0–34.9	1633	162.6	6.2	152.9	155.2	156.4	158.4	162.4	166.8	169.2	171.2	173.1
35.0–39.9	1461	162.8	6.5	152.0	155.0	156.4	158.6	162.7	167.0	169.4	171.0	173.5
40.0–44.9	1399	162.6	6.4	151.6	154.3	156.2	158.1	162.7	166.7	168.8	170.5	173.2
45.0–49.9	969	162.0	6.3	151.7	154.0	155.4	157.9	162.0	166.3	168.4	169.9	172.2
50.0–54.9	1012	161.2	6.0	151.3	153.8	155.3	156.9	161.1	165.1	167.3	169.2	171.0
55.0–59.9	887	160.3	6.2	149.8	152.7	154.1	156.7	160.3	164.4	166.6	167.8	170.1
60.0–64.9	1392	159.6	6.4	149.2	151.4	153.0	155.6	160.0	163.7	166.1	167.3	169.8
65.0–69.9	1952	158.6	6.1	148.5	150.7	152.4	154.8	158.8	162.6	164.8	166.2	168.1
70.0–74.9	1467	157.6	6.1	147.2	150.0	151.7	153.7	157.4	161.5	163.8	165.5	167.5

Table IV. 2.
Means, standard deviations, and percentiles of weight (kg) by age for males and females of 1 to 74 years

Age (yrs)	N	Mean	SD	Percentiles								
				5	10	15	25	50	75	85	90	95
Males												
1.0–1.9	681	11.8	1.7	9.6	10.0	10.3	10.7	11.6	12.6	13.1	13.7	14.4
2.0–2.9	677	13.6	1.7	11.1	11.6	11.9	12.5	13.6	14.6	15.2	15.8	16.6
3.0–3.9	717	15.7	2.1	12.8	13.4	13.8	14.4	15.5	16.8	17.5	18.1	19.4
4.0–4.9	709	17.7	2.4	14.1	15.0	15.4	16.1	17.5	19.0	20.0	20.6	21.5
5.0–5.9	676	19.9	3.0	16.0	16.7	17.1	17.8	19.6	21.4	22.4	23.5	25.4
6.0–6.9	298	22.6	3.7	17.5	18.8	19.4	20.2	21.9	24.0	26.0	27.7	30.0
7.0–7.9	312	25.1	4.2	19.0	20.4	21.2	22.2	24.7	27.2	28.7	29.9	33.1
8.0–8.9	296	27.7	5.2	21.5	22.7	23.5	24.5	26.8	29.7	31.8	33.6	37.3
9.0–9.9	322	31.3	6.3	23.6	24.7	25.7	27.1	30.3	33.6	37.1	40.3	43.2
10.0–10.9	334	35.4	7.8	26.2	27.7	28.5	30.2	33.8	38.6	42.1	45.6	53.1
11.0–11.9	324	39.8	10.0	28.3	30.0	31.5	33.4	37.6	43.3	48.6	52.3	58.6
12.0–12.9	349	44.2	11.1	30.8	32.8	34.4	36.6	42.2	49.0	53.9	59.0	66.9
13.0–13.9	348	49.8	11.6	34.6	37.1	38.7	41.6	48.5	56.1	60.3	65.2	69.6
14.0–14.9	359	56.9	11.9	41.3	44.0	45.9	49.2	55.3	63.0	66.4	70.1	76.9
15.0–15.9	359	61.0	11.2	44.7	48.6	50.8	54.2	60.0	66.2	70.4	74.4	81.3
16.0–16.9	349	66.8	11.9	51.7	54.2	55.7	59.0	64.8	72.9	77.8	81.6	89.0
17.0–17.9	339	67.5	12.2	51.1	54.1	56.5	59.3	65.7	72.5	78.0	83.3	91.4
18.0–24.9	1758	73.9	13.4	56.4	59.8	61.6	64.8	71.4	80.5	86.3	91.5	99.9
25.0–29.9	1256	77.9	14.6	58.7	61.8	64.5	68.1	76.0	84.8	90.6	95.1	103.4
30.0–34.9	948	79.8	14.4	59.8	63.3	66.3	69.8	78.4	87.4	93.4	96.8	103.0
35.0–39.9	840	80.3	13.6	58.4	62.9	66.6	72.2	79.8	87.8	92.4	96.7	102.8
40.0–44.9	830	81.0	13.8	60.7	64.3	67.9	71.9	79.6	89.4	94.3	98.8	104.8
45.0–49.9	871	80.8	14.0	60.0	64.0	66.8	71.4	79.7	89.2	94.0	97.2	103.6
50.0–54.9	882	79.5	13.9	58.7	63.3	66.2	70.0	78.0	87.4	93.3	99.3	103.6
55.0–59.9	808	79.4	13.9	58.2	63.0	66.4	70.2	78.5	86.8	92.9	97.1	103.5
60.0–64.9	1263	77.3	13.1	57.9	61.8	64.5	68.8	76.8	84.9	89.3	92.5	100.0
65.0–69.9	1774	75.0	13.0	55.1	58.5	61.5	66.4	74.5	83.2	88.0	91.8	97.2
70.0–74.9	1257	73.7	12.9	53.9	57.5	60.4	65.2	73.0	81.3	86.3	90.4	95.9
Females												
1.0–1.9	622	10.9	1.4	8.7	9.2	9.5	9.9	10.8	11.8	12.4	12.8	13.4
2.0–2.9	615	13.0	1.6	10.8	11.2	11.6	12.0	12.8	13.9	14.6	15.1	15.9
3.0–3.9	653	15.0	2.1	11.8	12.6	13.0	13.6	14.7	16.2	17.1	17.6	18.6
4.0–4.9	682	17.1	2.4	13.7	14.3	14.7	15.5	16.8	18.4	19.4	20.1	21.3
5.0–5.9	674	19.5	3.2	15.3	16.2	16.8	17.3	19.0	21.0	22.4	23.6	25.3
6.0–6.9	296	21.8	3.6	17.0	17.7	18.6	19.4	21.3	23.7	24.8	26.5	28.9
7.0–7.9	331	24.7	4.5	19.2	19.8	20.6	21.9	23.8	26.5	28.7	29.9	32.7
8.0–8.9	276	28.1	6.3	20.9	21.9	22.6	24.0	26.9	30.4	33.3	35.1	39.9
9.0–9.9	322	32.0	7.5	23.7	24.8	25.6	26.8	30.7	34.7	38.9	41.7	46.5
10.0–10.9	330	35.7	8.4	25.6	27.0	27.9	29.6	33.9	39.2	44.1	46.5	52.4
11.0–11.9	303	41.8	11.0	29.1	30.5	31.6	34.3	39.8	46.3	52.8	56.9	61.9
12.0–12.9	324	47.1	10.7	32.5	34.3	36.3	39.1	45.9	53.0	58.5	61.2	66.7
13.0–13.9	361	51.5	11.7	37.2	39.3	40.6	44.3	49.6	55.7	61.6	66.8	76.2
14.0–14.9	370	54.7	11.2	40.3	42.9	44.8	47.3	52.7	60.0	64.9	69.5	75.6
15.0–15.9	309	56.4	11.6	43.4	45.3	46.6	48.6	54.2	60.3	65.2	69.5	79.4
16.0–16.9	343	58.2	11.7	43.4	46.1	47.5	50.8	55.7	62.8	68.9	73.1	80.8
17.0–17.9	293	59.7	13.3	43.2	46.4	49.2	51.9	57.4	63.3	69.4	74.7	86.0
18.0–24.9	2592	60.8	12.8	45.6	48.4	50.0	52.6	58.3	65.4	71.5	76.1	84.3
25.0–29.9	1935	62.8	14.2	46.6	49.0	50.7	53.4	59.4	68.4	76.1	81.6	90.8
30.0–34.9	1633	65.6	16.1	47.5	50.1	52.0	54.9	61.5	72.2	80.5	86.5	97.9
35.0–39.9	1461	67.1	15.8	48.6	51.7	53.1	56.4	63.3	73.7	82.0	88.1	98.2
40.0–44.9	1399	67.8	16.1	49.2	51.8	54.0	57.0	64.0	75.1	83.3	89.8	99.1
45.0–49.9	969	68.2	16.3	47.8	51.4	53.5	57.1	64.9	75.9	83.0	87.4	98.4
50.0–54.9	1012	68.3	14.8	48.8	51.9	54.4	58.1	65.8	75.8	83.1	88.4	97.1
55.0–59.9	888	69.2	16.3	48.6	52.2	54.5	58.2	66.3	77.2	85.2	89.4	98.5
60.0–64.9	1393	68.0	14.2	48.5	51.7	54.1	58.1	66.0	75.8	82.1	86.0	94.1
65.0–69.9	1954	67.5	14.2	47.8	51.4	53.9	57.7	65.7	74.8	80.8	86.1	93.9
70.0–74.9	1468	66.0	13.6	46.5	50.1	52.4	57.0	64.5	74.4	79.7	83.3	88.8

Table IV. 3.
Means, standard deviations, and percentiles of weight (kg) by height (cm) for males of 2 to 74 years

Height (cm)	N	Mean	SD	Percentiles								
				5	10	15	25	50	75	85	90	95
boys: 2 to 11 years												
84–086	75	12.1	1.1	10.7	10.9	11.1	11.3	11.9	12.8	13.1	13.5	14.3
87–089	170	12.8	1.1	11.2	11.4	11.7	12.0	12.7	13.4	13.8	14.2	14.6
90–092	207	13.5	1.0	11.9	12.1	12.5	12.8	13.6	14.2	14.6	14.9	15.2
93–095	278	14.4	1.2	12.7	13.0	13.4	13.6	14.3	15.1	15.5	15.8	16.3
96–098	310	15.0	1.3	13.3	13.6	13.8	14.2	15.0	15.6	16.1	16.4	17.0
99–101	300	16.0	1.3	13.9	14.4	14.7	15.1	15.9	16.7	17.2	17.6	18.3
102–104	290	16.9	1.4	15.1	15.4	15.6	15.9	16.8	17.7	18.0	18.5	19.3
105–107	291	17.6	1.6	15.4	15.9	16.2	16.6	17.5	18.4	19.0	19.4	19.8
108–110	298	18.7	1.7	16.7	17.0	17.1	17.6	18.5	19.6	20.1	20.5	21.3
111–113	274	20.0	2.2	17.0	17.8	18.1	18.7	19.6	21.0	21.7	22.4	23.4
114–116	223	20.9	2.2	18.6	19.0	19.2	19.6	20.5	21.7	22.3	22.7	23.6
117–119	199	21.9	2.3	19.0	19.6	20.2	20.5	21.5	23.0	23.8	24.3	26.0
120–122	177	23.3	2.4	19.8	20.8	21.2	21.9	23.1	24.5	25.4	26.0	27.3
123–125	174	25.0	2.8	21.5	22.0	22.7	23.4	24.5	26.2	27.0	28.2	30.0
126–128	185	26.5	3.8	22.6	23.1	23.8	24.3	25.9	27.8	29.4	30.6	32.0
129–131	174	27.6	3.1	23.5	24.4	24.7	25.6	27.3	28.9	30.0	31.0	32.9
132–134	180	29.3	3.5	25.1	25.7	25.8	26.8	28.5	31.0	33.0	34.4	35.4
135–137	175	31.4	4.6	26.2	27.1	27.6	28.5	30.4	33.0	34.9	37.4	41.5
138–140	150	33.5	4.7	28.2	28.9	29.4	30.5	32.3	35.1	37.8	39.9	42.0
141–143	153	36.1	5.0	30.4	31.3	31.8	33.0	34.9	38.2	40.5	43.3	45.4
144–146	114	38.9	6.6	31.6	32.7	33.1	35.1	37.6	41.2	43.9	46.3	50.7
147–149	87	40.9	6.8	33.6	34.3	35.3	35.9	39.2	43.8	47.3	51.5	56.7
boys: 12 to 17 years												
144–146	59	38.1	5.5	31.1	32.4	33.6	34.6	36.5	40.3	42.1	46.1	53.0
147–149	77	40.9	7.1	33.6	34.0	34.7	36.5	38.3	43.8	47.4	49.4	59.8
150–152	103	43.4	6.6	36.3	37.2	38.0	38.7	41.4	46.5	51.5	54.7	56.7
153–155	106	45.9	7.9	36.5	38.1	39.1	40.6	43.7	49.7	51.9	55.2	60.9
156–158	113	48.5	9.2	39.9	40.7	41.3	42.5	45.8	50.0	57.9	62.0	67.3
159–161	146	51.1	9.2	40.8	42.9	43.9	45.6	48.6	53.6	60.9	65.4	68.4
162–164	177	54.8	8.9	44.7	45.9	46.9	49.1	53.2	58.4	61.8	64.3	69.1
165–167	197	57.3	9.2	47.1	48.8	49.9	51.3	55.3	61.0	64.8	68.6	73.3
168–170	235	61.4	10.4	49.2	51.4	52.4	55.0	59.9	65.5	69.6	72.5	79.1
171–173	233	62.8	8.8	51.4	53.4	54.8	56.9	61.3	66.1	71.2	73.7	78.2
174–176	202	66.7	10.9	52.3	55.7	57.4	60.0	64.8	71.2	75.5	81.4	89.9
177–179	166	68.8	12.0	55.8	58.7	59.6	61.6	66.3	72.3	75.5	79.6	88.0
180–182	103	71.8	9.7	60.2	60.9	62.1	64.0	70.1	79.5	82.2	85.2	88.7
183–185	64	73.5	9.1	62.4	63.6	65.4	67.8	72.1	77.3	79.4	89.9	91.1
Males: 18 to 74 years												
153–155	56	64.6	13.0	48.6	51.3	54.5	57.1	62.0	66.8	76.8	80.6	83.5
156–158	140	65.5	11.2	48.3	51.4	54.0	57.4	64.9	72.0	77.3	79.3	86.0
159–161	292	66.2	10.8	49.1	53.8	56.4	59.2	66.0	71.2	76.9	80.2	84.3
162–164	643	68.0	10.5	52.2	55.2	57.0	60.4	67.3	74.5	79.1	81.6	86.9
165–167	1147	70.8	11.6	53.0	56.6	59.6	62.7	72.7	80.2	82.3	85.2	90.1
168–170	1582	73.5	12.0	55.9	58.6	61.3	65.9	72.7	80.2	84.5	87.9	93.4
171–173	2047	76.1	12.5	58.2	61.3	63.6	67.6	75.1	83.2	88.1	92.0	97.8
174–176	2053	78.3	12.7	60.0	63.8	66.1	69.5	77.3	84.9	90.1	93.8	99.7
177–179	1750	80.3	12.8	61.9	65.1	67.5	71.4	79.4	87.3	92.6	96.5	102.6
180–182	1252	82.6	13.6	63.4	67.3	69.6	72.9	81.4	90.1	95.0	99.4	105.7
183–185	833	85.2	13.9	65.1	69.2	71.5	75.3	83.3	93.4	99.1	103.2	110.4
186–188	398	88.0	13.3	68.9	72.3	74.8	79.4	86.6	95.1	100.4	103.5	109.8
189–191	161	92.0	16.0	71.3	75.3	77.8	80.7	89.9	99.4	105.0	110.8	123.7
192–194	66	95.9	15.8	71.8	78.6	80.2	84.8	94.2	105.2	109.1	111.8	123.8

41

Table IV. 4.
Means, standard deviations, and percentiles of weight (kg) by height (cm) for females of 2 to 74 years

Height (cm)	N	Mean	SD	Percentiles								
				5	10	15	25	50	75	85	90	95
Girls: 2 to 10 years												
81–083	36	11.2	.8	10.1	10.2	10.3	10.4	11.0	11.7	12.1	12.6	12.6
84–086	118	11.9	.9	10.5	10.8	11.0	11.3	12.0	12.5	12.7	13.0	13.6
87–089	156	12.5	1.2	11.0	11.3	11.6	11.8	12.4	13.0	13.6	13.8	14.6
90–092	229	13.2	1.2	11.6	11.8	12.0	12.3	13.0	13.8	14.3	14.6	15.2
93–095	259	13.9	1.2	12.0	12.6	12.8	13.1	13.8	14.6	15.1	15.5	16.1
96–098	275	15.0	1.3	13.1	13.5	13.7	14.1	14.9	15.6	16.3	16.7	17.2
99–101	272	15.8	1.6	13.8	14.1	14.3	14.6	15.5	16.6	17.2	17.6	18.4
102–104	278	16.6	2.0	14.2	14.6	15.0	15.5	16.4	17.3	18.0	18.5	19.4
105–107	270	17.6	1.6	15.3	15.8	16.1	16.6	17.3	18.4	19.2	19.4	20.1
108–110	275	18.3	1.6	15.9	16.6	16.8	17.2	18.1	19.2	20.0	20.4	21.1
111–113	251	19.4	1.9	16.6	17.1	17.3	17.9	19.4	20.4	21.2	21.8	22.8
114–116	215	20.7	2.5	17.5	18.3	18.6	19.0	20.2	21.8	22.9	23.9	25.7
117–119	191	21.9	2.6	19.0	19.4	19.5	20.2	21.4	23.0	24.0	24.8	26.6
120–122	181	23.1	2.5	20.1	20.4	20.9	21.5	22.6	24.0	25.3	26.2	27.7
123–125	162	24.5	2.5	21.2	21.8	22.3	22.8	24.0	25.9	26.5	27.2	29.0
126–128	172	26.2	3.1	22.6	23.0	23.4	23.9	25.6	27.7	29.4	30.0	31.5
129–131	157	28.0	3.8	23.6	24.3	24.8	25.6	27.3	29.4	31.1	33.4	36.6
132–134	148	30.3	4.4	25.1	25.8	26.2	27.0	29.4	32.3	34.5	37.2	39.9
135–137	135	32.1	5.4	25.6	27.2	27.7	28.3	30.8	33.9	35.8	41.6	44.1
138–140	124	34.6	7.3	27.6	28.8	29.1	30.6	32.5	35.5	40.9	43.5	47.5
141–143	97	36.0	6.3	28.8	29.8	30.7	32.2	34.8	37.9	41.3	45.6	49.9
144–146	65	39.2	7.0	31.0	31.9	32.9	34.5	37.6	42.9	45.3	48.4	51.8
147–149	45	40.0	7.3	30.7	32.3	34.0	35.0	38.3	44.2	48.0	50.8	54.8
Girls: 11 to 17 years												
141–143	54	37.1	7.8	28.9	29.8	31.1	32.2	34.9	38.6	42.4	45.7	59.5
144–146	67	38.5	6.8	30.4	30.8	31.6	32.9	38.4	41.4	44.1	46.5	52.4
147–149	127	43.4	10.0	32.7	34.3	35.4	37.0	40.7	46.7	51.3	56.4	61.2
150–152	180	45.8	9.1	34.7	36.3	37.4	39.5	44.1	49.9	54.3	56.1	61.9
153–155	235	48.8	8.9	38.0	39.5	40.6	43.1	46.7	53.6	56.5	60.0	66.3
156–158	352	52.3	10.4	39.7	41.7	43.1	45.1	49.9	57.5	62.5	66.0	72.3
159–161	372	55.1	11.0	42.2	44.3	46.0	48.3	52.8	59.2	62.9	68.4	77.6
162–164	344	56.6	9.9	44.9	46.6	47.5	50.2	54.4	60.6	65.3	68.6	73.8
165–167	243	60.0	12.5	46.3	48.8	50.1	52.8	57.6	62.7	69.4	74.7	84.7
168–170	124	61.2	10.8	48.9	49.2	51.1	53.5	59.0	65.7	73.4	75.1	82.4
171–173	74	67.5	15.0	53.0	54.3	54.9	57.7	62.1	72.3	80.1	89.1	104.2
Females: 18 to 74 years												
141–143	64	55.9	10.2	39.2	41.3	43.9	49.0	56.5	63.3	64.9	67.7	76.6
144–146	178	57.1	14.2	38.7	42.0	44.3	48.1	54.3	64.4	71.3	74.6	82.0
147–149	430	59.4	13.2	41.5	44.6	46.8	50.1	56.9	66.9	71.9	76.1	84.8
150–152	928	61.1	13.2	43.1	46.5	48.1	51.5	59.0	68.3	74.3	78.4	86.2
153–155	1685	63.0	13.7	45.3	47.5	49.8	53.2	60.7	70.2	77.3	81.6	88.6
156–158	2670	63.8	14.6	46.6	49.1	50.8	53.5	60.7	70.9	77.1	82.3	90.0
159–161	3041	65.3	14.5	47.7	50.2	52.0	55.2	62.3	72.6	79.4	84.6	92.9
162–164	2849	66.9	14.6	49.4	51.5	53.4	56.6	63.5	74.2	81.4	86.0	94.9
165–167	2327	68.2	15.3	50.3	52.8	54.9	57.8	64.5	74.7	82.4	88.6	98.2
168–170	1327	69.5	15.1	52.5	54.7	56.5	59.2	65.4	76.1	83.5	90.1	99.4
171–173	685	71.8	15.8	54.1	55.9	57.9	60.5	67.6	78.9	86.1	93.9	105.0
174–176	334	72.9	17.3	56.1	57.9	59.6	62.3	68.4	77.6	85.7	93.1	106.9
177–179	97	75.3	16.5	57.6	59.9	60.7	64.4	71.2	81.8	89.6	102.1	112.8

Table IV. 5.

Means, standard deviations, and percentiles of body mass index (w/s^2) by age for males and females of 1 to 74 years

Age (yrs)	N	Mean	SD	Percentiles								
				5	10	15	25	50	75	85	90	95
Males												
1.0–1.9	366	17.3	2.4	15.2	15.6	15.9	16.4	17.1	18.0	18.6	19.0	19.6
2.0–2.9	664	16.2	1.3	14.3	14.6	15.0	15.4	16.2	17.1	17.5	17.8	18.4
3.0–3.9	716	16.0	1.4	14.2	14.6	14.8	15.1	15.8	16.6	17.1	17.5	18.2
4.0–4.9	709	15.7	1.3	13.9	14.2	14.5	14.9	15.6	16.4	16.8	17.2	17.8
5.0–5.9	675	15.6	1.5	13.8	14.1	14.3	14.7	15.5	16.3	16.8	17.2	18.1
6.0–6.9	298	15.8	1.9	13.7	14.1	14.3	14.8	15.3	16.4	17.2	18.0	19.3
7.0–7.9	312	16.0	1.8	13.7	14.1	14.3	14.9	15.6	16.7	17.5	18.2	19.5
8.0–8.9	296	16.3	2.2	13.8	14.3	14.6	15.0	15.9	17.1	18.0	19.1	20.1
9.0–9.9	322	16.9	2.4	14.1	14.6	14.8	15.3	16.3	17.7	19.0	19.9	21.8
10.0–10.9	334	17.7	2.8	14.6	15.0	15.3	15.8	17.1	18.7	19.8	21.2	23.4
11.0–11.9	324	18.4	3.6	14.7	15.1	15.7	16.2	17.4	19.8	21.5	22.5	25.3
12.0–12.9	349	18.9	3.5	15.2	15.7	16.1	16.7	17.9	20.2	21.7	23.7	25.8
13.0–13.9	348	19.5	3.5	15.6	16.4	16.6	17.2	18.7	20.7	22.2	24.0	25.9
14.0–14.9	359	20.3	3.3	16.5	17.0	17.5	18.1	19.5	21.6	23.1	24.2	26.4
15.0–15.9	359	20.8	3.1	16.8	17.5	18.0	19.0	20.4	22.0	23.4	24.1	26.6
16.0–16.9	349	21.9	3.3	18.0	18.5	19.0	19.6	21.3	23.0	24.8	25.9	27.3
17.0–17.9	338	21.8	3.5	17.8	18.4	18.9	19.5	21.1	23.4	24.9	26.1	28.3
18.0–24.9	1755	23.6	3.8	18.8	19.6	20.1	21.0	23.0	25.5	27.2	28.5	31.0
25.0–29.9	1255	24.9	4.3	19.5	20.4	21.1	21.9	24.3	27.0	28.5	30.0	32.8
30.0–34.9	947	25.7	4.2	19.9	21.0	21.9	23.0	25.1	27.8	29.3	30.5	32.9
35.0–39.9	839	25.9	4.0	19.7	21.0	21.9	23.3	25.6	28.0	29.5	30.6	32.8
40.0–44.9	829	26.2	4.0	20.4	21.5	22.2	23.4	26.0	28.5	29.9	31.0	32.5
45.0–49.9	871	26.3	4.2	20.1	21.5	22.4	23.5	26.0	28.6	30.1	31.2	33.4
50.0–54.9	882	26.1	4.2	19.9	21.1	22.0	23.3	25.9	28.2	30.1	31.3	33.3
55.0–59.9	807	26.2	4.3	19.8	21.3	22.1	23.5	26.1	28.5	30.2	31.6	33.6
60.0–64.9	1261	25.8	3.8	20.1	21.3	22.0	23.4	25.6	28.0	29.4	30.4	32.4
65.0–69.9	1773	25.5	4.0	19.1	20.5	21.4	22.7	25.5	27.8	29.6	30.7	32.3
70.0–74.9	1257	25.3	4.0	19.0	20.3	21.4	22.6	25.1	27.7	29.3	30.5	32.3
Females												
1.0–1.9	333	16.7	1.5	14.4	14.9	15.2	15.7	16.7	17.6	18.2	18.6	19.3
2.0–2.9	610	16.0	1.5	14.1	14.4	14.7	15.1	15.9	16.8	17.3	17.8	18.4
3.0–3.9	651	15.7	1.4	13.6	14.1	14.4	14.7	15.5	16.4	17.0	17.5	18.0
4.0–4.9	678	15.5	1.4	13.6	13.9	14.2	14.6	15.3	16.2	16.7	17.2	18.0
5.0–5.9	673	15.5	1.7	13.3	13.7	14.0	14.5	15.2	16.3	16.9	17.5	18.6
6.0–6.9	296	15.5	1.7	13.5	13.7	13.9	14.3	15.2	16.2	17.0	17.5	18.7
7.0–7.9	331	15.9	1.9	13.7	14.1	14.2	14.7	15.4	16.8	17.5	18.3	19.6
8.0–8.9	276	16.5	2.7	13.8	14.1	14.4	14.9	15.8	17.4	18.7	19.8	21.7
9.0–9.9	322	17.3	3.1	14.0	14.6	14.8	15.3	16.5	18.1	19.8	21.5	23.3
10.0–10.9	330	17.7	3.1	14.0	14.5	15.0	15.6	16.9	18.9	20.7	22.0	24.1
11.0–11.9	303	18.9	3.8	14.8	15.3	15.6	16.3	18.1	20.3	21.8	23.4	26.2
12.0–12.9	324	19.6	3.7	15.0	15.6	16.2	17.0	18.9	21.2	23.1	24.6	27.0
13.0–13.9	361	20.4	4.1	15.4	16.3	16.7	17.7	19.4	22.2	23.8	25.2	28.6
14.0–14.9	370	21.1	3.9	16.5	17.1	17.7	18.4	20.3	22.8	24.7	26.2	28.9
15.0–15.9	309	21.1	3.8	17.0	17.5	18.0	18.8	20.3	22.4	24.1	25.6	28.7
16.0–16.9	343	22.1	4.0	17.7	18.3	18.7	19.3	21.1	23.5	25.7	26.8	30.1
17.0–17.9	293	22.5	4.7	17.1	17.9	18.7	19.6	21.4	24.0	26.2	27.5	32.1
18.0–24.9	2592	22.9	4.6	17.7	18.4	19.0	19.9	21.8	24.5	26.5	28.6	32.1
25.0–29.9	1935	23.7	5.2	18.0	18.8	19.2	20.1	22.3	25.6	28.4	30.8	34.3
30.0–34.9	1633	24.8	5.9	18.5	19.4	19.9	20.8	23.1	27.2	30.4	33.0	36.6
35.0–39.9	1461	25.3	5.8	18.7	19.5	20.2	21.3	23.8	28.0	31.0	33.1	36.9
40.0–44.9	1399	25.7	5.9	18.8	19.8	20.5	21.5	24.2	28.3	31.6	33.7	36.6
45.0–49.9	969	26.0	6.2	19.0	20.1	20.8	21.9	24.5	28.6	31.4	33.4	37.1
50.0–54.9	1012	26.3	5.5	19.2	20.3	21.0	22.4	25.2	29.2	32.1	33.8	36.5
55.0–59.9	887	26.9	6.1	19.2	20.5	21.3	22.8	25.7	30.1	32.7	34.7	38.2
60.0–64.9	1392	26.7	5.5	19.3	20.7	21.4	22.9	25.8	29.7	32.1	33.8	36.6
65.0–69.9	1952	26.8	5.5	19.5	20.7	21.7	23.0	26.0	29.6	32.0	33.8	36.6
70.0–74.9	1467	26.6	5.3	19.3	20.5	21.5	23.0	26.0	29.5	31.7	33.1	35.8

Table IV. 6.

Means, standard deviations, and percentiles of standards of sitting height (cm) by age for males and females of 1 to 74 years

Age (yrs)	N	Mean	SD	Percentiles								
				5	10	15	25	50	75	85	90	95
Males												
2.0–2.9	525	54.0	2.6	50.0	51.0	51.3	52.0	54.0	56.0	57.0	57.0	58.0
3.0–3.9	715	56.9	2.7	52.1	54.0	54.0	55.0	57.0	58.8	59.6	60.0	61.0
4.0–4.9	709	59.8	3.0	55.0	56.0	57.0	58.0	60.0	61.7	63.0	63.0	64.3
5.0–5.9	676	62.3	2.9	57.9	59.0	59.3	60.0	62.3	64.0	65.0	66.0	67.0
6.0–6.9	298	65.0	3.0	59.5	61.0	62.0	63.0	65.0	67.0	68.0	69.0	69.4
7.0–7.9	312	67.2	3.3	62.0	63.2	64.0	65.3	67.2	69.2	70.0	71.0	72.0
8.0–8.9	296	69.3	3.4	64.1	65.4	66.0	67.5	69.0	71.4	72.6	73.0	74.6
9.0–9.9	322	71.6	3.2	66.0	67.5	68.0	69.0	71.4	74.0	75.0	75.6	76.7
10.0–10.9	332	73.7	3.4	68.0	69.0	70.0	71.6	73.8	76.0	77.0	78.0	79.4
11.0–11.9	324	75.7	3.8	69.3	71.0	71.9	73.0	76.0	78.0	79.6	80.4	82.0
12.0–12.9	349	78.2	4.4	71.7	72.9	74.0	75.1	78.0	81.0	82.3	84.2	86.0
13.0–13.9	349	81.7	5.1	74.0	75.0	76.0	78.0	81.7	85.3	87.2	88.5	90.5
14.0–14.9	358	85.5	4.8	76.7	79.3	80.5	82.5	86.0	88.9	90.5	91.5	92.9
15.0–15.9	358	88.0	4.3	80.4	82.0	83.5	85.4	88.1	91.1	92.6	93.8	95.0
16.0–16.9	347	90.4	3.9	84.1	85.2	86.1	87.6	90.5	93.4	94.5	95.1	96.5
17.0–17.9	339	91.0	4.0	84.3	86.0	87.0	88.4	91.1	93.5	94.7	95.9	97.3
18.0–24.9	1751	92.3	3.8	86.2	87.6	88.5	90.0	92.4	94.7	96.3	97.2	98.5
25.0–29.9	1254	92.8	3.7	86.5	88.0	89.0	90.3	92.9	95.2	96.7	97.6	98.8
30.0–34.9	943	92.7	3.8	86.7	87.9	88.8	90.3	92.7	95.1	96.4	97.4	98.7
35.0–39.9	837	92.4	3.7	86.4	87.6	88.6	90.0	92.5	95.1	96.4	97.0	98.3
40.0–44.9	827	92.3	3.6	86.3	87.8	88.8	90.1	92.4	94.5	96.0	96.9	98.2
45.0–49.9	871	91.9	3.6	85.5	87.2	88.3	89.6	92.1	94.2	95.6	96.4	97.8
50.0–54.9	880	91.4	3.6	85.3	86.8	87.6	89.2	91.6	93.8	95.1	96.0	97.3
55.0–59.9	805	91.0	3.6	84.9	86.2	87.3	88.6	91.1	93.5	94.6	95.4	96.6
60.0–64.9	1257	90.5	3.6	84.8	86.1	86.8	88.0	90.5	92.9	94.1	94.8	96.1
65.0–69.9	1772	89.3	3.7	83.3	84.5	85.5	86.7	89.4	91.7	93.3	94.1	95.2
70.0–74.9	1251	88.6	3.8	81.9	83.6	84.8	86.2	88.7	91.0	92.4	93.5	94.4
Females												
2.0–2.9	466	52.8	2.4	49.0	49.8	50.0	51.0	53.0	54.4	55.0	56.0	56.7
3.0–3.9	651	55.6	2.6	51.0	52.3	53.0	54.0	55.7	57.2	58.3	59.0	60.0
4.0–4.9	678	58.7	2.7	54.0	55.0	56.0	57.0	58.8	60.7	61.3	62.0	63.0
5.0–5.9	672	61.6	3.0	56.6	58.0	58.9	60.0	61.6	63.1	64.2	65.0	66.0
6.0–6.9	296	64.0	3.2	59.2	60.0	61.0	62.0	64.0	66.0	67.0	68.0	69.0
7.0–7.9	331	66.5	3.1	62.0	62.8	63.1	64.5	66.1	68.4	69.8	70.2	71.8
8.0–8.9	276	69.0	3.2	64.0	64.7	65.9	67.0	69.0	71.0	72.0	73.0	74.1
9.0–9.9	322	71.2	3.7	65.5	66.7	67.8	69.0	71.0	73.5	75.0	76.0	77.2
10.0–10.9	330	73.7	3.7	68.0	69.2	70.1	71.4	73.5	75.8	77.3	78.9	81.0
11.0–11.9	302	76.8	4.3	70.0	71.6	72.2	74.0	76.6	80.0	81.2	82.3	83.9
12.0–12.9	324	80.2	4.2	73.0	74.0	75.1	77.2	80.5	83.1	84.6	85.5	86.4
13.0–13.9	361	82.5	3.6	76.2	77.7	78.7	80.1	82.7	85.0	86.3	86.9	87.8
14.0–14.9	369	84.1	3.6	78.1	79.1	80.4	81.7	84.3	86.9	87.8	88.6	89.5
15.0–15.9	308	85.5	3.4	79.8	81.1	82.2	83.3	85.3	87.5	88.5	89.9	91.5
16.0–16.9	342	85.7	3.5	79.3	81.0	81.9	83.5	85.8	88.0	88.8	89.8	91.5
17.0–17.9	293	85.9	3.5	80.0	81.1	82.4	83.8	86.0	88.1	89.4	90.3	92.0
18.0–24.9	2590	86.3	3.5	80.4	81.9	82.8	84.0	86.4	88.5	89.8	90.6	91.9
25.0–29.9	1934	86.5	3.4	80.9	82.2	83.1	84.4	86.5	88.7	89.9	90.6	92.0
30.0–34.9	1627	86.6	3.5	81.0	82.3	83.1	84.4	86.5	89.0	90.1	91.1	92.3
35.0–39.9	1455	86.6	3.5	81.0	82.1	83.1	84.5	86.7	88.8	90.2	91.0	92.0
40.0–44.9	1398	86.3	3.3	80.6	82.0	82.8	84.1	86.3	88.4	89.7	90.5	91.7
45.0–49.9	967	86.2	3.3	80.5	82.0	83.0	84.2	86.4	88.3	89.4	90.3	91.6
50.0–54.9	1011	85.5	3.2	80.5	81.6	82.4	83.4	85.5	87.7	88.8	89.7	90.7
55.0–59.9	887	84.8	3.4	78.9	80.5	81.5	82.6	85.0	87.1	88.3	89.1	90.0
60.0–64.9	1389	84.2	3.5	78.6	80.0	80.9	82.1	84.4	86.5	87.7	88.4	89.7
65.0–69.9	1945	83.2	3.5	77.4	78.8	79.7	81.0	83.3	85.5	86.7	87.4	88.6
70.0–74.9	1463	82.2	3.5	76.5	77.9	78.7	80.0	82.4	84.4	85.7	86.5	87.6

Table IV. 7.
Means, standard deviations, and percentiles of sitting height index (sitting
height/stature x 100) by age for males and females of 1 to 74 years

Age (yrs)	N	Mean	SD	Percentiles								
				5	10	15	25	50	75	85	90	95
Males												
2.0–2.9	520	58.9	1.9	55.9	56.7	57.0	57.8	59.1	60.1	60.6	61.0	61.7
3.0–3.9	714	57.5	1.9	54.6	55.4	55.8	56.4	57.5	58.6	59.1	59.5	60.4
4.0–4.9	709	56.4	2.1	53.3	54.1	54.6	55.3	56.6	57.4	57.9	58.2	58.8
5.0–5.9	674	55.4	1.8	52.5	53.3	53.7	54.4	55.5	56.5	57.0	57.3	58.0
6.0–6.9	298	54.5	1.5	52.2	52.6	52.9	53.7	54.5	55.4	56.0	56.2	56.7
7.0–7.9	312	53.7	1.7	51.5	52.1	52.3	52.8	53.8	54.7	55.2	55.5	55.9
8.0–8.9	296	53.5	1.9	51.0	51.4	51.8	52.4	53.6	54.4	55.0	55.4	55.7
9.0–9.9	322	52.7	1.5	50.3	50.8	51.1	51.8	52.8	53.8	54.2	54.4	54.8
10.0–10.9	332	52.3	1.7	49.6	50.6	50.8	51.4	52.4	53.3	53.6	54.0	54.3
11.0–11.9	324	51.7	1.5	49.4	50.0	50.3	50.8	51.7	52.7	53.2	53.6	53.9
12.0–12.9	349	51.4	1.4	49.3	49.8	49.9	50.5	51.4	52.3	52.8	53.1	53.6
13.0–13.9	349	51.3	1.4	49.0	49.6	49.8	50.3	51.3	52.2	52.7	53.1	53.6
14.0–14.9	358	51.2	1.6	48.6	49.5	49.8	50.3	51.2	52.2	52.7	53.1	53.6
15.0–15.9	358	51.5	1.6	49.0	49.6	49.9	50.6	51.6	52.6	53.0	53.6	54.1
16.0–16.9	346	51.8	1.6	49.3	49.8	50.2	50.9	51.9	52.9	53.3	53.6	54.1
17.0–17.9	338	51.8	1.5	49.4	49.9	50.4	50.9	51.8	52.8	53.3	53.6	54.3
18.0–24.9	1749	52.3	1.5	49.7	50.4	50.8	51.4	52.4	53.2	53.8	54.1	54.7
25.0–29.9	1253	52.5	1.4	50.2	50.8	51.2	51.7	52.6	53.5	53.9	54.3	54.8
30.0–34.9	943	52.6	1.5	50.3	50.9	51.3	51.8	52.6	53.5	54.0	54.3	54.8
35.0–39.9	837	52.5	1.4	50.3	50.8	51.1	51.6	52.5	53.4	53.9	54.2	54.6
40.0–44.9	826	52.5	1.4	50.2	50.7	51.1	51.7	52.6	53.5	53.9	54.2	54.6
45.0–49.9	871	52.5	1.5	50.1	50.7	51.0	51.6	52.6	53.4	53.8	54.2	54.7
50.0–54.9	880	52.4	1.4	50.0	50.5	50.9	51.5	52.4	53.4	53.8	54.2	54.7
55.0–59.9	805	52.3	1.4	50.0	50.5	50.8	51.4	52.4	53.3	53.7	54.1	54.7
60.0–64.9	1257	52.3	1.4	49.9	50.5	51.0	51.5	52.4	53.2	53.7	54.0	54.5
65.0–69.9	1770	52.1	1.5	49.6	50.2	50.6	51.1	52.2	53.1	53.5	53.9	54.4
70.0–74.9	1251	51.9	1.6	49.2	50.0	50.4	51.0	52.1	53.0	53.4	53.8	54.3
Females												
2.0–2.9	463	58.5	1.8	55.6	56.4	56.7	57.5	58.6	59.8	60.2	60.6	61.2
3.0–3.9	651	57.0	1.7	54.1	54.9	55.4	56.0	57.1	58.2	58.7	58.9	59.5
4.0–4.9	677	55.9	1.6	53.3	53.9	54.3	55.0	56.0	56.9	57.4	57.7	58.4
5.0–5.9	671	55.0	1.9	52.2	52.8	53.3	53.9	55.1	56.0	56.5	56.9	57.4
6.0–6.9	296	54.1	2.0	51.3	52.1	52.6	53.3	54.3	55.1	55.6	55.8	56.3
7.0–7.9	331	53.5	1.6	50.8	51.5	52.0	52.7	53.6	54.5	55.0	55.4	55.8
8.0–8.9	276	53.2	1.6	50.7	51.2	51.7	52.1	53.2	54.0	54.6	55.0	55.7
9.0–9.9	322	52.5	2.1	49.5	50.4	50.8	51.5	52.5	53.5	54.0	54.5	54.8
10.0–10.9	330	52.1	1.3	49.9	50.2	50.7	51.2	52.1	53.0	53.5	53.7	54.1
11.0–11.9	302	51.9	1.4	49.4	50.1	50.5	51.0	51.9	52.8	53.2	53.6	53.9
12.0–12.9	324	51.9	1.6	49.1	49.8	50.2	50.8	51.9	52.8	53.5	53.9	54.5
13.0–13.9	361	52.0	1.5	49.5	50.0	50.3	51.0	52.0	53.0	53.5	53.9	54.4
14.0–14.9	369	52.3	1.5	49.6	50.4	50.8	51.4	52.3	53.4	53.9	54.3	54.8
15.0–15.9	308	52.4	1.5	49.8	50.6	51.0	51.5	52.4	53.3	53.9	54.2	55.1
16.0–16.9	342	52.8	1.4	50.5	51.0	51.4	51.8	52.9	53.8	54.2	54.5	55.0
17.0–17.9	293	52.8	1.5	50.1	51.0	51.4	51.9	52.9	53.7	54.2	54.7	55.1
18.0–24.9	2590	52.9	1.5	50.4	51.0	51.5	52.1	53.0	53.9	54.4	54.8	55.3
25.0–29.9	1934	53.1	1.5	50.8	51.4	51.8	52.3	53.1	54.0	54.4	54.9	55.5
30.0–34.9	1627	53.3	1.5	50.9	51.5	51.9	52.4	53.3	54.2	54.7	55.0	55.5
35.0–39.9	1455	53.2	1.5	50.8	51.4	51.8	52.3	53.2	54.1	54.7	55.0	55.6
40.0–44.9	1398	53.1	1.5	50.6	51.2	51.6	52.1	53.1	54.1	54.6	54.9	55.5
45.0–49.9	967	53.2	1.4	50.9	51.4	51.8	52.3	53.3	54.2	54.6	55.0	55.4
50.0–54.9	1011	53.1	1.5	50.8	51.3	51.7	52.1	53.1	54.0	54.5	54.9	55.3
55.0–59.9	887	52.9	1.5	50.4	51.1	51.4	52.0	53.0	54.0	54.5	54.7	55.3
60.0–64.9	1387	52.8	1.5	50.4	51.1	51.4	52.0	52.8	53.7	54.2	54.6	55.1
65.0–69.9	1945	52.5	1.5	49.8	50.5	50.9	51.5	52.5	53.5	53.9	54.3	54.8
70.0–74.9	1462	52.2	1.6	49.7	50.2	50.6	51.2	52.2	53.2	53.8	54.1	54.6

Table IV. 8.

Means, standard deviations, and percentiles of bitrochanteric breadth (cm) by age for males and females of 1 to 74 years

Age (yrs)	N	Mean	SD	Percentiles								
				5	10	15	25	50	75	85	90	95
Males												
1.0–1.9	679	14.8	2.3	12.6	13.3	13.6	14.0	14.7	15.5	16.0	16.2	16.6
2.0–2.9	669	15.8	1.2	13.8	14.3	14.6	15.0	15.7	16.5	16.9	17.3	17.6
3.0–3.9	710	16.8	1.2	14.7	15.3	15.6	16.1	16.8	17.5	17.9	18.2	18.7
4.0–4.9	706	17.7	1.2	15.7	16.2	16.5	16.9	17.7	18.5	18.9	19.3	19.6
5.0–5.9	675	18.6	1.3	16.6	17.1	17.3	17.8	18.6	19.4	19.9	20.2	20.8
6.0–6.9	297	19.6	1.4	17.4	18.0	18.4	18.9	19.5	20.3	20.9	21.2	22.0
7.0–7.9	312	20.5	1.4	18.3	18.8	19.0	19.5	20.3	21.4	21.8	22.1	22.7
8.0–8.9	295	21.3	1.6	19.0	19.5	19.8	20.3	21.3	22.3	22.9	23.4	24.2
9.0–9.9	322	22.4	1.8	19.9	20.5	20.7	21.2	22.3	23.4	24.0	24.5	25.1
10.0–10.9	334	23.6	1.9	20.8	21.3	21.9	22.4	23.5	24.7	25.4	26.0	26.8
11.0–11.9	324	24.7	2.3	21.3	22.0	22.6	23.2	24.4	25.9	26.8	27.5	28.8
12.0–12.9	348	25.8	2.4	22.4	23.1	23.6	24.4	25.6	27.2	28.1	28.8	30.1
13.0–13.9	350	27.3	2.4	23.4	24.1	24.8	25.6	27.3	28.8	29.8	30.3	31.3
14.0–14.9	359	28.9	2.4	24.9	25.9	26.5	27.3	29.0	30.5	31.3	31.8	32.3
15.0–15.9	359	29.8	2.1	26.3	27.1	27.6	28.4	29.9	31.2	31.9	32.4	33.0
16.0–16.9	350	30.7	2.0	27.4	28.2	28.7	29.4	30.5	32.0	32.6	33.1	33.9
17.0–17.9	339	30.8	2.0	27.8	28.4	28.9	29.6	30.8	32.0	32.8	33.3	34.0
18.0–24.9	1757	31.6	2.0	28.5	29.1	29.5	30.3	31.5	32.8	33.5	34.0	34.8
25.0–29.9	1256	32.1	2.0	29.0	29.6	30.1	30.8	32.1	33.2	34.0	34.4	35.5
30.0–34.9	946	32.2	2.1	29.2	29.9	30.3	30.9	32.1	33.4	34.2	34.7	35.5
35.0–39.9	838	32.5	1.9	29.3	30.0	30.5	31.2	32.5	33.8	34.5	35.0	35.7
40.0–44.9	830	32.7	2.0	29.4	30.1	30.7	31.4	32.8	33.9	34.5	35.0	35.9
45.0–49.9	871	32.7	1.9	29.7	30.4	30.9	31.5	32.7	34.0	34.6	35.1	35.9
50.0–54.9	882	32.8	2.0	29.6	30.4	30.9	31.5	32.8	34.0	34.6	35.0	35.8
55.0–59.9	808	32.9	3.4	29.8	30.4	31.0	31.5	32.7	34.1	34.6	35.1	36.0
60.0–64.9	1261	32.9	2.4	29.9	30.6	31.0	31.8	32.8	33.9	34.5	34.9	35.8
65.0–69.9	1772	32.9	2.4	29.6	30.4	30.9	31.6	32.9	34.1	34.9	35.4	36.0
70.0–74.9	1252	33.0	2.9	30.0	30.6	31.1	31.7	32.9	34.2	34.8	35.3	36.2
Females												
1.0–1.9	619	14.4	1.3	12.4	12.8	13.1	13.6	14.4	15.3	15.7	16.0	16.5
2.0–2.9	609	15.6	1.1	13.9	14.3	14.5	14.9	15.6	16.4	16.7	17.1	17.5
3.0–3.9	651	16.7	1.2	14.6	15.1	15.4	15.9	16.8	17.5	17.9	18.2	18.6
4.0–4.9	673	17.6	1.3	15.5	16.1	16.4	16.8	17.7	18.4	18.9	19.2	19.6
5.0–5.9	671	18.6	1.5	16.4	17.0	17.4	17.7	18.5	19.4	19.9	20.4	20.9
6.0–6.9	295	19.6	1.3	17.4	18.0	18.2	18.6	19.5	20.4	20.9	21.3	21.8
7.0–7.9	331	20.6	1.7	18.2	18.7	19.2	19.6	20.5	21.4	21.9	22.4	23.4
8.0–8.9	275	21.7	1.8	19.2	19.8	20.1	20.6	21.6	22.6	23.3	23.8	24.6
9.0–9.9	322	23.0	2.3	19.9	20.8	21.1	21.5	22.7	24.0	24.9	25.6	26.5
10.0–10.9	330	24.1	2.2	21.1	21.6	22.0	22.6	23.8	25.4	26.2	27.1	28.5
11.0–11.9	302	25.8	2.5	22.0	22.5	23.1	24.0	25.7	27.4	28.4	29.1	30.2
12.0–12.9	324	27.5	2.5	23.2	24.1	24.7	25.8	27.5	29.2	30.0	30.5	31.3
13.0–13.9	361	28.6	2.2	25.0	25.8	26.4	27.2	28.6	30.1	30.9	31.4	31.9
14.0–14.9	370	29.4	2.2	26.2	26.8	27.3	28.0	29.4	30.7	31.2	31.9	33.0
15.0–15.9	309	29.8	1.9	26.9	27.5	27.8	28.6	29.7	31.0	31.6	31.9	33.0
16.0–16.9	343	30.5	2.2	27.5	28.0	28.3	29.0	30.1	31.6	32.6	33.4	34.2
17.0–17.9	293	30.7	2.1	27.3	28.0	28.6	29.4	30.6	31.9	32.7	33.5	34.2
18.0–24.9	2592	31.1	2.2	28.0	28.6	29.0	29.7	31.0	32.4	33.2	33.6	35.0
25.0–29.9	1936	31.6	2.9	28.3	29.0	29.5	30.2	31.3	32.8	33.8	34.4	35.5
30.0–34.9	1632	32.0	3.1	28.4	29.2	29.7	30.5	31.7	33.3	34.3	35.0	36.4
35.0–39.9	1460	32.1	2.3	28.6	29.4	29.9	30.6	32.0	33.5	34.3	35.0	36.0
40.0–44.9	1399	32.3	2.3	28.8	29.5	30.0	30.7	32.1	33.6	34.5	35.2	36.2
45.0–49.9	969	32.3	2.3	28.8	29.5	29.9	30.8	32.2	33.6	34.4	35.2	36.1
50.0–54.9	1912	32.5	2.3	28.9	29.8	30.3	31.0	32.3	33.9	34.6	35.4	36.6
55.0–59.9	885	32.3	2.9	28.8	29.6	30.1	30.9	32.2	33.5	34.3	35.0	35.9
60.0–64.9	1393	32.2	2.1	29.0	29.6	30.1	30.8	32.2	33.6	34.4	35.0	35.8
65.0–69.9	1949	32.3	2.5	29.0	29.6	30.2	30.9	32.3	33.6	34.5	35.1	35.9
70.0–74.9	1467	32.4	3.0	28.9	29.7	30.2	31.0	32.3	33.7	34.4	35.0	35.8

Table IV. 9.
Means, standard deviations, and percentiles of elbow breadth (mm) by age for males and females of 1 to 74 years

Age (yrs)	N	Mean	SD	Percentiles								
				5	10	15	25	50	75	85	90	95
Males												
1.0–1.9	681	40.4	2.9	36.0	37.0	37.0	39.0	40.0	42.0	43.0	44.0	45.0
2.0–2.9	677	42.5	2.7	38.0	39.0	40.0	41.0	42.0	44.0	45.0	46.0	47.0
3.0–3.9	717	44.5	2.8	40.0	41.0	42.0	43.0	44.0	46.0	47.0	48.0	50.0
4.0–4.9	709	46.4	3.0	42.0	43.0	43.0	44.0	46.0	48.0	50.0	50.0	52.0
5.0–5.9	676	48.3	3.3	43.0	44.0	45.0	46.0	48.0	50.0	51.0	52.0	53.0
6.0–6.9	298	50.4	3.3	45.0	46.0	47.0	48.0	51.0	52.0	54.0	55.0	56.0
7.0–7.9	312	51.9	3.6	47.0	48.0	49.0	49.0	52.0	54.0	56.0	56.0	57.0
8.0–8.9	296	53.7	3.7	48.0	49.0	50.0	51.0	54.0	56.0	57.0	59.0	60.0
9.0–9.9	322	55.7	3.8	50.0	51.0	52.0	53.0	56.0	58.0	60.0	61.0	62.0
10.0–10.9	334	58.1	4.2	52.0	53.0	54.0	55.0	58.0	61.0	62.0	64.0	65.0
11.0–11.9	324	59.9	4.4	53.0	55.0	56.0	57.0	60.0	62.0	64.0	65.0	67.0
12.0–12.9	349	62.8	5.0	55.0	57.0	58.0	60.0	63.0	66.0	68.0	69.0	72.0
13.0–13.9	350	65.8	4.8	58.0	60.0	61.0	62.0	66.0	69.0	71.0	72.0	74.0
14.0–14.9	358	68.4	4.4	61.0	63.0	64.0	66.0	68.0	71.0	73.0	74.0	76.0
15.0–15.9	359	69.8	4.1	63.0	64.0	65.0	67.0	70.0	72.0	74.0	75.0	77.0
16.0–16.9	350	70.5	4.0	64.0	66.0	66.0	68.0	71.0	73.0	74.0	76.0	77.0
17.0–17.9	339	70.7	4.0	64.0	66.0	67.0	68.0	71.0	73.0	75.0	76.0	77.0
18.0–24.9	1757	71.2	4.1	64.0	66.0	67.0	69.0	71.0	74.0	75.0	76.0	78.0
25.0–29.9	1256	71.6	4.1	65.0	67.0	67.0	69.0	71.0	74.0	76.0	77.0	79.0
30.0–34.9	946	71.8	4.2	65.0	67.0	68.0	69.0	72.0	74.0	76.0	77.0	79.0
35.0–39.9	838	72.3	4.2	65.0	67.0	68.0	70.0	72.0	75.0	77.0	77.0	80.0
40.0–44.9	830	72.8	4.0	66.0	68.0	69.0	70.0	73.0	75.0	77.0	78.0	80.0
45.0–49.9	871	73.1	4.3	66.0	68.0	69.0	70.0	73.0	76.0	78.0	79.0	80.0
50.0–54.9	882	73.3	4.2	66.0	68.0	69.0	71.0	73.0	76.0	77.0	78.0	80.0
55.0–59.9	809	73.7	4.5	67.0	68.0	69.0	71.0	73.0	77.0	78.0	80.0	81.0
60.0–64.9	1263	73.5	4.3	67.0	68.0	69.0	71.0	73.0	76.0	78.0	79.0	81.0
65.0–69.9	1774	73.2	4.4	66.0	68.0	69.0	70.0	73.0	76.0	78.0	79.0	81.0
70.0–74.9	1252	73.5	4.3	67.0	68.0	69.0	71.0	73.0	76.0	78.0	79.0	81.0
Females												
1.0–1.9	622	38.7	2.8	34.0	35.0	36.0	37.0	39.0	41.0	42.0	42.0	43.0
2.0–2.9	615	40.7	2.8	36.0	37.0	38.0	39.0	41.0	42.0	44.0	44.0	45.0
3.0–3.9	652	42.5	2.9	38.0	39.0	40.0	41.0	42.0	44.0	45.0	46.0	47.0
4.0–4.9	681	44.2	2.9	40.0	41.0	41.0	42.0	44.0	46.0	47.0	48.0	49.0
5.0–5.9	674	46.4	3.1	42.0	43.0	43.0	44.0	46.0	48.0	50.0	50.0	52.0
6.0–6.9	296	47.9	3.2	43.0	44.0	45.0	46.0	48.0	50.0	51.0	52.0	53.0
7.0–7.9	331	50.1	3.4	45.0	46.0	47.0	48.0	50.0	52.0	53.0	54.0	55.0
8.0–8.9	276	51.5	3.7	46.0	47.0	48.0	49.0	51.0	54.0	55.0	56.0	58.0
9.0–9.9	322	54.0	3.9	48.0	50.0	50.0	51.0	54.0	56.0	57.0	59.0	60.0
10.0–10.9	330	55.6	3.9	50.0	51.0	52.0	53.0	56.0	58.0	60.0	61.0	62.0
11.0–11.9	302	57.8	4.0	52.0	53.0	54.0	55.0	58.0	60.0	62.0	63.0	64.0
12.0–12.9	324	59.2	3.7	53.0	55.0	55.0	57.0	59.0	62.0	63.0	64.0	66.0
13.0–13.9	361	60.1	3.8	54.0	56.0	56.0	58.0	60.0	62.0	64.0	65.0	66.0
14.0–14.9	370	60.4	3.5	54.0	56.0	57.0	58.0	60.0	63.0	64.0	65.0	66.0
15.0–15.9	309	60.7	4.0	54.0	56.0	57.0	58.0	61.0	63.0	65.0	66.0	67.0
16.0–16.9	343	61.0	3.8	55.0	56.0	57.0	59.0	61.0	64.0	65.0	66.0	67.0
17.0–17.9	293	61.3	4.0	55.0	56.0	57.0	59.0	61.0	64.0	65.0	66.0	68.0
18.0–24.9	2591	61.0	3.8	55.0	56.0	57.0	59.0	61.0	63.0	65.0	66.0	67.0
25.0–29.9	1934	61.5	3.9	56.0	57.0	58.0	59.0	61.0	64.0	65.0	66.0	68.0
30.0–34.9	1630	62.1	4.3	56.0	57.0	58.0	59.0	62.0	64.0	66.0	67.0	70.0
35.0–39.9	1460	62.7	4.4	56.0	58.0	59.0	60.0	62.0	65.0	67.0	68.0	71.0
40.0–44.9	1399	63.2	4.4	57.0	58.0	59.0	60.0	63.0	66.0	67.0	69.0	71.0
45.0–49.9	968	63.7	4.4	57.0	59.0	59.0	61.0	63.0	66.0	68.0	69.0	72.0
50.0–54.9	1011	64.1	4.7	57.0	59.0	60.0	61.0	64.0	67.0	69.0	70.0	73.0
55.0–59.9	887	64.7	4.8	58.0	59.0	60.0	61.0	64.0	67.0	70.0	71.0	73.0
60.0–64.9	1394	64.6	4.4	58.0	60.0	61.0	62.0	64.0	67.0	69.0	70.0	72.0
65.0–69.9	1950	64.7	4.5	58.0	59.0	60.0	62.0	64.0	67.0	69.0	71.0	73.0
70.0–74.9	1464	64.8	4.4	58.0	60.0	60.0	62.0	64.0	68.0	69.0	71.0	72.0

Table IV.10.
Means, standard deviations, and percentiles of upper arm circumference (cm) by age for males and females of 1 to 74 years

Age (yrs)	N	Mean	SD	Percentiles								
				5	10	15	25	50	75	85	90	95
Males												
1.0–1.9	681	16.1	1.2	14.2	14.7	14.9	15.2	16.0	16.9	17.4	17.7	18.2
2.0–2.9	672	16.4	1.4	14.3	14.8	15.1	15.5	16.3	17.1	17.6	17.9	18.6
3.0–3.9	715	16.9	1.4	15.0	15.3	15.5	16.0	16.8	17.6	18.1	18.4	19.0
4.0–4.9	708	17.2	1.4	15.1	15.5	15.8	16.2	17.1	18.0	18.5	18.7	19.3
5.0–5.9	676	17.7	1.8	15.5	16.0	16.1	16.6	17.5	18.5	19.1	19.5	20.5
6.0–6.9	298	18.3	2.1	15.8	16.1	16.5	17.0	18.0	19.1	19.8	20.7	22.8
7.0–7.9	312	19.0	2.1	16.1	16.8	17.0	17.6	18.7	20.0	21.0	21.8	22.9
8.0–8.9	296	19.6	2.3	16.5	17.2	17.5	18.1	19.2	20.5	21.6	22.6	24.0
9.0–9.9	322	20.7	2.7	17.5	18.0	18.4	19.0	20.1	21.8	23.2	24.5	26.0
10.0–10.9	333	21.8	3.0	18.1	18.6	19.1	19.7	21.1	23.1	24.8	26.0	27.9
11.0–11.9	324	22.8	3.4	18.5	19.3	19.8	20.6	22.1	24.5	26.1	27.6	29.4
12.0–12.9	349	23.8	3.5	19.3	20.1	20.7	21.5	23.1	25.4	27.1	28.5	30.3
13.0–13.9	350	24.8	3.3	20.0	20.8	21.6	22.5	24.5	26.6	28.2	29.0	30.8
14.0–14.9	358	26.2	3.5	21.6	22.5	23.2	23.8	25.7	28.1	29.1	30.0	32.3
15.0–15.9	359	27.3	3.2	22.5	23.4	24.0	25.1	27.2	29.0	30.3	31.2	32.7
16.0–16.9	350	28.7	3.2	24.1	25.0	25.7	26.7	28.3	30.6	32.1	32.7	34.7
17.0–17.9	339	29.0	3.4	24.3	25.1	25.9	26.8	28.6	30.8	32.2	33.3	34.7
18.0–24.9	1757	31.0	3.5	26.0	27.1	27.7	28.7	30.7	33.0	34.4	35.4	37.2
25.0–29.9	1255	32.1	3.5	27.0	28.0	28.7	29.8	31.8	34.2	35.5	36.6	38.3
30.0–34.9	945	32.7	3.4	27.7	28.7	29.3	30.5	32.5	34.9	35.9	36.7	38.2
35.0–39.9	838	32.9	3.3	27.4	28.6	29.5	30.7	32.9	35.1	36.2	36.9	38.2
40.0–44.9	830	32.9	3.2	27.8	28.9	29.7	31.0	32.8	34.9	36.1	36.9	38.1
45.0–49.9	871	32.7	3.4	27.2	28.6	29.4	30.6	32.6	34.9	36.1	36.9	38.2
50.0–54.9	882	32.4	3.4	27.1	28.3	29.1	30.2	32.3	34.5	35.8	36.8	38.3
55.0–59.9	809	32.3	3.3	26.8	28.1	29.2	30.4	32.3	34.3	35.5	36.6	37.8
60.0–64.9	1263	31.9	3.4	26.6	27.8	28.6	29.7	32.0	34.0	35.1	36.0	37.5
65.0–69.9	1773	31.1	3.4	25.4	26.7	27.7	29.0	31.1	33.2	34.5	35.3	36.6
70.0–74.9	1251	30.6	3.4	25.1	26.2	27.1	28.5	30.7	32.6	33.7	34.8	36.0
Females												
1.0–1.9	622	15.7	1.3	13.6	14.1	14.4	14.8	15.7	16.4	17.0	17.2	17.8
2.0–2.9	615	16.2	1.3	14.2	14.6	15.0	15.4	16.1	17.0	17.4	18.0	18.5
3.0–3.9	651	16.6	1.4	14.4	15.0	15.2	15.7	16.6	17.4	18.0	18.4	19.0
4.0–4.9	680	17.1	1.5	14.8	15.3	15.7	16.1	17.0	18.0	18.5	19.0	19.5
5.0–5.9	673	17.7	1.8	15.2	15.7	16.1	16.5	17.5	18.5	19.4	20.0	21.0
6.0–6.9	296	18.2	2.0	15.7	16.2	16.5	17.0	17.8	19.0	19.9	20.5	22.0
7.0–7.9	330	19.0	2.2	16.4	16.7	17.0	17.5	18.6	20.1	20.9	21.6	23.3
8.0–8.9	275	20.0	2.6	16.7	17.2	17.6	18.2	19.5	21.2	22.2	23.2	25.1
9.0–9.9	321	21.1	2.8	17.6	18.1	18.6	19.1	20.6	22.2	23.8	25.0	26.7
10.0–10.9	330	21.8	3.1	17.8	18.4	18.9	19.5	21.2	23.4	25.0	26.1	27.3
11.0–11.9	302	23.2	3.6	18.8	19.6	20.0	20.6	22.2	25.1	26.5	27.9	30.0
12.0–12.9	324	24.0	3.4	19.2	20.0	20.5	21.5	23.7	25.8	27.6	28.3	30.2
13.0–13.9	361	25.0	3.7	20.1	21.0	21.5	22.5	24.3	26.7	28.3	30.1	32.7
14.0–14.9	370	25.9	3.6	21.2	21.8	22.5	23.5	25.1	27.4	29.5	30.9	32.9
15.0–15.9	309	25.9	3.5	21.6	22.2	22.9	23.5	25.2	27.7	28.8	30.0	32.2
16.0–16.9	343	26.8	3.5	22.3	23.2	23.5	24.4	26.1	28.5	29.9	31.6	33.5
17.0–17.9	293	27.3	4.1	22.0	23.1	23.6	24.5	26.6	29.0	30.7	32.8	35.4
18.0–24.9	2591	27.5	4.0	22.4	23.3	24.0	24.8	26.8	29.2	31.2	32.4	35.2
25.0–29.9	1934	28.5	4.3	23.1	24.0	24.5	25.5	27.6	30.6	32.5	34.3	37.1
30.0–34.9	1630	29.6	4.7	23.8	24.7	25.4	26.4	28.6	32.0	34.1	36.0	38.5
35.0–39.9	1460	30.2	4.8	24.1	25.2	25.8	26.8	29.4	32.6	35.0	36.8	39.0
40.0–44.9	1398	30.6	4.8	24.3	25.4	26.2	27.2	29.7	33.2	35.5	37.2	38.8
45.0–49.9	968	30.9	5.0	24.2	25.5	26.3	27.4	30.1	33.5	35.6	37.2	40.0
50.0–54.9	1010	31.2	4.5	24.8	26.0	26.8	28.0	30.6	33.8	35.9	37.5	39.3
55.0–59.9	887	31.6	5.1	24.8	26.1	27.0	28.2	30.9	34.3	36.7	38.0	40.0
60.0–64.9	1394	31.4	4.6	25.0	26.1	27.1	28.4	30.8	34.0	35.7	37.3	39.6
65.0–69.9	1950	30.9	4.4	24.3	25.7	26.7	28.0	30.5	33.4	35.2	36.5	38.5
70.0–74.9	1465	30.5	4.3	23.8	25.3	26.3	27.6	30.3	33.1	34.7	35.8	37.5

Table IV.11.

Means, standard deviations, and percentiles of total upper arm area (cm^2) by age for males and females of 1 to 74 years

Age (yrs)	N	Mean	SD	Percentiles								
				5	10	15	25	50	75	85	90	95
Males												
1.0–1.9	681	20.7	3.2	16.0	17.2	17.7	18.4	20.4	22.7	24.1	24.9	26.4
2.0–2.9	672	21.6	4.2	16.3	17.4	18.1	19.1	21.1	23.3	24.6	25.5	27.5
3.0–3.9	715	22.8	4.2	17.9	18.6	19.1	20.4	22.5	24.6	26.1	26.9	28.7
4.0–4.9	708	23.6	3.9	18.1	19.1	19.9	20.9	23.3	25.8	27.2	27.8	29.6
5.0–5.9	676	25.2	5.5	19.1	20.4	20.6	21.9	24.4	27.2	29.0	30.3	33.4
6.0–6.9	298	27.0	6.7	19.9	20.6	21.7	23.0	25.8	29.0	31.2	34.1	41.4
7.0–7.9	312	29.1	6.7	20.6	22.5	23.0	24.6	27.8	31.8	35.1	37.8	41.7
8.0–8.9	296	31.0	7.7	21.7	23.5	24.4	26.1	29.3	33.4	37.1	40.6	45.8
9.0–9.9	322	34.6	9.5	24.4	25.8	26.9	28.7	32.2	37.8	42.8	47.8	53.8
10.0–10.9	333	38.6	11.4	26.1	27.5	29.0	30.9	35.4	42.5	48.9	53.8	61.9
11.0–11.9	324	42.4	13.7	27.2	29.6	31.2	33.8	38.9	47.8	54.2	60.6	68.8
12.0–12.9	349	45.9	14.4	29.6	32.2	34.1	36.8	42.5	51.3	58.4	64.6	73.1
13.0–13.9	350	49.8	13.8	31.8	34.4	37.1	40.3	47.8	56.3	63.3	66.9	75.5
14.0–14.9	358	55.7	15.8	37.1	40.3	42.8	45.1	52.6	62.8	67.4	71.6	83.0
15.0–15.9	359	60.1	14.8	40.3	43.6	45.8	50.1	58.9	66.9	73.1	77.5	85.1
16.0–16.9	350	66.4	15.2	46.2	49.7	52.6	56.7	63.7	74.5	82.0	85.1	95.8
17.0–17.9	339	67.9	16.6	47.0	50.1	53.4	57.2	65.1	75.5	82.5	88.2	95.8
18.0–24.9	1757	77.5	17.8	53.8	58.4	61.1	65.5	75.0	86.7	94.2	99.7	110.1
25.0–29.9	1255	83.1	18.9	58.0	62.4	65.5	70.7	80.5	93.1	100.3	106.6	116.7
30.0–34.9	945	86.2	18.5	61.1	65.5	68.3	74.0	84.1	96.9	102.6	107.2	116.1
35.0–39.9	838	86.9	17.5	59.7	65.1	69.3	75.0	86.1	98.0	104.3	108.4	116.1
40.0–44.9	830	87.1	17.1	61.5	66.5	70.2	76.5	85.6	96.9	103.7	108.4	115.5
45.0–49.9	871	86.2	17.9	58.9	65.1	68.8	74.5	84.6	96.9	103.7	108.4	116.1
50.0–54.9	882	84.5	17.8	58.4	63.7	67.4	72.6	83.0	94.7	102.0	107.8	116.7
55.0–59.9	809	84.0	17.3	57.2	62.8	67.9	73.5	83.0	93.6	100.3	106.6	113.7
60.0–64.9	1263	82.0	17.4	56.3	61.5	65.1	70.2	81.5	92.0	98.0	103.1	111.9
65.0–69.9	1773	77.8	17.0	51.3	56.7	61.1	66.9	77.0	87.7	94.7	99.2	106.6
70.0–74.9	1251	75.3	16.5	50.1	54.6	58.4	64.6	75.0	84.6	90.4	96.4	103.1
Females												
1.0–1.9	622	19.7	3.2	14.7	15.8	16.5	17.4	19.6	21.4	23.0	23.5	25.2
2.0–2.9	615	21.0	3.4	16.0	17.0	17.9	18.9	20.6	23.0	24.1	25.8	27.2
3.0–3.9	651	22.2	3.7	16.5	17.9	18.4	19.6	21.9	24.1	25.8	26.9	28.7
4.0–4.9	680	23.3	4.1	17.4	18.6	19.6	20.6	23.0	25.8	27.2	28.7	30.3
5.0–5.9	673	25.2	5.3	18.4	19.6	20.6	21.7	24.4	27.2	29.9	31.8	35.1
6.0–6.9	296	26.7	6.4	19.6	20.9	21.7	23.0	25.2	28.7	31.5	33.4	38.5
7.0–7.9	330	29.1	7.2	21.4	22.2	23.0	24.4	27.5	32.2	34.8	37.1	43.2
8.0–8.9	275	32.4	9.3	22.2	23.5	24.6	26.4	30.3	35.8	39.2	42.8	50.1
9.0–9.9	321	36.0	10.2	24.6	26.1	27.5	29.0	33.8	39.2	45.1	49.7	56.7
10.0–10.9	330	38.4	11.4	25.2	26.9	28.4	30.3	35.8	43.6	49.7	54.2	59.3
11.0–11.9	302	43.9	14.6	28.1	30.6	31.8	33.8	39.2	50.1	55.9	61.9	71.6
12.0–12.9	324	46.7	13.9	29.3	31.8	33.4	36.8	44.7	53.0	60.6	63.7	72.6
13.0–13.9	361	50.9	16.0	32.2	35.1	36.8	40.3	47.0	56.7	63.7	72.1	85.1
14.0–14.9	370	54.3	16.1	35.8	37.8	40.3	43.9	50.1	59.7	69.3	76.0	86.1
15.0–15.9	309	54.5	15.8	37.1	39.2	41.7	43.9	50.5	61.1	66.0	71.6	82.5
16.0–16.9	343	58.3	16.2	39.6	42.8	43.9	47.4	54.2	64.6	71.1	79.5	89.3
17.0–17.9	293	60.4	19.6	38.5	42.5	44.3	47.8	56.3	66.9	75.0	85.6	99.7
18.0–24.9	2591	61.5	19.2	39.9	43.2	45.8	48.9	57.2	67.9	77.5	83.5	98.6
25.0–29.9	1934	66.0	21.2	42.5	45.8	47.8	51.7	60.6	74.5	84.1	93.6	109.5
30.0–34.9	1630	71.4	24.3	45.1	48.5	51.3	55.5	65.1	81.5	92.5	103.1	118.0
35.0–39.9	1460	74.5	25.3	46.2	50.5	53.0	57.2	68.8	84.6	97.5	107.8	121.0
40.0–44.9	1398	76.1	25.9	47.0	51.3	54.6	58.9	70.2	87.7	100.3	110.1	119.8
45.0–49.9	968	77.9	26.5	46.6	51.7	55.0	59.7	72.1	89.3	100.9	110.1	127.3
50.0–54.9	1010	79.0	23.6	48.9	53.8	57.2	62.4	74.5	90.9	102.6	111.9	122.9
55.0–59.9	887	81.7	28.5	48.9	54.2	58.0	63.3	76.0	93.6	107.2	114.9	127.3
60.0–64.9	1394	80.1	24.4	49.7	54.2	58.4	64.2	75.5	92.0	101.4	110.7	124.8
65.0–69.9	1950	77.5	23.0	47.0	52.6	56.7	62.4	74.0	88.8	98.6	106.0	118.0
70.0–74.9	1465	75.5	21.9	45.1	50.9	55.0	60.6	73.1	87.2	95.8	102.0	111.9

Table IV.12.

Means, standard deviations, and percentiles of upper arm muscle area (cm^2) by age for males and females of 1 to 74 years

Age (yrs)	N	Mean	SD	Percentiles								
				5	10	15	25	50	75	85	90	95
Males												
1.0–1.9	681	13.2	2.3	9.7	10.4	10.8	11.6	13.0	14.6	15.4	16.3	17.2
2.0–2.9	672	14.1	3.2	10.1	10.9	11.3	12.4	13.9	15.6	16.4	16.9	18.4
3.0–3.9	715	15.2	3.1	11.2	12.0	12.6	13.5	15.0	16.4	17.4	18.3	19.5
4.0–4.9	707	16.3	2.7	12.0	12.9	13.5	14.5	16.2	17.9	18.8	19.8	20.9
5.0–5.9	676	17.8	3.7	13.2	14.2	14.7	15.7	17.6	19.5	20.7	21.7	23.2
6.0–6.9	298	19.3	4.0	14.4	15.3	15.8	16.8	18.7	21.3	22.9	23.8	25.7
7.0–7.9	312	21.0	4.5	15.1	16.2	17.0	18.5	20.6	22.6	24.5	25.2	29.0
8.0–8.9	296	22.1	4.2	16.3	17.8	18.5	19.5	21.6	24.0	25.5	26.6	29.0
9.0–9.9	322	24.5	5.1	18.2	19.3	20.3	21.7	23.5	26.7	28.7	30.4	32.9
10.0–10.9	333	26.7	5.9	19.6	20.7	21.6	23.0	25.7	29.0	32.2	34.0	37.1
11.0–11.9	324	28.8	6.7	21.0	22.0	23.0	24.8	27.7	31.6	33.6	36.1	40.3
12.0–12.9	348	31.9	7.4	22.6	24.1	25.3	26.9	30.4	35.9	39.3	40.9	44.9
13.0–13.9	350	36.8	9.0	24.5	26.7	28.1	30.4	35.7	41.3	45.3	48.1	52.5
14.0–14.9	358	42.4	9.1	28.3	31.3	33.1	36.1	41.9	47.4	51.3	54.0	57.5
15.0–15.9	356	46.8	9.6	31.9	34.9	36.9	40.3	46.3	53.1	56.3	57.7	63.0
16.0–16.9	350	52.6	10.0	37.0	40.9	42.4	45.9	51.9	57.8	63.6	66.2	70.5
17.0–17.9	337	54.7	10.5	39.6	42.6	44.8	48.0	53.4	60.4	64.3	67.9	73.1
18.0–24.9	1752	50.5	11.6	34.2	37.3	39.6	42.7	49.4	57.1	61.8	65.0	72.0
25.0–29.9	1250	54.1	11.9	36.6	39.9	42.4	46.0	53.0	61.4	66.1	68.9	74.5
30.0–34.9	940	55.6	12.1	37.9	40.9	43.4	47.3	54.4	63.2	67.6	70.8	76.1
35.0–39.9	832	56.5	12.4	38.5	42.6	44.6	47.9	55.3	64.0	69.1	72.7	77.6
40.0–44.9	828	56.6	11.7	38.4	42.1	45.1	48.7	56.0	64.0	68.5	71.6	77.0
45.0–49.9	867	55.9	12.3	37.7	41.3	43.7	47.9	55.2	63.3	68.4	72.2	76.2
50.0–54.9	879	55.0	12.5	36.0	40.0	42.7	46.6	54.0	62.7	67.0	70.4	77.4
55.0–59.9	807	54.7	11.8	36.5	40.8	42.7	46.7	54.3	61.9	66.4	69.6	75.1
60.0–64.9	1259	52.8	11.7	34.5	38.7	41.2	44.9	52.1	60.0	64.8	67.5	71.6
65.0–69.9	1773	49.8	11.6	31.4	35.8	38.4	42.3	49.1	57.3	61.2	64.3	69.4
70.0–74.9	1250	47.8	11.5	29.7	33.8	36.1	40.2	47.0	54.6	59.1	62.1	67.3
Females												
1.0–1.9	622	12.3	2.3	8.9	9.7	10.1	10.8	12.3	13.8	14.6	15.3	16.2
2.0–2.9	614	13.3	2.3	10.1	10.6	10.9	11.8	13.2	14.7	15.6	16.4	17.3
3.0–3.9	651	14.3	2.4	10.8	11.4	11.8	12.6	14.3	15.8	16.7	17.4	18.8
4.0–4.9	680	15.4	2.8	11.2	12.2	12.7	13.6	15.3	17.0	18.0	18.6	19.8
5.0–5.9	672	16.7	3.1	12.4	13.2	13.9	14.8	16.4	18.3	19.4	20.6	22.1
6.0–6.9	296	18.0	3.9	13.5	14.1	14.6	15.6	17.4	19.5	21.0	22.0	24.2
7.0–7.9	329	19.3	4.0	14.4	15.2	15.8	16.7	18.9	21.2	22.6	23.9	25.3
8.0–8.9	275	21.1	4.7	15.2	16.0	16.8	18.2	20.8	23.2	24.6	26.5	28.0
9.0–9.9	321	22.9	4.6	17.0	17.9	18.7	19.8	21.9	25.4	27.2	28.3	31.1
10.0–10.9	329	24.3	5.5	17.6	18.5	19.3	20.9	23.8	27.0	29.1	31.0	33.1
11.0–11.9	302	27.6	6.7	19.5	21.0	21.7	23.2	26.4	30.7	33.5	35.7	39.2
12.0–12.9	323	29.7	6.5	20.4	21.8	23.1	25.5	29.0	33.2	36.3	37.8	40.5
13.0–13.9	360	31.9	7.4	22.8	24.5	25.4	27.1	30.8	35.3	38.1	39.6	43.7
14.0–14.9	370	33.9	7.7	24.0	26.2	27.1	29.0	32.8	36.9	39.8	42.3	47.5
15.0–15.9	309	33.8	7.0	24.4	25.8	27.5	29.2	33.0	37.3	40.2	41.7	45.9
16.0–16.9	343	34.8	8.0	25.2	26.8	28.2	30.0	33.6	38.0	40.2	43.7	48.3
17.0–17.9	291	36.1	8.8	25.9	27.5	28.9	30.7	34.3	39.6	43.4	46.2	50.8
18.0–24.9	2588	29.8	8.4	19.5	21.5	22.8	24.5	28.3	33.1	36.4	39.0	44.2
25.0–29.9	1921	31.1	9.1	20.5	21.9	23.1	25.2	29.4	34.9	38.5	41.9	47.8
30.0–34.9	1619	32.8	10.4	21.1	23.0	24.2	26.3	30.9	36.8	41.2	44.7	51.3
35.0–39.9	1453	34.2	11.5	21.1	23.4	24.7	27.3	31.8	38.7	45.8	49.5	55.8
40.0–44.9	1390	35.2	13.3	21.3	23.4	25.5	27.5	32.3	39.8	44.7	48.4	56.1
45.0–49.9	961	34.9	11.8	21.6	23.1	24.8	27.4	32.5	39.5	44.7	48.4	55.6
50.0–54.9	1004	35.6	11.0	22.2	24.6	25.7	28.3	33.4	40.4	46.1	49.6	55.6
55.0–59.9	879	37.1	13.3	22.8	24.8	26.5	28.7	34.7	42.3	47.3	52.1	58.8
60.0–64.9	1389	36.3	11.3	22.4	24.5	26.3	29.2	34.5	41.1	45.6	49.1	55.1
65.0–69.9	1946	36.3	11.3	21.9	24.5	26.2	28.9	34.6	41.6	46.3	49.6	56.5
70.0–74.9	1463	36.0	10.8	22.2	24.4	26.0	28.8	34.3	41.8	46.4	49.2	54.6

Note: Values for males and females aged 18 years and older have been adjusted for bone area by subtracting 10.0 cm^2 and 6.5 cm^2 respectively from the calculated mid upper arm muscle area.

Table IV.13.

Means, standard deviations, and percentiles of upper arm muscle area (cm^2) by height (cm) for boys and girls of 2 to 17 years

Height (cm)	N	Mean	SD	Percentiles								
				5	10	15	25	50	75	85	90	95
Boys: 2 to 11 years												
87–092	94	12.9	2.2	9.3	10.4	10.6	11.2	12.9	14.2	15.0	15.8	16.5
93–098	373	13.7	2.4	10.2	10.9	11.2	12.1	13.5	15.3	15.9	16.5	17.0
99–104	587	14.6	3.1	10.9	11.7	12.2	13.0	14.5	15.9	16.5	17.1	18.4
105–110	587	15.7	3.1	12.0	12.8	13.3	14.1	15.4	17.0	17.8	18.6	19.8
111–116	588	16.7	2.9	12.6	13.6	14.3	15.0	16.6	18.1	18.9	19.6	20.7
117–122	496	18.1	3.5	14.1	14.5	15.0	16.1	17.7	19.7	20.7	21.6	23.4
123–128	376	19.5	3.6	15.0	15.9	16.3	17.4	19.2	21.2	22.3	23.2	24.2
129–134	359	21.6	4.3	16.1	17.3	18.4	19.3	21.1	23.2	24.7	25.3	27.9
135–140	354	22.9	4.2	17.2	18.1	18.9	20.4	22.6	24.9	26.1	27.2	30.2
141–146	325	25.1	5.2	19.3	20.1	20.8	21.9	24.0	27.2	29.0	30.5	34.0
147–152	266	27.5	4.8	21.2	22.4	23.2	24.8	27.0	29.8	31.8	32.9	34.4
153–158	150	29.8	7.2	22.3	23.2	24.3	25.4	28.4	32.2	34.8	36.9	40.1
159–164	65	32.5	6.5	23.7	24.5	25.3	27.5	31.9	35.6	39.7	41.4	44.5
Boys: 12 to 17 years												
141–146	31	26.8	4.7	20.7	21.4	22.7	24.1	25.6	30.3	32.8	33.9	36.3
147–152	90	28.2	4.1	22.4	23.4	24.1	25.6	27.5	30.2	33.1	34.2	36.1
153–158	181	31.4	6.4	22.7	24.9	26.1	27.5	30.4	34.1	36.4	39.1	41.5
159–164	218	35.0	7.7	23.7	26.7	27.8	30.2	34.1	38.6	41.5	44.3	48.4
165–170	323	40.8	9.3	28.1	29.7	31.5	34.2	40.0	45.6	49.0	52.9	58.9
171–176	431	46.6	9.9	32.8	35.2	36.6	39.5	45.8	52.6	56.0	59.1	66.0
177–182	431	50.3	9.3	36.1	38.7	40.8	43.4	49.5	56.4	59.4	62.6	65.9
183–188	269	53.4	11.2	38.3	41.3	42.8	46.1	52.6	57.8	63.0	67.5	74.3
189–194	99	55.4	9.9	41.4	44.2	45.7	48.9	53.9	60.3	65.0	68.5	74.0
Girls: 2 to 10 years												
87–092	154	12.6	2.1	9.5	10.1	10.5	11.0	12.6	14.2	14.8	15.5	16.2
93–098	384	13.2	2.1	10.1	10.7	11.0	11.8	13.2	14.4	15.3	15.5	16.2
99–104	533	14.1	2.3	10.6	11.2	11.7	12.5	14.0	15.5	16.4	15.8	16.9
105–110	550	14.8	2.4	11.3	11.9	12.4	13.2	14.6	16.3	16.4	16.9	18.0
111–116	543	15.9	2.8	12.3	13.0	13.5	14.2	15.7	17.4	18.4	17.9	18.9
117–122	465	17.0	2.8	13.0	13.9	14.4	15.2	16.7	18.5	19.6	19.1	20.3
123–128	372	18.2	2.8	14.2	15.0	15.5	16.2	17.9	19.6	20.8	20.3	21.4
129–134	333	20.1	4.6	15.3	16.1	16.8	17.6	19.7	21.7	22.9	21.6	22.9
135–140	303	21.6	4.2	16.1	17.4	18.1	19.2	21.1	23.8	24.8	23.8	25.4
141–146	258	23.3	4.0	17.6	18.5	19.5	20.5	23.0	25.8	27.9	26.3	27.9
147–152	161	25.2	5.2	18.5	20.0	20.7	21.7	24.4	27.8	30.0	28.8	30.6
153–158	66	26.7	6.7	19.4	20.1	22.4	23.0	25.4	29.2	31.8	31.2	32.9
Girls: 11 to 17 years												
141–146	53	23.8	4.4	17.1	19.3	19.5	21.0	23.4	25.5	27.9	28.6	33.4
147–152	119	25.2	4.6	18.5	19.7	20.9	22.0	24.3	28.0	29.8	30.3	34.4
153–158	305	29.1	6.4	20.8	22.0	23.0	24.7	28.3	32.9	35.0	37.5	39.2
159–164	587	32.2	7.1	23.3	24.8	26.0	27.7	31.2	35.7	38.0	40.1	43.5
165–170	715	34.2	7.4	25.0	26.6	27.8	29.5	33.2	37.6	40.2	42.8	46.9
171–176	367	34.9	8.0	25.9	27.1	28.0	29.9	33.7	38.0	41.2	43.5	47.6
177–182	113	37.8	8.4	28.6	29.5	30.5	31.7	35.9	41.1	45.9	47.8	58.2

Table IV.14.

Means, standard deviations, and percentiles of upper arm fat area (cm^2) by age for males and females of 1 to 74 years

Age (yrs)	N	Mean	SD	Percentiles								
				5	10	15	25	50	75	85	90	95
Males												
1.0–1.9	681	7.5	2.2	4.5	4.9	5.3	5.9	7.4	8.9	9.6	10.3	11.7
2.0–2.9	672	7.4	2.3	4.2	4.8	5.1	5.8	7.3	8.6	9.7	10.6	11.6
3.0–3.9	715	7.6	2.4	4.5	5.0	5.4	5.9	7.2	8.8	9.8	10.6	11.8
4.0–4.9	707	7.3	2.5	4.1	4.7	5.2	5.7	6.9	8.5	9.3	10.0	11.4
5.0–5.9	676	7.4	3.1	4.0	4.5	4.9	5.5	6.7	8.3	9.8	10.9	12.7
6.0–6.9	298	7.7	4.1	3.7	4.3	4.6	5.2	6.7	8.6	10.3	11.2	15.2
7.0–7.9	312	8.1	4.2	3.8	4.3	4.7	5.4	7.1	9.6	11.6	12.8	15.5
8.0–8.9	296	8.9	5.0	4.1	4.8	5.1	5.8	7.6	10.4	12.4	15.6	18.6
9.0–9.9	322	10.1	6.2	4.2	4.8	5.4	6.1	8.3	11.8	15.8	18.2	21.7
10.0–10.9	333	12.0	7.3	4.7	5.3	5.7	6.9	9.8	14.7	18.3	21.5	27.0
11.0–11.9	324	13.6	9.4	4.9	5.5	6.2	7.3	10.4	16.9	22.3	26.0	32.5
12.0–12.9	348	13.9	9.6	4.7	5.6	6.3	7.6	11.3	15.8	21.1	27.3	35.0
13.0–13.9	350	13.0	9.2	4.7	5.7	6.3	7.6	10.1	14.9	21.2	25.4	32.1
14.0–14.9	358	13.3	10.2	4.6	5.6	6.3	7.4	10.1	15.9	19.5	25.5	31.8
15.0–15.9	356	12.8	9.0	5.6	6.1	6.5	7.3	9.6	14.6	20.2	24.5	31.3
16.0–16.9	350	13.9	9.5	5.6	6.1	6.9	8.3	10.5	16.6	20.6	24.8	33.5
17.0–17.9	337	12.9	8.9	5.4	6.1	6.7	7.4	9.9	15.6	19.7	23.7	28.9
18.0–24.9	1752	16.9	10.8	5.5	6.9	7.7	9.2	13.9	21.5	26.8	30.7	37.2
25.0–29.9	1250	18.8	11.6	6.0	7.3	8.4	10.2	16.3	23.9	29.7	33.3	40.4
30.0–34.9	940	20.4	11.4	6.2	8.4	9.7	11.9	18.4	25.6	31.6	34.8	41.9
35.0–39.9	832	20.1	10.5	6.5	8.1	9.6	12.8	18.8	25.2	29.6	33.4	39.4
40.0–44.9	828	20.4	11.2	7.1	8.7	9.9	12.4	18.0	25.3	30.1	35.3	42.1
45.0–49.9	867	20.1	11.0	7.4	9.0	10.2	12.3	18.1	24.9	29.7	33.7	40.4
50.0–54.9	879	19.4	10.3	7.0	8.6	10.1	12.3	17.3	23.9	29.0	32.4	40.0
55.0–59.9	807	19.2	10.2	6.4	8.2	9.7	12.3	17.4	23.8	28.4	33.3	39.1
60.0–64.9	1259	19.1	10.2	6.9	8.7	9.9	12.1	17.0	23.5	28.3	31.8	38.7
65.0–69.9	1773	18.0	9.8	5.8	7.4	8.5	10.9	16.5	22.8	27.2	30.7	36.3
70.0–74.9	1250	17.5	9.4	6.0	7.5	8.9	11.0	15.9	22.0	25.7	29.1	34.9
Females												
1.0–1.9	622	7.3	2.3	4.1	4.6	5.0	5.6	7.1	8.6	9.5	10.4	11.7
2.0–2.9	614	7.7	2.3	4.4	5.0	5.4	6.1	7.5	9.0	10.0	10.8	12.0
3.0–3.9	651	7.8	2.5	4.3	5.0	5.4	6.1	7.6	9.2	10.2	10.8	12.2
4.0–4.9	680	8.0	2.6	4.3	4.9	5.4	6.2	7.7	9.3	10.4	11.3	12.8
5.0–5.9	672	8.5	3.4	4.4	5.0	5.4	6.3	7.8	9.8	11.3	12.5	14.5
6.0–6.9	296	8.7	3.9	4.5	5.0	5.6	6.2	8.1	10.0	11.2	13.3	16.5
7.0–7.9	329	9.8	4.5	4.8	5.5	6.0	7.0	8.8	11.0	13.2	14.7	19.0
8.0–8.9	275	11.3	6.5	5.2	5.7	6.4	7.2	9.8	13.3	15.8	18.0	23.7
9.0–9.9	321	13.1	7.3	5.4	6.2	6.8	8.1	11.5	15.6	18.8	22.0	27.5
10.0–10.9	329	14.1	7.7	6.1	6.9	7.2	8.4	11.9	18.0	21.5	25.3	29.9
11.0–11.9	302	16.3	9.7	6.6	7.5	8.2	9.8	13.1	19.9	24.4	28.2	36.8
12.0–12.9	323	16.9	8.9	6.7	8.0	8.8	10.8	14.8	20.8	24.8	29.4	34.0
13.0–13.9	360	19.1	11.0	6.7	7.7	9.4	11.6	16.5	23.7	28.7	32.7	40.8
14.0–14.9	370	20.4	11.0	8.3	9.6	10.9	12.4	17.7	25.1	29.5	34.6	41.2
15.0–15.9	309	20.7	11.4	8.6	10.0	11.4	12.8	18.2	24.4	29.2	32.9	44.3
16.0–16.9	343	23.5	10.9	11.3	12.8	13.7	15.9	20.5	28.0	32.7	37.0	46.0
17.0–17.9	291	23.9	13.0	9.5	11.7	13.0	14.6	21.0	29.5	33.5	38.0	51.6
18.0–24.9	2588	25.2	13.4	10.0	12.0	13.5	16.1	21.9	30.6	37.2	42.0	51.6
25.0–29.9	1921	28.1	14.7	11.0	13.3	15.1	17.7	24.5	34.8	42.1	47.1	57.5
30.0–34.9	1619	31.6	16.1	12.2	14.8	17.2	20.4	28.2	39.0	46.8	52.3	64.5
35.0–39.9	1453	33.6	16.8	13.0	15.8	18.0	21.8	29.7	41.7	49.2	55.5	64.9
40.0–44.9	1390	34.3	16.2	13.8	16.7	19.2	23.0	31.3	42.6	51.0	56.3	64.5
45.0–49.9	961	36.0	17.2	13.6	17.1	19.8	24.3	33.0	44.4	52.3	58.4	68.8
50.0–54.9	1004	36.7	15.9	14.3	18.3	21.4	25.7	34.1	45.6	53.9	57.7	65.7
55.0–59.9	879	37.6	17.7	13.7	18.2	20.7	26.0	34.5	46.4	53.9	59.1	69.7
60.0–64.9	1389	37.1	16.0	15.3	19.1	21.9	26.0	34.8	45.7	51.7	58.3	68.3
65.0–69.9	1946	34.7	15.1	13.9	17.6	20.0	24.1	32.7	42.7	49.2	53.6	62.4
70.0–74.9	1463	32.9	14.6	13.0	16.2	18.8	22.7	31.2	41.0	46.4	51.4	57.7

Table IV.15.
Means, standard deviations, and percentiles of arm fat index (arm fat area/
total arm area x 100) by age for males and females of 1 to 74 years

Age (yrs)	N	Mean	SD	Percentiles								
				5	10	15	25	50	75	85	90	95
Males												
1.0–1.9	681	36.2	7.9	24.5	26.1	27.9	30.3	36.1	41.4	44.6	46.2	48.7
2.0–2.9	672	34.4	8.0	22.3	24.3	26.1	28.2	34.0	39.4	42.7	44.9	49.0
3.0–3.9	715	33.1	7.3	22.5	24.6	25.8	28.0	32.9	37.3	40.9	43.1	46.1
4.0–4.9	707	30.7	7.0	20.3	22.4	23.7	25.5	30.0	35.2	37.8	39.4	43.5
5.0–5.9	676	28.8	7.3	17.9	20.5	21.7	23.8	27.7	33.2	36.4	38.4	42.1
6.0–6.9	298	27.5	7.9	15.7	18.3	20.0	22.0	26.2	32.6	35.8	37.5	40.4
7.0–7.9	312	26.9	8.6	15.0	17.2	19.2	20.8	25.2	31.2	35.8	38.7	43.8
8.0–8.9	296	27.5	8.6	16.3	17.4	19.2	21.1	26.0	31.3	35.4	39.4	44.4
9.0–9.9	322	27.6	9.3	15.3	17.3	18.8	20.8	25.9	33.5	38.1	40.1	44.9
10.0–10.9	333	29.1	9.8	15.8	17.5	19.0	21.6	27.6	34.9	40.0	44.1	48.4
11.0–11.9	324	29.8	11.1	14.3	16.8	18.7	21.5	26.7	36.4	42.6	45.2	50.3
12.0–12.9	348	28.3	11.0	12.9	16.2	17.6	20.0	26.9	34.3	39.2	45.6	50.3
13.0–13.9	350	24.7	10.8	11.8	12.9	14.4	16.8	22.3	29.9	35.4	40.3	44.9
14.0–14.9	358	22.3	10.0	10.5	11.8	12.7	15.4	20.1	27.2	32.5	37.4	42.8
15.0–15.9	356	20.5	10.0	10.8	11.7	12.7	13.8	17.4	23.4	30.0	34.3	42.1
16.0–16.9	350	19.8	8.9	9.5	10.7	11.8	13.7	17.3	23.8	27.5	32.2	39.6
17.0–17.9	337	18.1	7.9	9.6	10.4	11.0	12.9	15.7	21.8	25.6	28.8	34.1
18.0–24.9	1752	20.7	9.3	9.2	10.5	11.6	13.6	19.1	26.3	30.6	33.4	38.3
25.0–29.9	1250	21.6	9.4	8.7	10.7	12.1	14.2	20.1	27.4	31.7	34.6	39.6
30.0–34.9	940	22.8	9.4	9.2	11.6	13.0	15.7	21.9	28.5	32.6	35.3	40.0
35.0–39.9	832	22.4	8.8	9.4	11.3	13.4	16.0	21.6	27.7	30.9	33.9	38.7
40.0–44.9	828	22.6	9.1	10.5	12.1	13.4	15.7	21.2	27.7	31.9	35.2	40.0
45.0–49.9	867	22.5	8.9	10.4	12.2	13.5	16.0	21.2	27.6	31.8	34.6	39.1
50.0–54.9	879	22.2	8.6	10.6	12.5	13.8	16.1	20.9	26.7	31.3	34.9	39.1
55.0–59.9	807	22.1	8.6	9.7	11.8	13.3	15.9	21.1	26.9	30.7	33.6	39.1
60.0–64.9	1259	22.5	8.5	10.6	12.6	14.1	16.3	21.3	27.9	31.1	34.2	38.2
65.0–69.9	1773	22.2	8.7	9.8	11.9	13.5	15.7	21.3	27.4	31.1	33.7	38.5
70.0–74.9	1250	22.4	8.5	10.5	12.3	14.0	16.3	21.5	27.1	30.7	33.4	37.8
Females												
1.0–1.9	622	36.9	8.4	24.0	26.2	28.2	30.5	36.8	41.8	45.5	47.8	51.2
2.0–2.9	614	36.3	7.7	24.0	26.4	28.1	30.9	36.1	41.1	44.2	45.8	49.9
3.0–3.9	651	35.0	7.4	23.7	25.6	27.1	29.6	35.0	39.8	42.4	44.3	47.8
4.0–4.9	680	33.9	7.8	22.0	24.5	25.9	28.4	33.6	38.8	41.3	43.5	46.0
5.0–5.9	672	32.9	7.8	20.5	23.6	25.2	27.2	32.2	37.7	40.3	42.8	46.6
6.0–6.9	296	31.9	7.9	20.1	22.7	24.5	26.2	31.3	37.2	39.8	41.8	45.5
7.0–7.9	329	32.7	8.4	20.1	22.8	24.3	26.5	32.3	37.0	41.0	44.3	48.2
8.0–8.9	275	33.4	9.5	19.4	22.3	24.1	26.4	32.8	38.5	43.3	45.3	51.6
9.0–9.9	321	34.7	9.9	20.6	22.6	23.7	27.6	33.8	41.0	45.5	48.1	52.3
10.0–10.9	329	35.0	10.1	20.7	23.3	24.1	26.9	33.7	41.9	46.8	49.6	52.6
11.0–11.9	302	35.0	9.9	20.2	22.9	24.7	27.6	34.0	41.0	46.1	48.0	52.3
12.0–12.9	323	34.6	9.1	20.3	23.2	25.1	28.2	33.6	41.0	45.3	47.5	50.3
13.0–13.9	360	35.4	10.2	19.4	21.4	23.8	28.0	35.3	42.2	46.1	48.5	52.3
14.0–14.9	370	35.9	9.9	21.3	23.9	25.5	28.9	34.9	42.6	46.4	49.4	53.0
15.0–15.9	309	36.2	9.9	20.7	23.4	25.5	28.5	36.2	42.7	46.6	48.7	53.5
16.0–16.9	343	39.0	9.1	24.8	26.9	28.8	32.4	39.2	45.0	48.0	51.3	53.9
17.0–17.9	291	38.1	10.3	22.0	25.3	27.0	30.5	38.4	45.1	48.7	51.6	55.2
18.0–24.9	2588	39.1	10.2	22.5	26.0	28.2	32.0	38.8	46.2	50.1	53.0	56.0
25.0–29.9	1921	40.9	10.3	24.1	27.4	29.7	33.6	40.8	48.4	52.4	54.3	57.4
30.0–34.9	1619	42.7	10.4	24.7	28.7	31.9	35.7	43.4	50.0	53.6	55.6	59.2
35.0–39.9	1453	43.5	10.1	25.9	29.8	32.9	37.0	43.9	50.6	54.0	56.5	59.2
40.0–44.9	1390	43.7	10.0	27.1	30.1	33.2	37.5	44.8	50.8	53.6	55.6	59.1
45.0–49.9	961	44.9	10.0	27.4	31.7	34.5	38.4	45.5	52.1	55.4	57.2	59.3
50.0–54.9	1004	45.1	9.7	26.8	31.7	35.0	39.7	45.8	51.7	55.0	57.0	59.5
55.0–59.9	879	44.8	9.8	26.7	31.2	34.3	38.9	45.4	52.0	54.9	56.5	59.0
60.0–64.9	1389	45.1	9.4	28.1	32.6	35.2	39.2	45.7	51.4	54.6	56.5	59.0
65.0–69.9	1946	43.5	9.5	27.0	30.6	33.4	37.3	43.9	50.2	53.0	54.7	57.6
70.0–74.9	1463	42.2	9.7	25.2	29.4	32.1	36.0	43.0	49.0	51.9	53.8	57.6

Table IV.16.
Means, standard deviations, and percentiles of triceps skinfold thickness (mm) by age for males and females of 1 to 74 years

Age (yrs)	N	Mean	SD	Percentiles								
				5	10	15	25	50	75	85	90	95
Males												
1.0–1.9	681	10.4	2.9	6.5	7.0	7.5	8.0	10.0	12.0	13.0	14.0	15.5
2.0–2.9	677	10.0	2.9	6.0	6.5	7.0	8.0	10.0	12.0	13.0	14.0	15.0
3.0–3.9	717	9.9	2.7	6.0	7.0	7.0	8.0	9.5	11.5	12.5	13.5	15.0
4.0–4.9	708	9.2	2.7	5.5	6.5	7.0	7.5	9.0	11.0	12.0	12.5	14.0
5.0–5.9	677	8.9	3.1	5.0	6.0	6.0	7.0	8.0	10.0	11.5	13.0	14.5
6.0–6.9	298	8.9	3.8	5.0	5.5	6.0	6.5	8.0	10.0	12.0	13.0	16.0
7.0–7.9	312	9.0	4.0	4.5	5.0	6.0	6.0	8.0	10.5	12.5	14.0	16.0
8.0–8.9	296	9.6	4.4	5.0	5.5	6.0	7.0	8.5	11.0	13.0	16.0	19.0
9.0–9.9	322	10.2	5.1	5.0	5.5	6.0	6.5	9.0	12.5	15.5	17.0	20.0
10.0–10.9	334	11.5	5.7	5.0	6.0	6.0	7.5	10.0	14.0	17.0	20.0	24.0
11.0–11.9	324	12.5	7.0	5.0	6.0	6.5	7.5	10.0	16.0	19.5	23.0	27.0
12.0–12.9	348	12.2	6.8	4.5	6.0	6.0	7.5	10.5	14.5	18.0	22.5	27.5
13.0–13.9	350	11.0	6.7	4.5	5.0	5.5	7.0	9.0	13.0	17.0	20.5	25.0
14.0–14.9	358	10.4	6.5	4.0	5.0	5.0	6.0	8.5	12.5	15.0	18.0	23.5
15.0–15.9	356	9.8	6.5	5.0	5.0	5.0	6.0	7.5	11.0	15.0	18.0	23.5
16.0–16.9	350	10.0	5.9	4.0	5.0	5.1	6.0	8.0	12.0	14.0	17.0	23.0
17.0–17.9	337	9.1	5.3	4.0	5.0	5.0	6.0	7.0	11.0	13.5	16.0	19.5
18.0–24.9	1752	11.3	6.4	4.0	5.0	5.5	6.5	10.0	14.5	17.5	20.0	23.5
25.0–29.9	1251	12.2	6.7	4.0	5.0	6.0	7.0	11.0	15.5	19.0	21.5	25.0
30.0–34.9	941	13.1	6.7	4.5	6.0	6.5	8.0	12.0	16.5	20.0	22.0	25.0
35.0–39.9	832	12.9	6.2	4.5	6.0	7.0	8.5	12.0	16.0	18.5	20.5	24.5
40.0–44.9	828	13.0	6.6	5.0	6.0	6.9	8.0	12.0	16.0	19.0	21.5	26.0
45.0–49.9	867	12.9	6.4	5.0	6.0	7.0	8.0	12.0	16.0	19.0	21.0	25.0
50.0–54.9	879	12.6	6.1	5.0	6.0	7.0	8.0	11.5	15.0	18.5	20.8	25.0
55.0–59.9	807	12.4	6.0	5.0	6.0	6.5	8.0	11.5	15.0	18.0	20.5	25.0
60.0–64.9	1259	12.5	6.0	5.0	6.0	7.0	8.0	11.5	15.5	18.5	20.5	24.0
65.0–69.9	1774	12.1	5.9	4.5	5.0	6.5	8.0	11.0	15.0	18.0	20.0	23.5
70.0–74.9	1251	12.0	5.8	4.5	6.0	6.5	8.0	11.0	15.0	17.0	19.0	23.0
Females												
1.0–1.9	622	10.4	3.1	6.0	7.0	7.0	8.0	10.0	12.0	13.0	14.0	16.0
2.0–2.9	614	10.5	2.9	6.0	7.0	7.5	8.5	10.0	12.0	13.5	14.5	16.0
3.0–3.9	652	10.4	2.9	6.0	7.0	7.5	8.5	10.0	12.0	13.0	14.0	16.0
4.0–4.9	681	10.3	3.0	6.0	7.0	7.5	8.0	10.0	12.0	13.0	14.0	15.5
5.0–5.9	673	10.4	3.5	5.5	7.0	7.0	8.0	10.0	12.0	13.5	15.0	17.0
6.0–6.9	296	10.4	3.7	6.0	6.5	7.0	8.0	10.0	12.0	13.0	15.0	17.0
7.0–7.9	330	11.1	4.2	6.0	7.0	7.0	8.0	10.5	12.5	15.0	16.0	19.0
8.0–8.9	276	12.1	5.4	6.0	7.0	7.5	8.5	11.0	14.5	17.0	18.0	22.5
9.0–9.9	322	13.4	5.9	6.5	7.0	8.0	9.0	12.0	16.0	19.0	21.0	25.0
10.0–10.9	329	13.9	6.1	7.0	8.0	8.0	9.0	12.5	17.5	20.0	22.5	27.0
11.0–11.9	302	15.0	6.8	7.0	8.0	8.5	10.0	13.0	18.0	21.5	24.0	29.0
12.0–12.9	323	15.1	6.3	7.0	8.0	9.0	11.0	14.0	18.5	21.5	24.0	27.5
13.0–13.9	360	16.4	7.4	7.0	8.0	9.0	11.0	15.0	20.0	24.0	25.0	30.0
14.0–14.9	370	17.1	7.3	8.0	9.0	10.0	11.5	16.0	21.0	23.5	26.5	32.0
15.0–15.9	309	17.3	7.4	8.0	9.5	10.5	12.0	16.5	20.5	23.0	26.0	32.5
16.0–16.9	343	19.2	7.0	10.5	11.5	12.0	14.0	18.0	23.0	26.0	29.0	32.5
17.0–17.9	291	19.1	8.0	9.0	10.0	12.0	13.0	18.0	24.0	26.5	29.0	34.5
18.0–24.9	2588	20.0	8.2	9.0	11.0	12.0	14.0	18.5	24.5	28.5	31.0	36.0
25.0–29.9	1921	21.7	8.8	10.0	12.0	13.0	15.0	20.0	26.5	31.0	34.0	38.0
30.0–34.9	1619	23.7	9.2	10.5	13.0	15.0	17.0	22.5	29.5	33.0	35.5	41.5
35.0–39.9	1453	24.7	9.3	11.0	13.0	15.5	18.0	23.5	30.0	35.0	37.0	41.0
40.0–44.9	1391	25.1	9.0	12.0	14.0	16.0	19.0	24.5	30.5	35.0	37.0	41.0
45.0–49.9	962	26.1	9.3	12.0	14.5	16.5	19.5	25.5	32.0	35.5	38.0	42.5
50.0–54.9	1006	26.5	9.0	12.0	15.0	17.5	20.5	25.5	32.0	36.0	38.5	42.0
55.0–59.9	880	26.6	9.4	12.0	15.0	17.0	20.5	26.0	32.0	36.0	39.0	42.5
60.0–64.9	1389	26.6	8.8	12.5	16.0	17.5	20.5	26.0	32.0	35.5	38.0	42.5
65.0–69.9	1946	25.1	8.5	12.0	14.5	16.0	19.0	25.0	30.0	33.5	36.0	40.0
70.0–74.9	1463	24.0	8.5	11.0	13.5	15.5	18.0	24.0	29.5	32.0	35.0	38.5

Table IV.17.
Means, standard deviations, and percentiles of subscapular skinfold
thickness (mm) by age for males and females of 1 to 74 years

Age (yrs)	N	Mean	SD	Percentiles								
				5	10	15	25	50	75	85	90	95
Males												
1.0–1.9	681	6.3	1.9	4.0	4.0	4.5	5.0	6.0	7.0	8.0	8.5	10.0
2.0–2.9	677	5.9	2.0	3.5	4.0	4.0	4.5	5.5	7.0	7.5	8.5	10.0
3.0–3.9	716	5.5	1.8	3.5	4.0	4.0	4.5	5.0	6.0	7.0	7.0	9.0
4.0–4.9	708	5.3	1.8	3.0	3.5	4.0	4.0	5.0	6.0	6.5	7.0	8.0
5.0–5.9	677	5.2	2.4	3.0	3.5	4.0	4.0	5.0	5.5	6.5	7.0	8.0
6.0–6.9	298	5.5	3.3	3.0	3.5	3.5	4.0	4.5	5.5	6.5	8.0	13.0
7.0–7.9	312	5.7	3.3	3.0	3.5	4.0	4.0	5.0	6.0	7.0	8.0	12.0
8.0–8.9	296	6.0	3.8	3.0	3.5	4.0	4.0	5.0	6.0	7.5	9.0	12.5
9.0–9.9	322	6.8	4.8	3.0	3.5	4.0	4.0	5.0	7.0	9.5	12.0	14.5
10.0–10.9	334	7.6	5.5	3.5	4.0	4.0	4.5	6.0	8.0	11.0	14.0	19.5
11.0–11.9	324	9.0	7.6	4.0	4.0	4.0	5.0	6.0	9.0	15.0	18.5	26.0
12.0–12.9	349	8.9	7.1	4.0	4.0	4.5	5.0	6.0	9.5	15.0	19.0	24.0
13.0–13.9	350	8.8	7.0	4.0	4.0	5.0	5.0	6.5	9.0	13.0	17.0	25.0
14.0–14.9	358	9.0	6.5	4.0	5.0	5.0	5.5	7.0	9.0	12.0	15.5	22.5
15.0–15.9	357	9.4	6.8	5.0	5.0	5.5	6.0	7.0	10.0	13.0	16.0	22.0
16.0–16.9	349	10.1	6.2	5.0	6.0	6.0	7.0	8.0	11.0	14.0	16.0	22.0
17.0–17.9	339	10.1	6.0	5.0	6.0	6.0	7.0	8.0	11.0	14.0	17.0	21.5
18.0–24.9	1750	13.4	7.6	6.0	7.0	7.0	8.0	11.0	16.0	20.0	24.0	30.0
25.0–29.9	1247	15.5	8.2	7.0	7.0	8.0	9.0	13.0	20.0	24.5	26.5	31.0
30.0–34.9	938	17.3	8.5	7.0	8.0	9.0	11.0	15.5	22.0	25.5	29.0	33.0
35.0–39.9	835	17.6	8.3	7.0	8.0	9.5	11.0	16.0	22.5	25.5	28.0	33.0
40.0–44.9	818	17.4	8.2	7.0	8.0	9.0	11.5	16.0	22.0	25.5	29.5	33.0
45.0–49.9	860	18.2	8.6	7.0	8.0	9.5	11.5	17.0	23.5	27.0	30.0	34.5
50.0–54.9	872	17.7	8.4	7.0	8.0	9.0	11.5	16.0	22.5	26.5	29.5	34.0
55.0–59.9	802	17.6	8.1	6.5	8.0	9.5	11.5	16.5	23.0	26.0	28.5	32.0
60.0–64.9	1251	18.1	8.4	7.0	8.0	10.0	12.0	17.0	23.0	26.0	29.0	34.0
65.0–69.9	1770	16.8	8.2	6.0	7.5	8.5	10.5	15.0	21.5	25.0	28.0	32.5
70.0–74.9	1247	16.3	7.8	6.5	7.0	8.0	10.3	15.0	21.0	25.0	27.5	31.0
Females												
1.0–1.9	622	6.5	2.0	4.0	4.0	4.5	5.0	6.0	7.5	8.5	9.0	10.0
2.0–2.9	615	6.4	2.3	4.0	4.0	4.5	5.0	6.0	7.0	8.0	9.0	10.5
3.0–3.9	652	6.1	2.2	3.5	4.0	4.0	5.0	5.5	7.0	7.5	8.5	10.0
4.0–4.9	681	6.0	2.3	3.5	4.0	4.0	4.5	5.5	7.0	8.0	9.0	10.5
5.0–5.9	672	6.2	3.0	3.5	4.0	4.0	4.5	5.0	7.0	8.0	9.0	12.0
6.0–6.9	296	6.3	3.4	3.5	4.0	4.0	4.5	5.5	7.0	8.0	10.0	11.5
7.0–7.9	330	6.7	3.5	3.5	4.0	4.0	4.5	6.0	7.5	9.5	11.0	13.0
8.0–8.9	276	7.8	5.8	3.5	4.0	4.0	5.0	6.0	8.0	11.5	14.5	21.0
9.0–9.9	322	9.0	6.5	4.0	4.5	5.0	5.0	6.5	9.5	13.0	18.0	24.0
10.0–10.9	329	9.7	6.5	4.0	4.5	5.0	5.5	7.0	11.5	16.0	19.5	24.0
11.0–11.9	300	10.7	7.6	4.5	5.0	5.0	6.0	8.0	12.0	16.0	20.0	28.5
12.0–12.9	323	11.5	7.7	5.0	5.5	6.0	6.5	9.0	13.0	17.0	22.0	30.0
13.0–13.9	360	12.3	7.8	5.0	6.0	6.0	7.0	10.0	15.5	19.0	23.0	26.5
14.0–14.9	370	13.0	7.7	6.0	6.0	7.0	7.5	10.0	16.0	20.5	25.0	30.0
15.0–15.9	308	13.0	7.5	6.0	7.0	7.5	8.0	10.0	15.0	20.0	23.0	28.0
16.0–16.9	343	14.7	8.7	7.0	7.5	8.0	9.0	11.5	16.5	24.0	26.0	34.0
17.0–17.9	291	15.4	8.9	6.0	7.0	7.5	9.0	12.5	19.0	24.5	28.0	34.0
18.0–24.9	2587	16.1	9.4	6.5	7.0	8.0	9.5	13.0	20.0	25.5	29.0	36.0
25.0–29.9	1913	17.5	10.4	6.5	7.0	8.0	10.0	14.0	23.0	29.0	33.0	38.5
30.0–34.9	1615	19.7	11.7	6.5	7.5	8.5	10.5	16.0	26.5	32.5	37.0	43.0
35.0–39.9	1446	20.6	11.6	7.0	8.0	9.0	11.0	18.0	28.5	34.0	36.5	43.0
40.0–44.9	1382	20.9	11.4	6.5	8.0	9.0	11.5	19.0	28.5	34.0	37.0	42.0
45.0–49.9	956	21.8	11.4	7.0	8.5	10.0	12.5	20.0	29.5	34.0	37.5	43.5
50.0–54.9	995	23.0	11.4	7.0	9.0	11.0	14.0	21.9	30.0	35.0	39.0	43.5
55.0–59.9	870	23.2	11.7	7.0	9.0	11.0	13.5	22.0	31.0	35.0	38.0	45.0
60.0–64.9	1376	22.8	11.3	7.5	9.0	11.0	14.0	21.5	30.5	35.0	38.0	43.0
65.0–69.9	1933	21.4	10.6	7.0	8.0	10.0	13.0	20.0	28.0	33.0	36.0	41.0
70.0–74.9	1460	20.5	10.1	6.5	8.5	10.0	12.0	19.5	27.0	32.0	35.0	38.5

Table IV.18.

Means, standard deviations, and percentiles of sum of skinfold thickness (mm) by age for males and females of 1 to 74 years

Age (yrs)	N	Mean	SD	Percentiles								
				5	10	15	25	50	75	85	90	95
Males												
1.0–1.9	681	16.8	4.1	11.0	12.0	12.5	14.0	16.5	19.0	21.0	22.0	24.0
2.0–2.9	677	16.0	4.3	10.0	11.0	12.0	13.0	15.5	18.0	20.0	21.5	24.0
3.0–3.9	716	15.4	4.1	10.5	11.0	12.0	13.0	14.5	17.5	19.0	20.5	23.0
4.0–4.9	707	14.5	4.2	9.5	10.5	11.0	12.0	14.0	16.5	18.0	19.0	21.5
5.0–5.9	677	14.2	5.0	9.0	10.0	10.0	11.0	13.0	16.0	18.0	19.0	22.0
6.0–6.9	298	14.3	6.7	8.0	9.0	10.0	10.5	13.0	15.2	18.0	20.0	28.0
7.0–7.9	312	14.8	6.9	8.5	9.0	9.5	10.5	13.0	16.0	19.5	23.0	26.6
8.0–8.9	296	15.6	7.8	8.5	9.0	10.0	11.0	13.5	17.0	20.0	24.5	30.5
9.0–9.9	322	17.0	9.4	8.5	9.5	10.0	11.0	14.0	19.0	24.0	29.0	34.0
10.0–10.9	334	19.1	10.6	9.0	10.0	11.0	12.0	15.5	22.0	27.0	33.5	42.0
11.0–11.9	324	21.4	13.9	9.0	10.0	11.0	12.5	16.5	25.0	33.0	40.0	53.5
12.0–12.9	348	21.0	13.2	9.0	10.0	11.0	12.5	17.0	24.0	34.0	40.5	53.0
13.0–13.9	350	19.8	13.3	8.5	10.5	11.0	12.5	15.0	21.0	29.0	37.0	48.0
14.0–14.9	358	19.4	12.6	9.0	10.0	11.0	12.0	15.0	22.0	27.0	33.0	45.0
15.0–15.9	356	19.3	12.8	10.0	10.5	11.0	12.0	15.0	21.0	27.0	32.5	43.0
16.0–16.9	349	20.0	11.4	10.0	11.5	12.0	13.0	16.0	22.5	27.5	33.5	44.0
17.0–17.9	337	19.1	10.8	10.0	11.0	12.0	13.0	16.0	22.0	27.0	31.5	41.0
18.0–24.9	1748	24.6	13.1	11.0	12.0	13.5	15.0	21.0	30.0	37.0	41.5	50.5
25.0–29.9	1246	27.6	13.9	11.5	13.0	14.0	17.0	24.5	35.0	41.0	46.0	54.5
30.0–34.9	938	30.4	14.1	12.0	14.5	16.5	20.0	28.0	38.0	44.0	49.0	58.0
35.0–39.9	829	30.3	13.3	12.0	14.5	16.5	21.0	29.0	37.0	42.4	47.0	54.5
40.0–44.9	816	30.1	13.3	13.0	15.0	16.5	20.5	28.5	37.0	42.5	47.5	55.0
45.0–49.9	856	30.9	13.6	12.5	15.0	17.5	20.5	29.0	39.0	44.0	48.0	55.0
50.0–54.9	872	30.1	13.1	13.0	15.0	17.0	20.5	28.0	37.5	43.0	48.0	55.5
55.0–59.9	802	29.9	12.7	12.0	15.0	17.0	21.0	28.5	37.0	43.0	47.0	53.5
60.0–64.9	1250	30.5	13.1	13.0	15.5	17.5	21.0	29.0	37.5	43.0	47.0	55.5
65.0–69.9	1770	28.9	13.1	11.0	13.5	16.0	19.5	27.0	36.0	42.0	46.5	53.5
70.0–74.9	1247	28.2	12.4	11.5	14.0	16.0	19.0	26.0	35.0	41.0	45.0	51.0
Females												
1.0–1.9	622	16.9	4.5	10.5	12.0	12.0	13.5	16.5	19.5	21.0	23.0	25.0
2.0–2.9	614	16.9	4.5	11.0	12.0	12.5	14.0	16.0	19.0	21.5	23.5	25.5
3.0–3.9	652	16.5	4.5	10.5	11.5	12.0	13.5	16.0	18.5	20.5	21.5	25.0
4.0–4.9	681	16.3	4.7	10.0	11.0	12.0	13.0	15.5	18.5	20.5	22.5	24.5
5.0–5.9	672	16.5	5.9	10.0	11.0	11.5	12.5	15.0	18.5	21.0	24.0	28.5
6.0–6.9	296	16.7	6.5	10.0	10.5	11.0	12.5	15.5	18.5	21.0	23.5	28.0
7.0–7.9	330	17.8	7.1	10.0	11.0	12.0	13.5	16.0	20.0	23.0	26.0	32.5
8.0–8.9	276	20.0	10.7	10.5	11.0	12.0	13.0	17.0	22.5	28.5	31.0	41.5
9.0–9.9	322	22.4	11.8	11.0	12.0	12.5	14.5	19.0	25.5	30.0	39.0	48.9
10.0–10.9	329	23.6	12.1	12.0	12.5	13.0	15.0	20.0	28.5	34.5	40.5	51.0
11.0–11.9	300	25.5	13.6	12.0	13.5	14.5	16.0	22.0	30.0	37.0	42.0	55.0
12.0–12.9	323	26.6	13.3	13.0	14.0	15.0	18.0	23.0	31.0	37.0	44.0	57.0
13.0–13.9	360	28.7	14.6	12.5	14.0	15.5	18.5	24.5	35.5	43.0	47.5	56.5
14.0–14.9	370	30.1	14.3	14.5	16.0	17.5	20.0	26.0	37.0	44.5	48.5	62.0
15.0–15.9	308	30.1	14.1	15.0	17.0	18.0	20.5	26.5	34.5	42.5	48.5	62.5
16.0–16.9	343	33.9	14.9	17.5	20.0	21.5	24.0	30.0	39.5	47.0	53.5	69.5
17.0–17.9	291	34.5	16.2	16.5	18.5	20.0	23.0	31.0	42.0	49.0	55.5	67.4
18.0–24.9	2586	36.1	16.6	16.7	19.0	21.0	24.0	32.0	44.0	52.0	58.5	70.0
25.0–29.9	1907	39.0	18.0	17.5	20.0	22.0	25.5	35.0	48.5	58.0	64.5	73.9
30.0–34.9	1613	43.3	19.8	18.0	22.0	24.5	28.5	39.0	55.0	64.0	71.0	83.0
35.0–39.9	1443	45.2	19.5	19.0	22.5	25.5	30.0	42.0	57.5	66.0	72.2	82.5
40.0–44.9	1378	45.8	18.9	20.0	23.5	27.0	31.0	43.0	58.0	67.0	73.0	80.0
45.0–49.9	953	47.7	19.2	21.0	24.0	27.5	33.5	45.0	59.5	69.0	74.5	81.0
50.0–54.9	992	49.3	18.9	21.0	26.0	30.0	35.5	47.0	61.0	70.0	75.3	83.5
55.0–59.9	868	49.5	19.5	21.0	26.0	29.0	35.0	47.5	62.0	69.5	75.0	85.0
60.0–64.9	1374	49.2	18.6	22.0	27.0	30.0	35.5	48.0	61.0	68.0	74.0	83.5
65.0–69.9	1930	46.3	17.6	21.0	25.0	28.5	34.0	44.0	57.0	64.0	70.0	78.0
70.0–74.9	1458	44.5	17.1	19.0	23.5	27.0	32.0	43.0	56.0	62.0	67.0	75.5

Table IV.19.

Means, standard deviations, and percentiles of percent fat weight (%) by age for males and females of 18 to 74 years

Age (yrs)	N	Mean	SD	Percentiles								
				5	10	15	25	50	75	85	90	95
Males												
18.0–24.9	1708	16.5	6.2	8.0	9.0	10.0	12.0	16.0	20.0	23.0	25.0	28.0
25.0–29.9	1217	18.2	6.2	9.0	10.0	11.0	13.0	18.0	23.0	25.0	26.0	29.0
30.0–34.9	916	22.6	4.2	16.0	17.0	18.0	20.0	23.0	26.0	27.0	28.0	30.0
35.0–39.9	817	22.5	4.1	15.0	17.0	18.0	20.0	23.0	25.0	27.0	27.0	29.0
40.0–44.9	805	25.3	6.6	14.0	16.0	18.0	21.0	26.0	30.0	32.0	34.0	36.0
45.0–49.9	842	25.7	6.6	15.0	17.0	19.0	21.0	26.0	30.0	32.0	34.0	36.0
50.0–54.9	858	26.4	6.7	15.0	17.0	19.0	22.0	27.0	31.0	33.0	35.0	37.0
55.0–59.9	780	26.6	6.4	15.0	18.0	20.0	22.0	27.0	31.0	33.0	35.0	37.0
60.0–64.9	1228	26.8	6.5	16.0	18.0	20.0	22.0	27.0	31.0	33.0	35.0	37.0
65.0–69.9	1725	25.8	6.9	13.0	16.0	18.0	21.0	26.0	30.0	33.0	35.0	37.0
70.0–74.9	1229	25.4	6.7	13.0	16.0	18.0	21.0	26.0	30.0	33.0	34.0	36.0
Females												
18.0–24.9	2585	27.9	7.0	17.0	19.0	21.0	23.0	27.0	33.0	35.0	37.0	40.0
25.0–29.9	1905	29.1	7.3	18.0	20.0	21.0	24.0	29.0	34.0	37.0	39.0	41.0
30.0–34.9	1613	31.4	6.4	21.0	23.0	25.0	27.0	31.0	36.0	38.0	40.0	42.0
35.0–39.9	1442	32.1	6.2	22.0	24.0	25.0	28.0	32.0	37.0	39.0	40.0	42.0
40.0–44.9	1376	34.9	5.7	25.0	28.0	29.0	31.0	35.0	39.0	41.0	42.0	43.0
45.0–49.9	952	35.5	5.6	26.0	28.0	29.0	32.0	36.0	39.0	41.0	42.0	44.0
50.0–54.9	991	38.9	6.4	27.0	30.0	32.0	35.0	39.0	43.0	46.0	47.0	48.0
55.0–59.9	867	38.9	6.5	27.0	30.0	32.0	35.0	39.0	44.0	45.0	47.0	49.0
60.0–64.9	1370	39.0	6.2	28.0	31.0	32.0	35.0	40.0	43.0	45.0	46.0	48.0
65.0–69.9	1927	38.0	6.2	27.0	30.0	32.0	34.0	38.0	42.0	44.0	46.0	47.0
70.0–74.9	1454	37.3	6.4	26.0	29.0	31.0	34.0	38.0	42.0	44.0	45.0	47.0

Table IV.20.

Mean percent fat weight by sum of triceps and subscapular skinfold thicknesses for adults ranging in age from 18 to 49 years

Males		Females	
Summed Skinfold Thicknesses Range (mm)	Percent Fat Weight (Mean ±SD)	Summed Skinfold Thicknesses Range (mm)	Percent Fat Weight (Mean ±SD)
Age Group: 18 to 24 years			
9 to 11	6.8 ± 1.0	8 to 17	15.5 ± 2.3
12 to 13	9.3 ± 0.7	18 to 21	19.8 ± 1.1
14 to 30	15.2 ± 3.1	22 to 44	27.0 ± 3.2
31 to 37	22.1 ± 0.8	45 to 52	34.1 ± 0.8
38 to 113	27.2 ± 3.0	53 to 130	39.5 ± 3.0
Age Group: 25 to 29 years			
9 to 12	7.9 ± 1.2	9 to 17	15.3 ± 2.2
13 to 14	10.2 ± 0.4	18 to 22	20.1 ± 1.2
15 to 35	17.1 ± 3.3	23 to 48	28.1 ± 3.5
36 to 42	23.9 ± 0.7	49 to 58	35.9 ± 0.9
43 to 100	28.2 ± 2.6	59 to 116	40.9 ± 2.7
Age Group: 30 to 34 years			
9 to 13	14.4 ± 1.1	9 to 18	18.4 ± 2.2
14 to 17	17.2 ± 0.9	19 to 24	23.3 ± 1.0
18 to 38	22.2 ± 2.1	25 to 55	30.6 ± 3.1
39 to 44	26.3 ± 0.5	56 to 64	37.2 ± 0.7
45 to 104	29.1 ± 1.7	65 to 117	41.3 ± 2.1
Age Group: 35 to 39 years			
8 to 12	13.9 ± 1.1	8 to 19	19.5 ± 2.3
13 to 17	16.7 ± 0.9	20 to 25	23.8 ± 1.1
18 to 37	22.3 ± 2.0	26 to 57	31.4 ± 3.1
38 to 42	26.0 ± 0.4	58 to 66	37.7 ± 0.6
43 to 114	28.6 ± 1.8	67 to 112	41.3 ± 2.0
Age Group: 40 to 44 years			
8 to 13	12.6 ± 1.6	8 to 20	22.9 ± 2.8
14 to 17	16.6 ± 1.1	21 to 27	27.8 ± 1.2
18 to 37	24.7 ± 3.1	28 to 58	34.5 ± 2.8
38 to 43	31.0 ± 0.8	59 to 67	40.2 ± 0.6
44 to 92	35.5 ± 2.7	68 to 115	43.2 ± 1.7
Age Group: 45 to 49 years			
9 to 14	12.8 ± 2.0	8 to 21	23.4 ± 2.5
15 to 18	17.5 ± 1.1	22 to 27	27.8 ± 1.0
19 to 39	25.3 ± 3.3	28 to 59	35.0 ± 2.8
40 to 44	31.7 ± 0.6	60 to 69	40.5 ± 0.6
45 to 98	35.6 ± 2.7	70 to 117	43.6 ± 1.6

Note: Includes the sum of triceps and subscapular skinfold thickness.

Table IV.21.

Mean percent fat weight by sum of triceps and subscapular skinfold thicknesses for adults ranging in age from 50 to 74 years

Males		Females	
Summmed Skinfold Thicknesses Range (mm)	Percent Fat Weight (Mean ±SD)	Summed Skinfold Thicknesses Range (mm)	Percent Fat Weight (Mean ±SD)
Age Group: 50 to 54 years			
8 to 13	12.9 ± 2.2	10 to 21	24.1 ± 3.1
14 to 17	17.5 ± 1.1	22 to 30	30.5 ± 1.5
18 to 37	25.7 ± 3.2	31 to 61	38.7 ± 3.0
38 to 43	32.3 ± 0.8	62 to 70	44.7 ± 0.7
44 to 94	36.8 ± 2.5	71 to 114	48.1 ± 1.8
Age Group: 55 to 59 years			
9 to 13	13.2 ± 1.5	12 to 21	24.5 ± 2.2
14 to 18	18.5 ± 1.3	22 to 29	30.3 ± 1.4
19 to 37	26.2 ± 3.0	30 to 62	38.6 ± 3.2
38 to 43	32.3 ± 0.8	63 to 69	44.6 ± 0.5
44 to 86	36.4 ± 2.4	70 to 125	48.1 ± 2.2
Age Group: 60 to 64 years			
9 to 14	14.1 ± 1.9	8 to 22	25.2 ± 2.7
15 to 18	18.6 ± 1.1	23 to 30	30.8 ± 1.3
19 to 37	26.1 ± 3.1	31 to 61	38.6 ± 3.0
38 to 43	32.2 ± 0.7	62 to 68	44.4 ± 0.5
44 to 94	36.9 ± 2.7	69 to 120	47.9 ± 1.9
Age Group: 65 to 69 years			
8 to 12	12.0 ± 1.6	8 to 21	24.0 ± 2.9
13 to 16	16.6 ± 1.1	22 to 29	30.1 ± 1.4
17 to 36	25.2 ± 3.4	30 to 57	37.7 ± 2.8
37 to 42	31.9 ± 0.8	58 to 64	43.4 ± 0.5
43 to 102	36.4 ± 2.7	65 to 118	46.9 ± 2.1
Age Group: 70 to 74 years			
9 to 12	12.0 ± 1.3	8 to 19	22.5 ± 2.9
13 to 16	16.6 ± 1.1	20 to 27	29.1 ± 1.4
17 to 35	24.7 ± 3.2	28 to 56	37.2 ± 3.1
36 to 41	31.3 ± 0.9	57 to 62	43.0 ± 0.6
42 to 90	35.8 ± 2.6	63 to 122	46.3 ± 2.0

Note: Includes the sum of triceps and subscapular skinfold thickness.

Table IV.22.
Means, standard deviations, and percentiles of weight (kg) by age for adult males of small, medium, and large frames

Age (yrs)	N	Mean	SD	Percentiles								
				5	10	15	25	50	75	85	90	95
Males with Small Frames												
18.0–24.9	444	69.9	11.5	54.5	57.4	59.0	62.3	68.3	76.1	80.5	83.8	89.8
25.0–29.9	318	73.4	12.0	56.7	60.3	61.9	65.1	71.8	79.4	84.7	87.5	97.9
30.0–34.9	239	75.7	12.5	57.9	61.6	63.2	67.0	74.6	83.1	87.8	92.9	98.0
35.0–39.9	212	75.5	12.0	56.0	59.9	62.1	66.6	75.9	83.5	87.8	91.4	96.0
40.0–44.9	210	78.3	12.4	58.8	62.8	65.4	70.3	76.1	86.3	92.3	94.8	101.0
45.0–49.9	220	76.3	11.7	57.7	60.9	63.2	67.6	76.2	83.6	89.0	92.1	95.8
50.0–54.9	225	75.4	11.9	57.3	60.2	64.5	67.1	74.7	82.8	88.2	90.5	99.3
55.0–59.9	204	74.5	12.0	54.7	58.2	61.5	66.7	74.8	81.9	87.2	90.6	94.7
60.0–64.9	318	74.0	12.3	54.2	59.2	62.5	65.9	73.4	80.7	85.7	88.4	93.8
65.0–69.9	446	70.7	12.1	50.8	55.4	57.8	61.9	70.3	79.0	83.3	86.8	92.4
70.0–74.9	315	70.5	12.5	49.9	54.4	57.3	61.9	70.1	78.4	83.0	85.5	92.8
Males with Medium Frames												
18.0–24.9	877	74.0	12.7	57.5	60.6	62.3	65.3	71.5	80.3	86.0	91.6	99.6
25.0–29.9	627	77.0	13.2	58.5	61.8	64.5	68.4	75.9	84.1	88.3	92.4	100.4
30.0–34.9	473	78.5	12.9	59.8	63.0	65.9	69.5	77.8	85.8	91.1	93.8	98.8
35.0–39.9	419	80.5	12.8	58.7	64.8	68.4	72.9	80.4	87.4	91.5	95.9	102.5
40.0–44.9	414	80.1	12.4	60.8	64.2	67.9	71.9	79.3	88.1	92.4	96.8	102.6
45.0–49.9	436	80.7	13.0	60.3	65.1	67.1	71.9	79.8	88.7	93.3	96.7	101.3
50.0–54.9	441	79.0	13.7	58.4	62.5	65.8	70.0	78.3	86.3	91.7	96.6	103.1
55.0–59.9	404	78.8	12.7	59.9	64.5	66.7	70.5	77.9	85.3	91.1	95.4	102.2
60.0–64.9	629	76.7	11.9	58.3	61.5	64.5	68.7	76.3	84.4	88.4	91.6	97.8
65.0–69.9	886	75.0	12.2	56.1	59.5	62.5	66.9	74.5	82.9	86.9	90.8	97.2
70.0–74.9	627	73.6	12.2	54.3	58.3	61.1	65.5	72.6	81.0	86.1	89.8	93.9
Males with Large Frames												
18.0–24.9	433	77.5	15.4	58.2	61.3	62.6	67.4	74.7	85.0	91.2	95.0	104.9
25.0–29.9	310	84.3	17.4	61.2	66.0	68.4	72.6	82.2	91.6	99.8	102.8	115.2
30.0–34.9	233	86.5	16.6	65.5	68.4	70.2	75.2	85.4	94.0	101.6	106.7	116.7
35.0–39.9	206	85.0	15.0	59.6	67.4	71.8	75.4	84.1	93.1	98.9	104.1	113.3
40.0–44.9	205	85.8	16.4	63.7	67.7	68.8	74.3	84.9	94.5	100.3	107.4	113.3
45.0–49.9	215	85.5	16.5	62.7	67.0	69.4	74.0	84.0	94.0	101.3	105.9	119.2
50.0–54.9	216	84.7	14.7	64.4	66.9	68.8	73.3	83.1	94.3	101.7	103.6	108.4
55.0–59.9	199	85.7	15.7	64.5	67.1	70.3	74.8	84.5	93.5	100.5	103.5	121.1
60.0–64.9	313	82.1	14.6	61.5	66.6	69.3	73.1	80.7	89.4	94.5	98.9	107.7
65.0–69.9	440	79.5	13.8	57.0	61.5	64.9	70.4	78.9	87.8	93.0	96.3	104.0
70.0–74.9	310	77.1	13.8	55.3	59.9	63.6	67.9	76.7	84.1	90.5	95.8	101.4

Table IV.23.

Means, standard deviations, and percentiles of weight (kg) by age for adult females of small, medium, and large frames

Age (yrs)	N	Mean	SD	Percentiles								
				5	10	15	25	50	75	85	90	95
Females with Small Frames												
18.0–24.9	652	56.2	8.7	44.0	46.1	48.0	50.3	55.1	60.9	64.4	66.9	71.5
25.0–29.9	487	56.9	9.5	44.1	47.3	48.6	50.9	55.6	61.1	64.5	67.6	72.6
30.0–34.9	413	59.1	10.0	45.7	48.2	50.0	52.7	57.6	63.4	68.1	71.8	77.7
35.0–39.9	369	61.1	11.4	45.8	48.2	50.8	53.4	59.5	66.7	71.9	76.0	79.5
40.0–44.9	353	60.6	9.4	48.1	50.3	51.8	54.5	59.1	66.1	70.0	73.6	80.3
45.0–49.9	244	61.4	11.1	46.3	47.8	50.8	53.6	60.3	67.3	71.4	75.1	80.8
50.0–54.9	257	61.3	10.8	46.3	49.1	51.7	54.5	60.3	66.9	71.0	73.1	78.4
55.0–59.9	224	61.3	11.1	47.3	49.5	52.2	54.7	59.9	65.3	70.2	73.6	81.5
60.0–64.9	351	61.9	11.0	46.4	48.9	50.6	54.2	60.9	68.5	71.7	74.0	82.2
65.0–69.9	491	61.1	10.7	44.9	48.4	50.7	53.6	60.2	67.4	71.7	74.0	79.3
70.0–74.9	369	60.6	12.1	42.6	45.9	48.5	51.6	60.2	67.0	72.3	75.4	81.0
Females with Medium Frames												
18.0–24.9	1297	59.5	10.4	46.0	48.4	50.0	52.5	58.1	64.4	69.5	72.8	78.4
25.0–29.9	967	60.9	11.5	46.9	49.1	50.6	53.0	58.6	66.3	72.2	76.9	83.0
30.0–34.9	815	63.5	13.4	47.2	50.0	51.7	54.3	60.7	69.3	76.7	80.6	87.2
35.0–39.9	730	64.1	12.1	49.2	51.7	53.0	56.1	61.8	69.8	74.7	79.4	87.9
40.0–44.9	700	65.6	13.3	48.8	51.3	53.6	57.0	62.8	71.8	77.3	82.4	92.1
45.0–49.9	484	65.8	13.4	48.3	51.4	53.3	56.4	63.4	72.2	77.8	83.1	91.6
50.0–54.9	504	66.4	12.2	48.9	52.0	54.4	57.7	64.4	73.1	79.3	82.8	89.7
55.0–59.9	444	68.0	15.3	48.2	51.1	54.3	58.1	66.3	74.8	81.0	86.2	92.1
60.0–64.9	695	66.2	12.4	49.1	52.3	54.0	57.5	64.5	73.5	78.1	82.2	89.0
65.0–69.9	973	66.2	12.7	48.1	51.4	53.6	57.1	64.9	73.1	78.7	82.4	88.8
70.0–74.9	731	64.3	11.9	46.8	50.5	52.5	56.8	62.9	70.8	76.9	80.2	84.7
Females with Large Frames												
18.0–24.9	642	68.0	17.2	48.9	51.3	53.1	56.3	62.9	76.2	83.8	89.0	102.7
25.0–29.9	480	72.6	17.7	49.9	53.4	55.6	59.3	68.7	82.9	90.9	98.8	105.0
30.0–34.9	402	76.4	19.7	51.1	54.9	57.7	61.1	72.7	88.4	97.3	102.8	111.9
35.0–39.9	361	79.1	19.5	52.8	56.1	59.1	64.5	76.7	90.4	98.1	106.0	117.9
40.0–44.9	346	79.7	19.8	53.4	57.3	60.7	65.7	77.1	91.3	99.2	104.9	114.2
45.0–49.9	240	80.1	19.6	54.5	60.1	63.2	66.7	76.8	86.6	97.6	105.0	116.9
50.0–54.9	250	79.4	16.9	55.6	60.0	63.0	67.8	77.7	88.8	97.1	103.3	112.1
55.0–59.9	218	79.8	17.5	56.4	60.2	62.5	67.6	77.6	89.9	97.0	101.6	111.3
60.0–64.9	346	77.8	15.6	56.0	59.4	62.8	66.8	76.8	85.7	92.8	100.0	104.8
65.0–69.9	484	76.6	15.4	55.3	59.4	62.0	65.8	74.5	84.6	91.7	97.8	105.0
70.0–74.9	363	74.9	14.0	53.5	57.9	60.9	65.8	74.5	82.7	87.9	91.3	99.1

Table IV.24.

Means, standard deviations, and percentiles of muscle area (cm^2) by age for adult males of small, medium, and large frames

Age (yrs)	N	Mean	SD	Percentiles								
				5	10	15	25	50	75	85	90	95
Males with Small Frames												
18.0–24.9	443	45.6	10.6	30.8	33.8	35.8	38.7	44.6	51.3	55.2	58.1	63.2
25.0–29.9	318	48.2	9.8	33.5	36.8	39.2	41.8	47.6	53.5	57.7	61.2	63.7
30.0–34.9	237	49.6	10.2	35.0	37.5	38.9	42.0	48.8	56.4	60.0	62.7	66.9
35.0–39.9	212	51.2	10.4	34.7	38.7	40.9	44.1	50.7	57.5	61.7	63.8	70.0
40.0–44.9	210	51.5	10.1	34.9	38.1	40.6	44.2	51.6	58.2	61.6	64.5	66.9
45.0–49.9	220	49.7	10.8	32.8	36.5	38.9	42.9	49.1	55.7	59.5	63.3	68.8
50.0–54.9	225	49.1	11.2	33.8	36.0	38.2	41.5	47.6	55.5	60.7	63.8	69.3
55.0–59.9	204	47.9	10.1	31.2	35.4	37.8	41.7	47.8	54.3	58.8	61.4	64.2
60.0–64.9	318	48.7	11.2	32.5	36.3	38.7	41.4	48.0	54.6	59.6	62.2	68.0
65.0–69.9	446	45.1	10.7	26.7	31.5	34.7	37.6	44.7	52.5	56.1	58.5	62.7
70.0–74.9	314	43.5	10.3	27.7	30.8	32.9	36.1	43.4	49.6	53.4	56.6	59.9
Males with Medium Frames												
18.0–24.9	875	50.5	10.5	35.5	38.2	40.8	43.6	49.5	56.5	60.8	63.2	69.3
25.0–29.9	626	54.0	11.3	37.0	40.1	42.9	46.8	53.2	60.9	65.6	67.7	73.0
30.0–34.9	472	55.0	10.4	38.5	42.2	44.8	48.0	54.3	61.8	65.7	68.6	72.7
35.0–39.9	416	56.7	11.7	39.9	43.1	45.2	48.8	55.9	64.0	69.0	71.6	75.6
40.0–44.9	413	56.7	11.0	39.2	42.6	45.8	49.2	56.3	64.0	68.0	71.1	74.4
45.0–49.9	433	56.6	11.2	39.0	42.6	45.6	49.4	55.9	63.7	69.6	72.8	76.2
50.0–54.9	440	55.3	11.7	37.6	41.8	44.5	47.7	54.2	62.5	65.9	69.6	74.1
55.0–59.9	403	55.4	10.8	39.2	42.5	44.4	48.5	54.8	62.2	66.7	69.5	75.0
60.0–64.9	627	52.3	10.8	34.5	38.3	41.6	45.0	52.1	59.2	63.3	66.3	70.4
65.0–69.9	886	49.8	10.5	33.4	37.2	39.6	43.0	49.2	56.7	60.1	62.4	68.1
70.0–74.9	626	47.8	10.8	30.8	34.6	36.9	40.6	47.5	54.4	59.1	62.0	66.8
Males with Large Frames												
18.0–24.9	431	55.7	12.2	37.6	40.8	43.0	47.3	54.6	63.5	67.0	71.6	76.7
25.0–29.9	305	60.3	12.0	42.6	45.7	48.4	52.6	60.4	67.3	72.8	75.8	81.2
30.0–34.9	230	62.8	13.4	44.2	46.9	49.2	53.3	62.6	70.6	75.3	78.8	84.0
35.0–39.9	203	61.6	13.3	43.2	46.0	48.9	51.8	59.9	70.3	76.6	79.4	82.8
40.0–44.9	204	61.8	12.3	44.9	47.4	49.6	53.2	60.0	69.8	74.4	79.4	83.7
45.0–49.9	214	61.1	13.0	42.9	46.3	48.1	52.4	59.6	67.5	71.1	74.9	86.4
50.0–54.9	214	60.5	12.8	41.8	46.0	47.8	51.6	59.4	67.6	72.5	77.6	85.4
55.0–59.9	198	60.2	12.0	42.3	45.0	47.9	52.9	59.8	66.9	71.8	75.3	83.8
60.0–64.9	311	57.9	12.1	38.9	43.9	46.8	50.1	57.5	65.8	69.0	71.8	77.4
65.0–69.9	439	54.5	12.7	35.6	39.4	41.7	46.0	53.7	62.7	66.9	70.7	75.6
70.0–74.9	310	52.0	12.4	33.2	38.3	40.3	43.6	51.6	59.0	63.8	67.2	72.2

Note: Values for males aged 18 years and older have been adjusted for bone area by subtracting 10.0 cm² from the calculated mid upper arm muscle area (see text).

Table IV.25.

Means, standard deviations, and percentiles of muscle area (cm^2) by age for adult females of small, medium, and large frames

Age (yrs)	N	Mean	SD	Percentiles								
				5	10	15	25	50	75	85	90	95
Females with Small Frames												
18.0–24.9	651	26.2	6.0	18.2	19.6	20.7	22.5	25.5	29.2	31.2	32.8	36.2
25.0–29.9	486	27.8	7.4	19.5	20.6	21.6	23.2	26.9	30.8	33.3	35.2	38.1
30.0–34.9	413	28.6	7.8	19.1	21.6	22.4	24.5	27.8	31.4	33.7	36.2	38.8
35.0–39.9	368	29.8	10.1	19.7	21.4	22.9	24.4	28.8	32.5	35.4	37.5	42.2
40.0–44.9	350	29.8	6.6	20.9	22.1	23.4	25.7	28.9	33.2	36.0	37.9	41.8
45.0–49.9	241	29.2	7.4	19.1	21.5	22.6	24.3	28.3	33.3	36.1	38.7	41.2
50.0–54.9	256	30.3	7.3	20.8	22.1	23.9	25.5	29.1	33.4	36.7	38.5	41.3
55.0–59.9	223	30.9	7.6	20.4	22.3	23.6	25.8	30.2	34.8	37.6	41.3	45.1
60.0–64.9	351	31.9	8.7	20.9	22.4	23.6	25.8	31.2	36.4	39.1	41.1	46.2
65.0–69.9	491	31.3	8.1	19.4	22.1	23.7	25.7	30.6	35.4	39.8	41.8	45.7
70.0–74.9	367	32.0	9.9	20.3	22.5	24.1	25.9	30.3	36.1	39.8	42.6	47.3
Females with Medium Frames												
18.0–24.9	1296	29.3	7.0	19.8	21.9	23.2	24.9	28.4	32.8	35.2	37.2	40.7
25.0–29.9	964	30.0	7.2	20.7	22.1	23.3	25.0	29.0	33.9	36.8	39.0	43.3
30.0–34.9	814	32.0	9.1	21.4	23.1	24.2	26.3	30.8	36.1	39.4	41.8	46.4
35.0–39.9	728	32.7	8.4	21.4	23.6	24.9	27.3	31.4	37.3	40.8	43.0	47.0
40.0–44.9	696	33.7	12.1	21.2	23.2	25.1	27.2	31.6	37.7	43.1	47.1	52.3
45.0–49.9	484	33.8	8.8	22.2	23.6	25.5	27.9	32.2	37.9	42.5	45.4	49.6
50.0–54.9	502	35.0	9.7	22.8	25.2	26.2	28.5	33.7	40.0	43.5	46.7	51.4
55.0–59.9	442	36.3	11.5	23.7	25.3	26.6	28.7	34.5	41.5	44.9	49.2	53.4
60.0–64.9	695	35.1	9.1	23.0	25.3	26.5	29.2	33.9	39.9	43.7	46.1	49.4
65.0–69.9	971	35.7	10.0	22.4	24.8	26.4	29.1	34.6	40.7	44.5	48.1	51.9
70.0–74.9	731	35.3	9.7	22.2	24.3	26.1	28.9	34.0	40.0	44.4	46.7	51.3
Females with Large Frames												
18.0–24.9	641	34.4	10.7	21.9	23.8	25.3	27.3	31.9	38.7	43.9	47.5	55.8
25.0–29.9	471	36.7	11.5	22.2	25.4	26.8	29.3	34.5	42.0	46.8	50.3	60.1
30.0–34.9	392	38.8	12.3	24.0	25.8	27.3	30.1	36.3	45.1	50.7	55.1	61.2
35.0–39.9	357	41.6	14.4	23.9	27.4	29.1	32.2	39.1	47.2	53.7	61.0	72.1
40.0–44.9	344	43.5	16.6	26.2	28.8	30.5	32.9	40.3	49.5	54.4	58.7	71.6
45.0–49.9	236	43.0	15.8	25.0	28.0	29.4	32.5	39.7	49.0	58.3	62.8	69.9
50.0–54.9	246	42.4	13.1	25.1	28.4	30.1	33.4	39.6	49.5	54.8	59.7	68.4
55.0–59.9	213	45.2	16.9	27.0	30.0	32.4	35.8	42.0	51.0	58.5	62.2	65.7
60.0–64.9	341	43.1	14.2	26.6	29.1	31.2	33.9	40.7	49.8	54.8	57.5	67.6
65.0–69.9	482	42.5	13.4	26.4	28.4	30.6	33.5	40.0	48.7	55.3	58.7	66.5
70.0–74.9	363	41.5	11.6	25.7	28.8	30.2	32.8	40.1	48.7	51.4	54.8	60.3

Note: Values for females aged 18 years and older have been adjusted for bone area by subtracting 6.5 cm² from the calculated mid upper arm muscle area (see text).

Anthropometric Graphs by Age, Sex, Height, and Frame Size

The anthropometric graphs presented in figures IV.1 to IV.54 have been designed so as to permit a rapid visual evaluation of growth, body size, and nutritional and fat status. These graphs have been smoothed with a two-floating-point method of cricket graph. We have refrained from using other methods such as splining or polynomials because the resulting smoothed curves tended to distort the naturally occurring differences in anthropometric dimensions.

Growth, Body Size, and Nutritional Status

The graphs describing growth in length are given in figures IV.1 to IV.4, growth in body mass in figures IV.5 to IV.16, growth in body proportion in figures IV.17 to IV.20, changes in body muscle for children and adults in figures IV.21 to IV.30. For adults, weight by age and frame size are given in figures IV.43 to IV.48 and arm muscle area by age and frame size are shown in figures IV.49 to IV.54. The trend lines presented in these graphs represent the five statistical categories derived from the percentile cutoffs of the anthropometric dimensions, which correspond to the following:

Category I = Below 5th percentile or Z-score is less than -1.650.
Category II = 5.0 to 15th percentile or Z-score is between -1.645 and -1.040.
Category III = 15.1 to 85th percentile or Z-score is between -1.036 and +1.030.
Category IV = 85.1 to 95th percentile or Z-score is between +1.036 and +1.640.
Category V = 95.1 to 100th percentile or Z-score is equal to or greater than +1.645.

Fat Status

The graphs on arm fat index and sum of skinfold thickness given in figures IV.31 to IV.42 have been designed to provide information on fat status. The trend lines presented in these graphs represent the five statistical categories derived from the percentile cutoffs for skinfold thickness and/or arm fat index. These categories use, as indicated in chapter III, instead of the 95th percentile, the 85th percentile as the upper limit of statistical normality as follows:

Category I = Below 5th percentile or Z-score is less than -1.650.
Category II = 5.1 to 15th percentile or Z-score is between -1.645 and -1.040.
Category III = 15.1 to 75th percentile or Z-score is between -1.036 and +0.670.
Category IV = 75.1 to 85th percentile or Z-score is between +0.675 and +1.030.
Category V = 85.1 to 100th percentile or Z-score is equal to or greater than +1.036

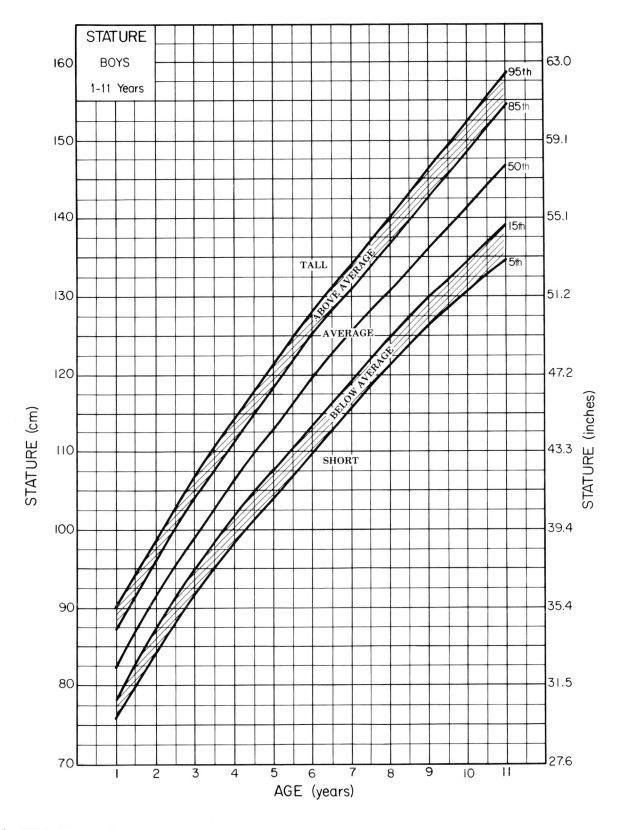

Fig. IV.1. Percentiles of stature in cm (and in.) by age for boys ranging in age from 1 to 11 years.

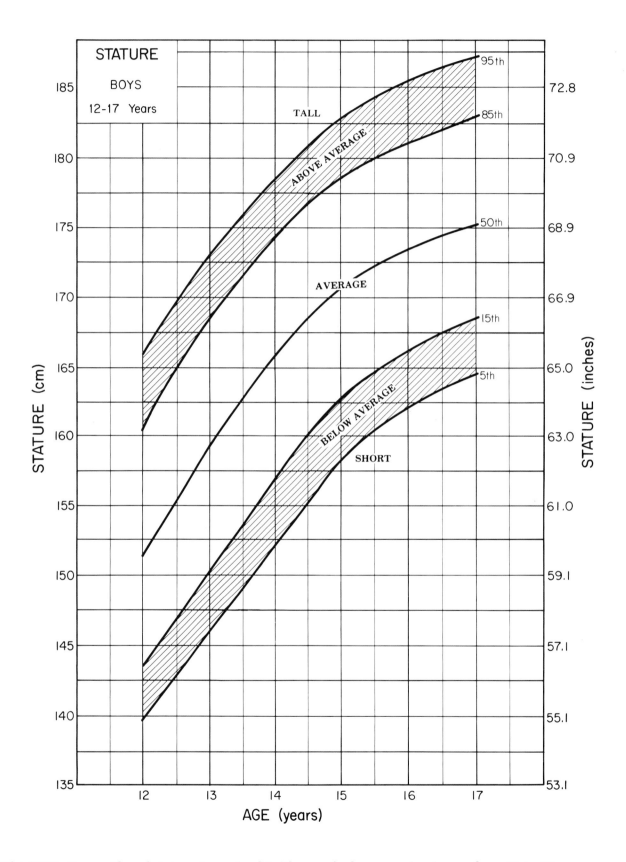

Fig. IV.2. Percentiles of stature in cm (and in.) by age for boys ranging in age from 12 to 17 years.

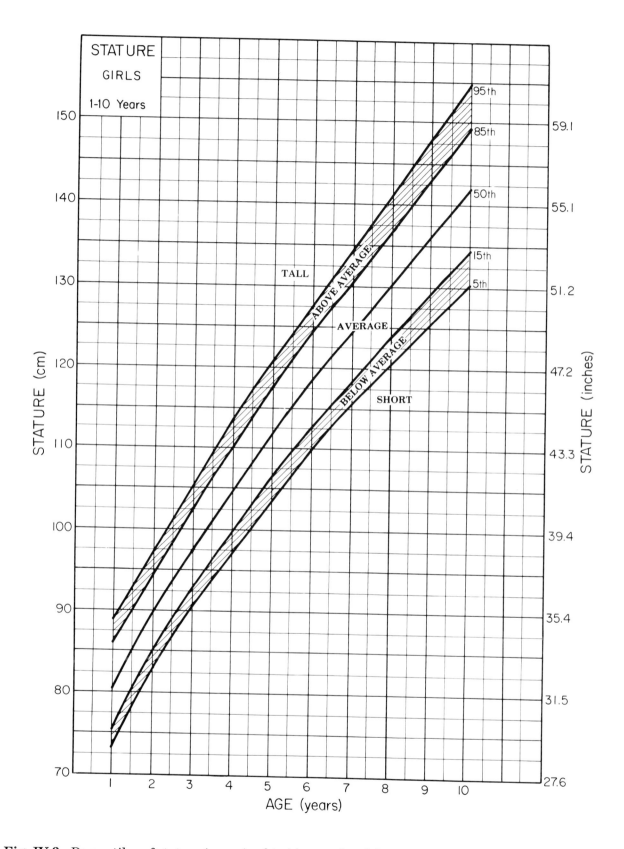

Fig. IV.3. Percentiles of stature in cm (and in.) by age for girls ranging in age from 1 to 10 years.

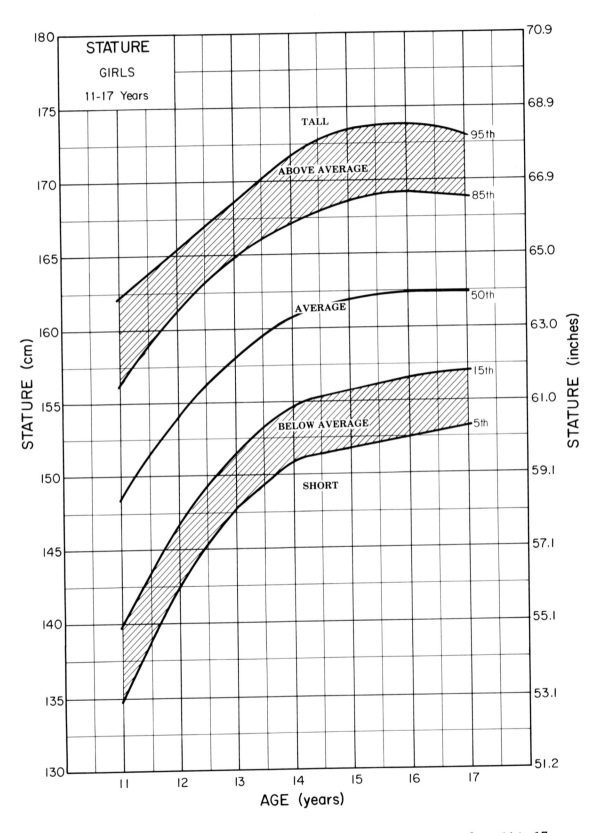

Fig. IV.4. Percentiles of stature in cm (and in.) by age for girls ranging in age from 11 to 17 years.

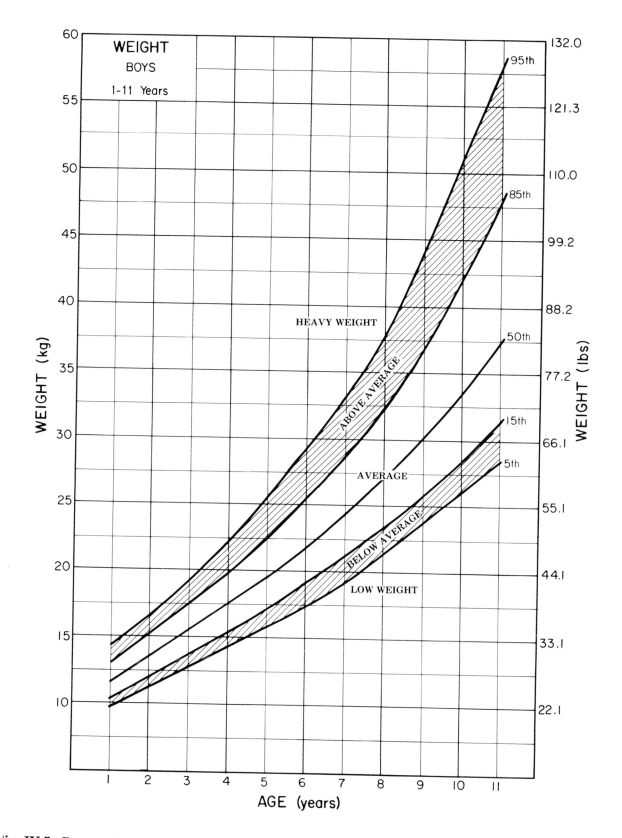

Fig. IV.5. Percentiles of weight in kg (and lb.) by age for boys ranging in age from 1 to 11 years.

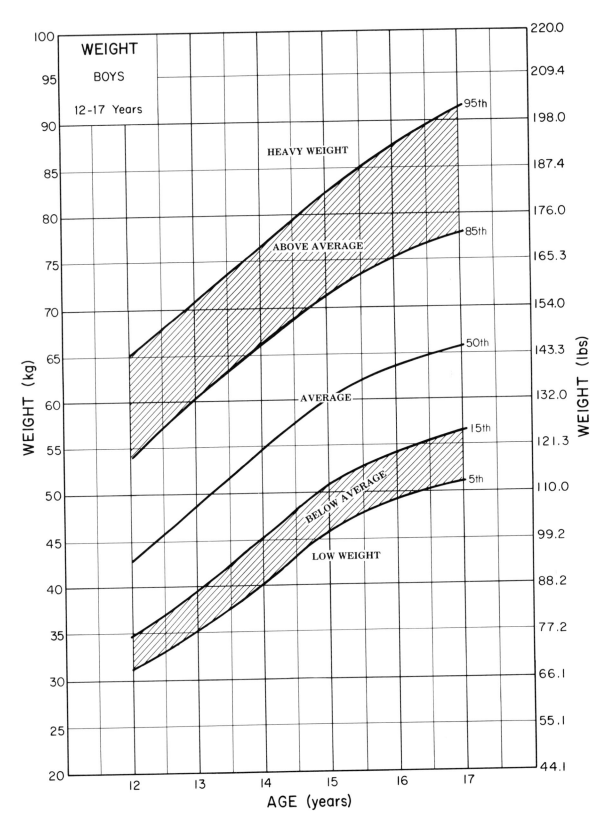

Fig. IV.6. Percentiles of weight in kg (and lb.) by age for boys ranging in age from 12 to 17 years.

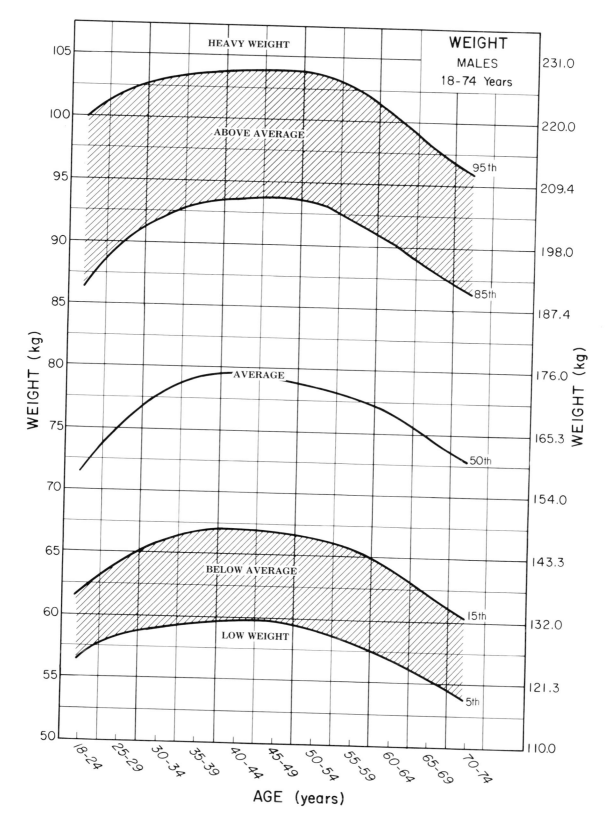

Fig. IV.7. Percentiles of weight in kg (and lb.) by age for males ranging in age from 18 to 74 years.

71

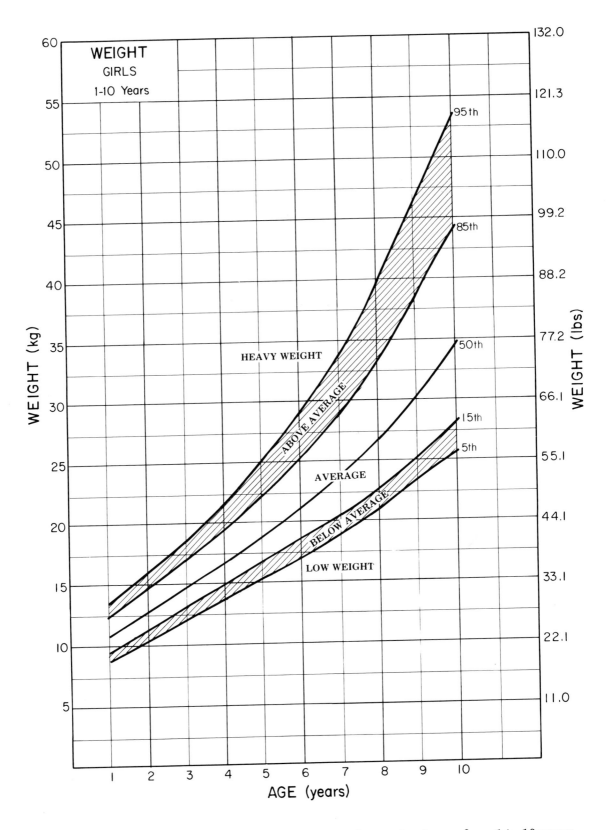

Fig. IV.8. Percentiles of weight in kg (and lb.) by age for girls ranging in age from 1 to 10 years.

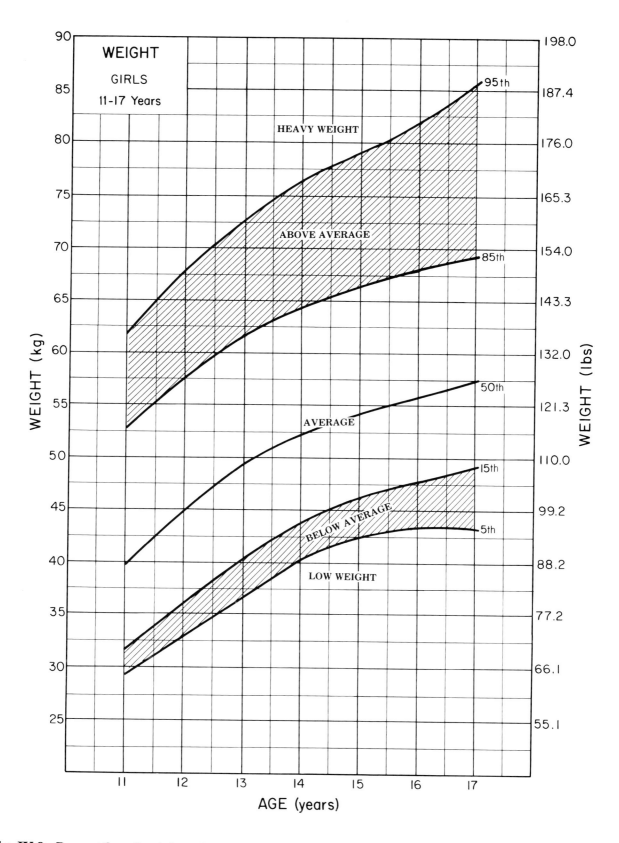

Fig. IV.9. Percentiles of weight in kg (and lb.) by age for girls ranging in age from 11 to 17 years.

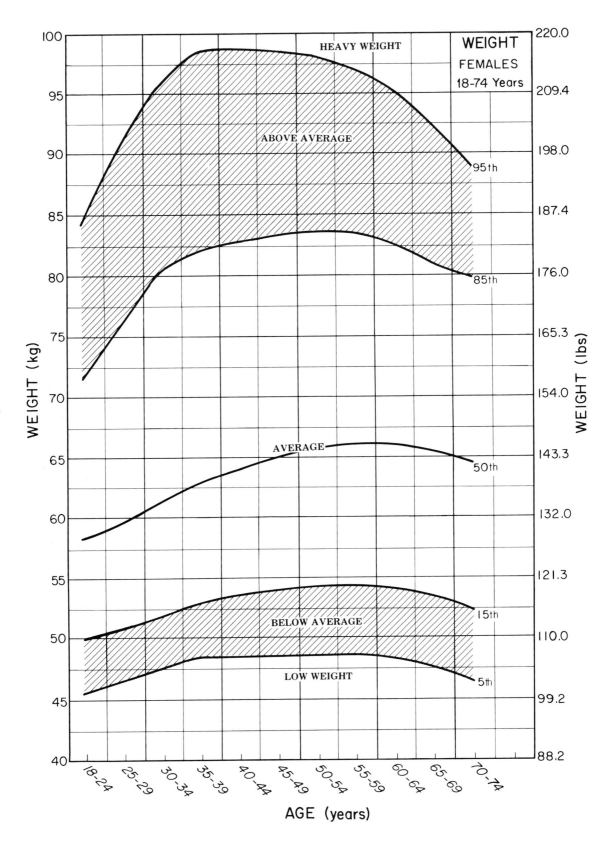

Fig. IV.10. Percentiles of weight in kg (and lb.) by age for females ranging in age from 18 to 74 years.

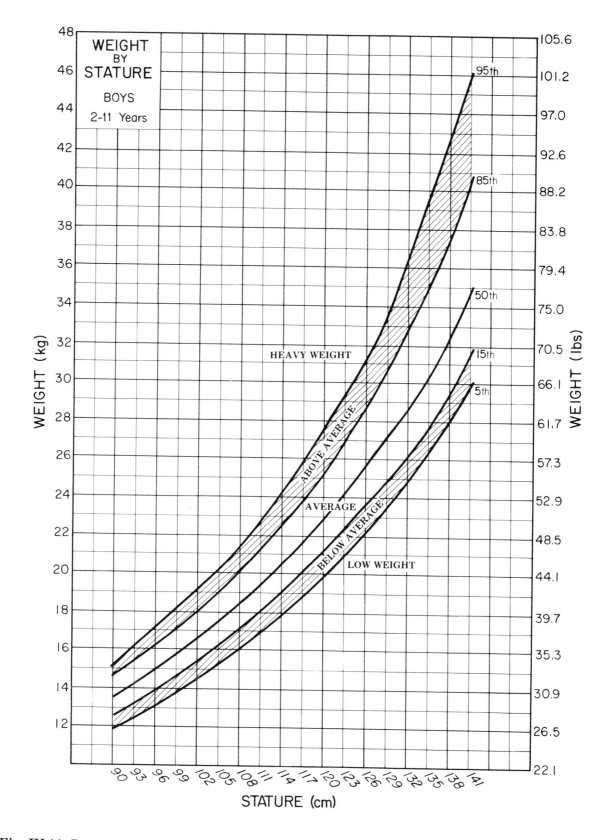

Fig. IV.11. Percentiles of weight in kg (and lb.) by height in cm (and in.) for boys ranging in age from 2 to 11 years.

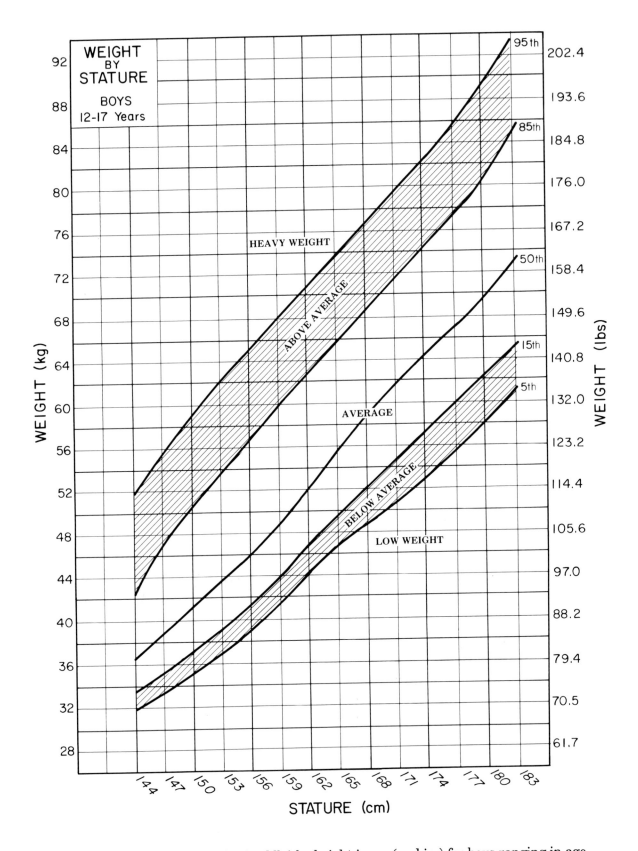

Fig. IV.12. Percentiles of weight in kg (and lb.) by height in cm (and in.) for boys ranging in age from 12 to 17 years.

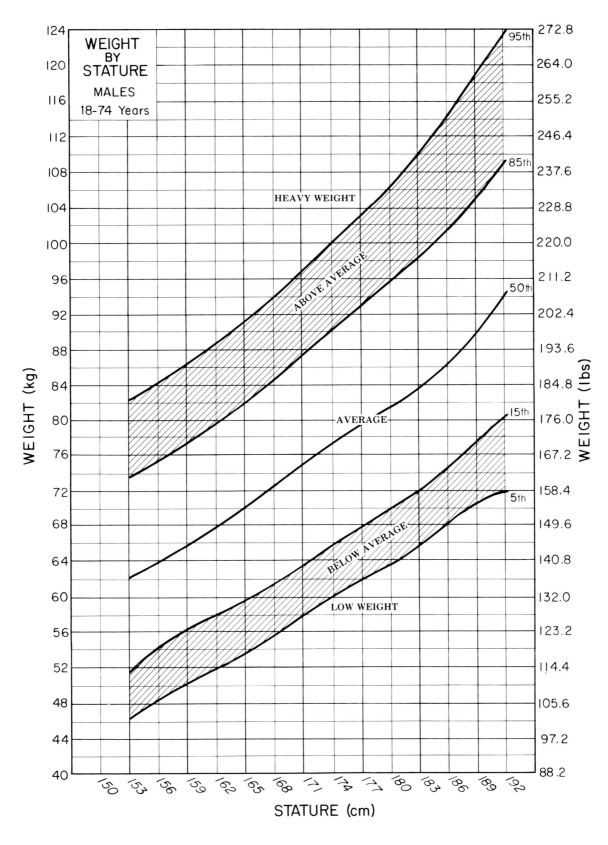

Fig. IV.13. Percentiles of weight in kg (and lb.) by height in cm (and in.) for males ranging in age from 18 to 74 years.

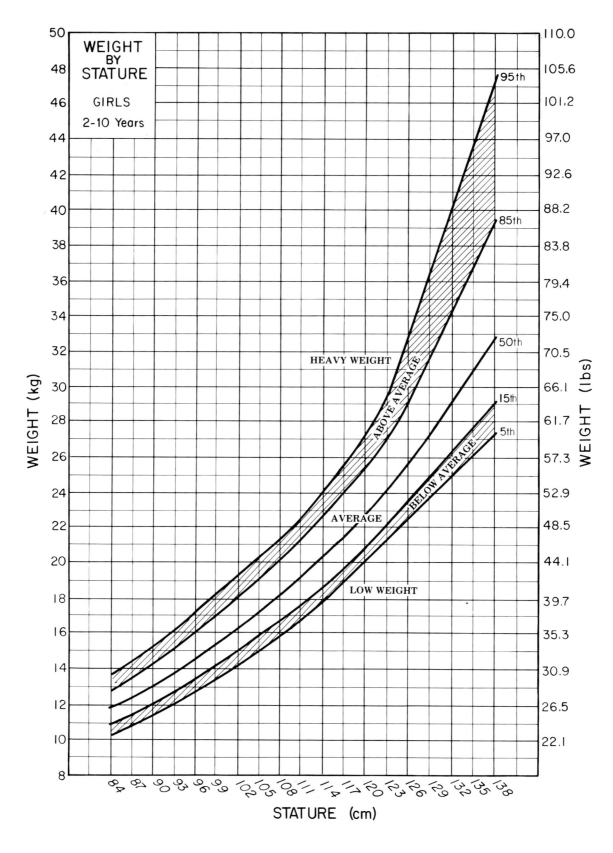

Fig. IV.14. Percentiles of weight in kg (and lb.) by height in cm (and in.) for girls ranging in age from 2 to 10 years.

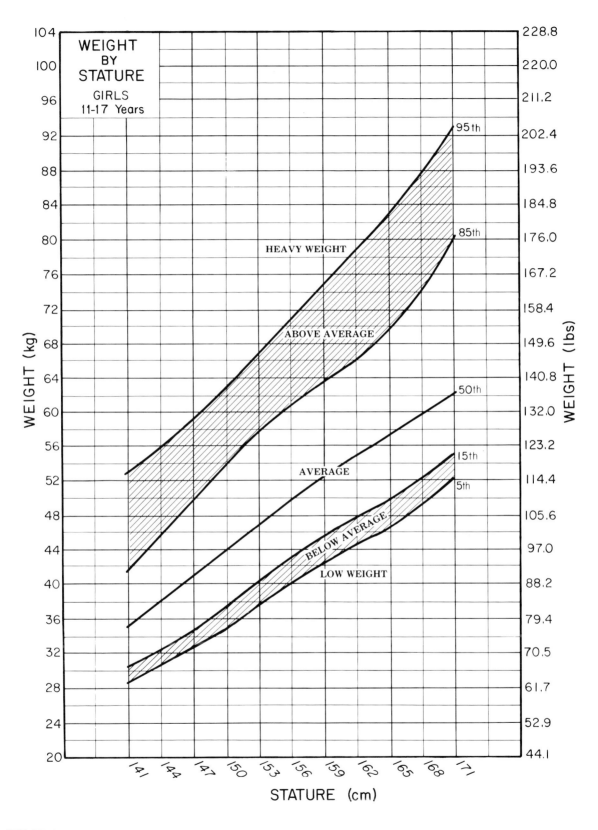

Fig. IV.15. Percentiles of weight in kg (and lb.) by height in cm (and in.) for girls ranging in age from 11 to 17 years.

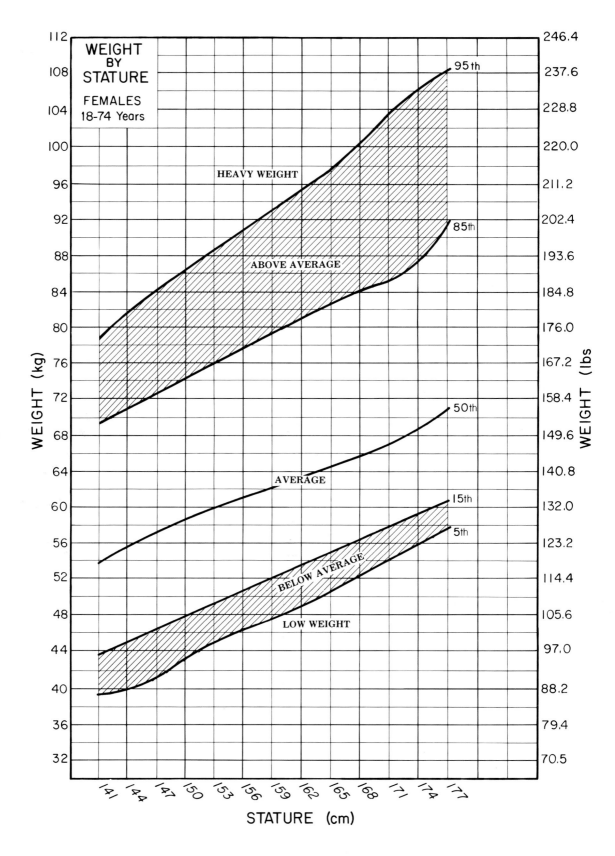

Fig. IV.16. Percentiles of weight in kg (and lb.) by height in cm (and in.) for females ranging in age from 18 to 74 years.

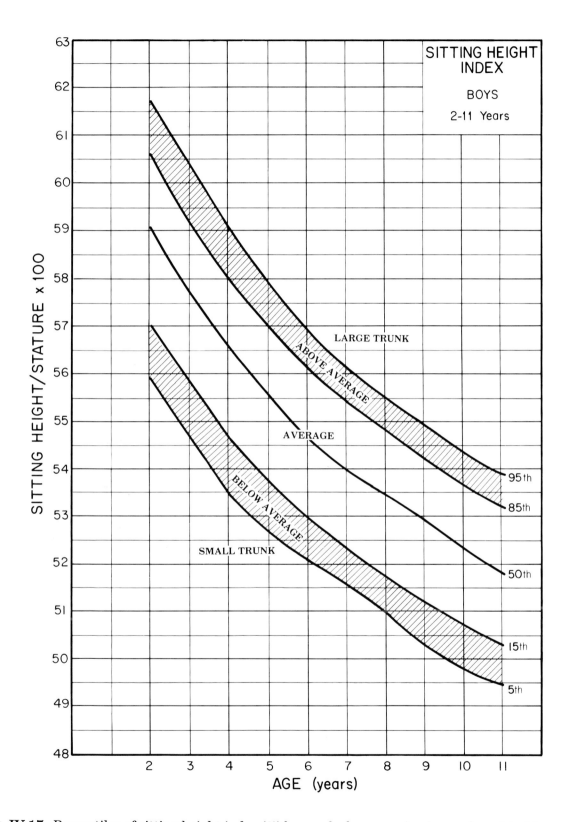

Fig. IV.17. Percentiles of sitting height index (%) by age for boys ranging in age from 2 to 11 years.

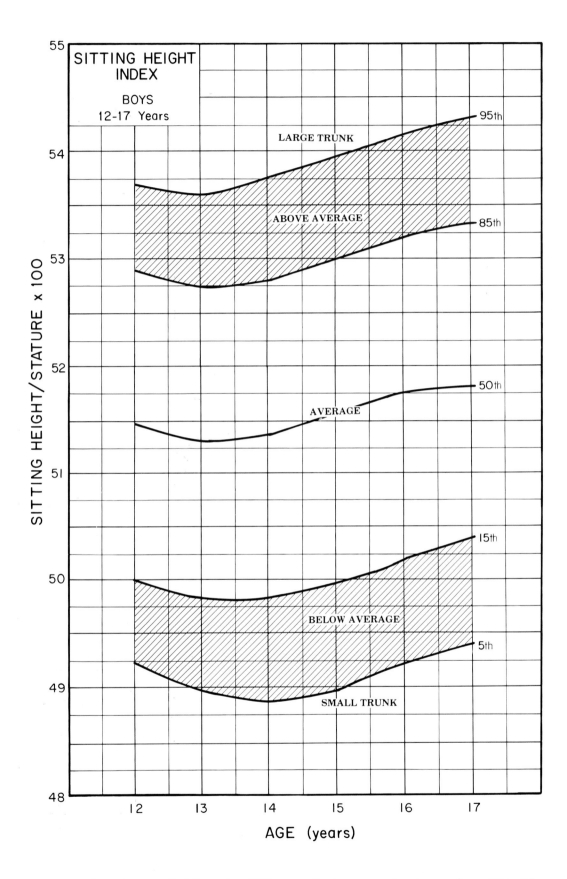

Fig. IV.18. Percentiles of sitting height index (%) by age for boys ranging in age from 12 to 17 years.

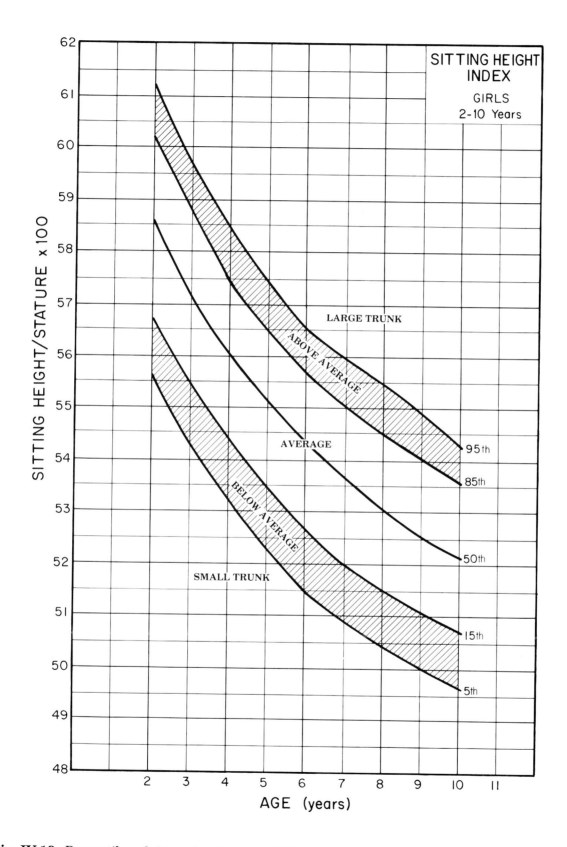

Fig. IV.19. Percentiles of sitting height index (%) by age for girls ranging in age from 2 to 10 years.

83

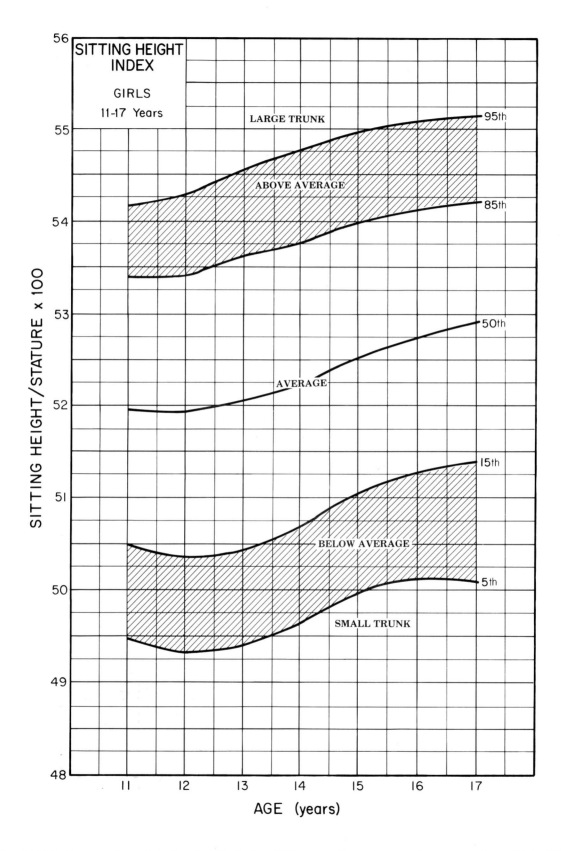

Fig. IV.20. Percentiles of sitting height index (%) by age for girls ranging in age from 11 to 17 years.

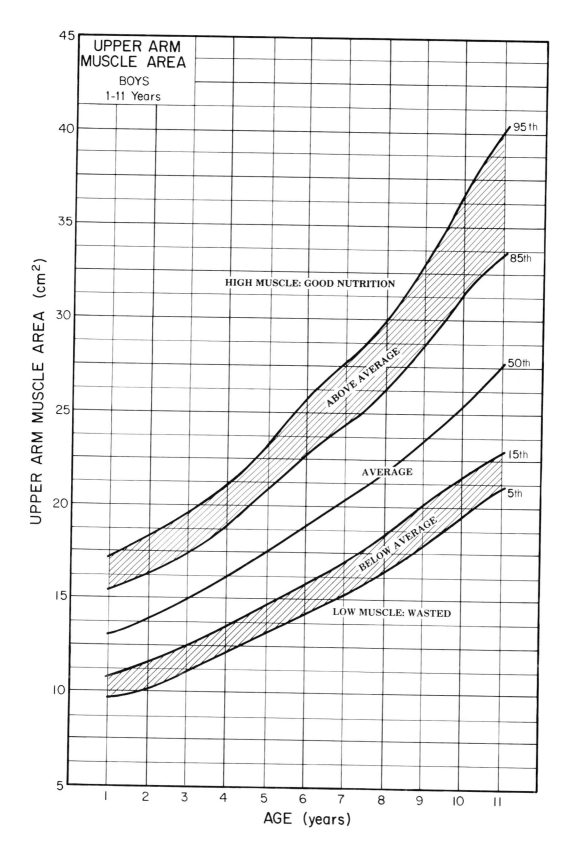

Fig. IV.21. Percentiles of upper arm muscle area (cm²) by age for boys ranging in age from 1 to 11 years.

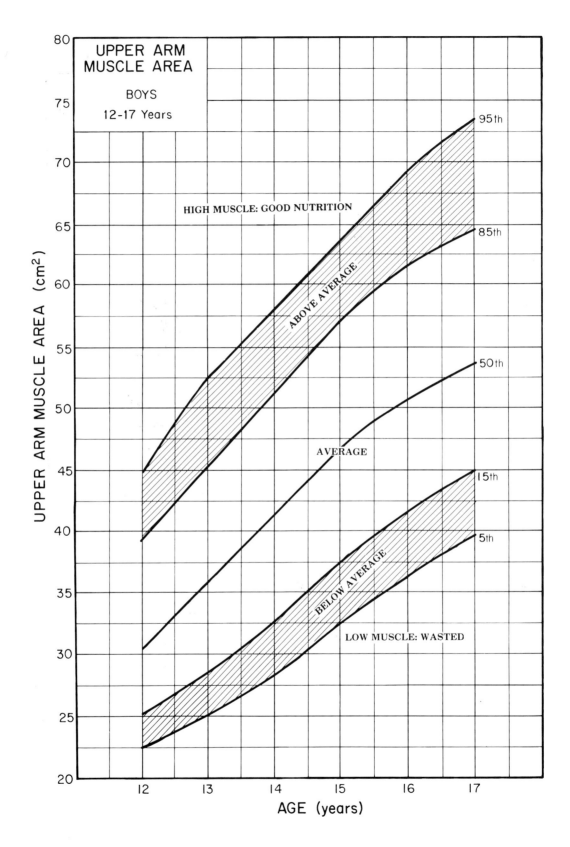

Fig. IV.22. Percentiles of upper arm muscle area (cm²) by age for boys ranging in age from 12 to 17 years.

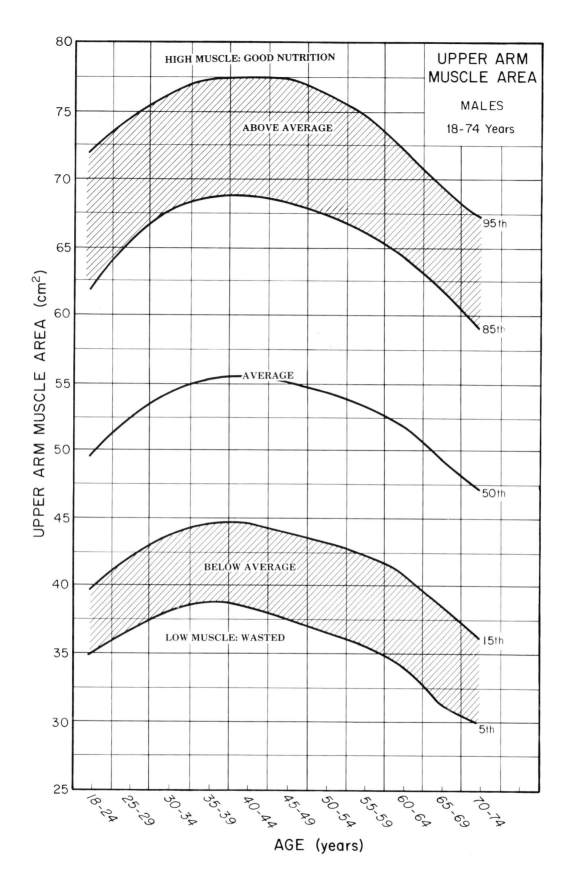

Fig. IV.23. Percentiles of upper arm muscle area (cm²) by age for males ranging in age from 18 to 74 years. Note: Values for males aged 18 years and older have been adjusted for bone area by subtracting 10.0 cm² from the calculated muscle area.

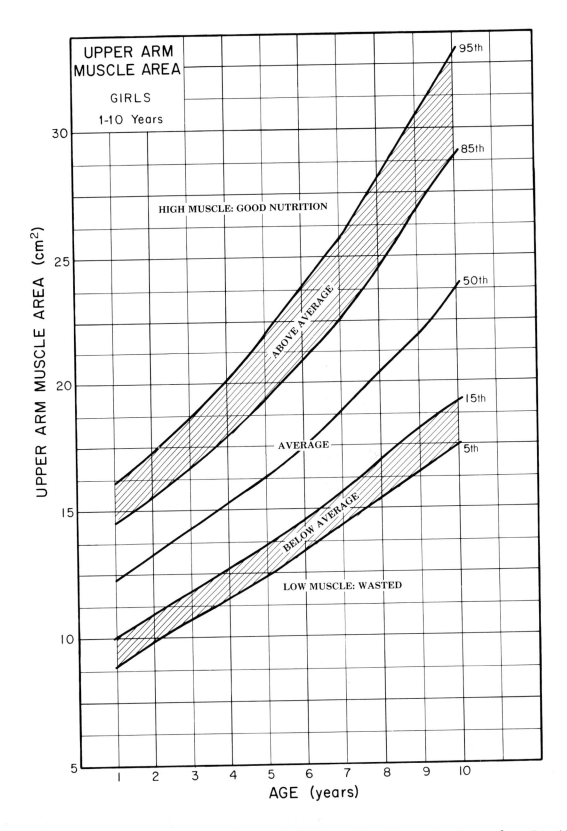

Fig. IV.24. Percentiles of upper arm muscle area (cm²) by age for girls ranging in age from 1 to 10 years.

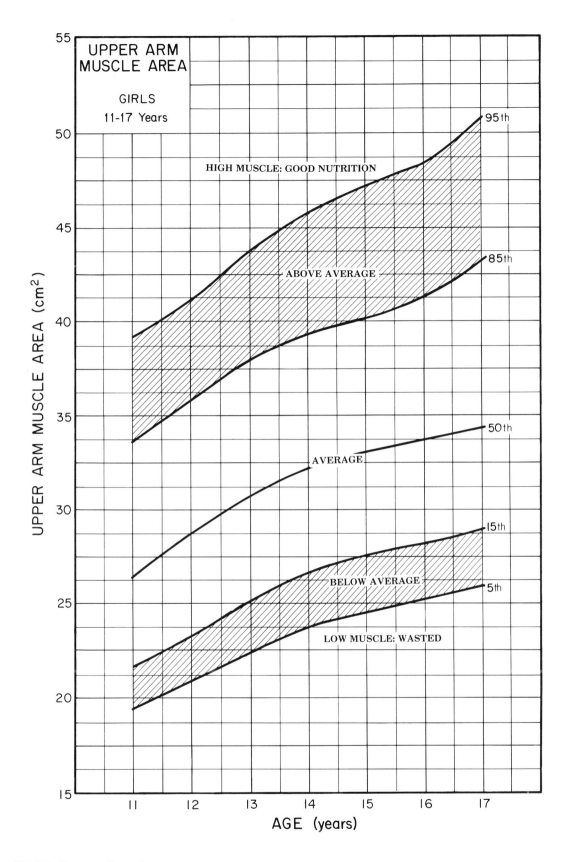

Fig. IV.25. Percentiles of upper arm muscle area (cm²) by age for girls ranging in age from 11 to 17 years.

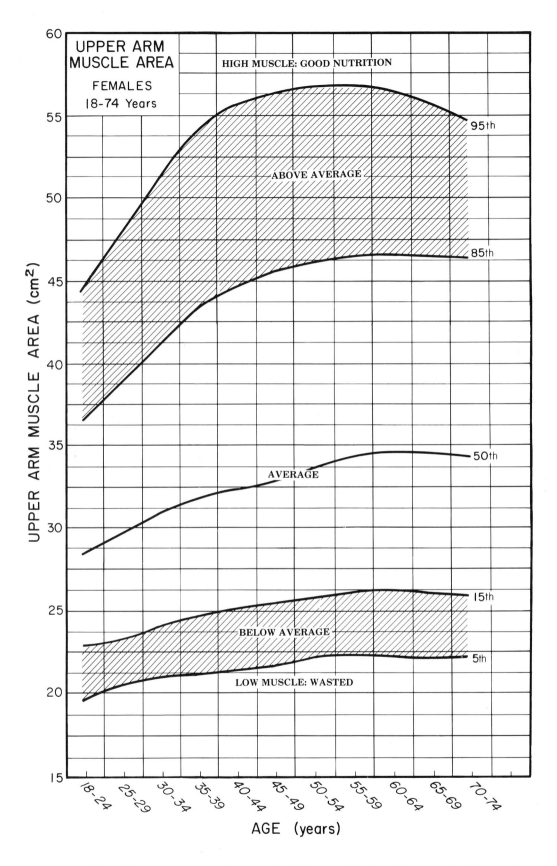

Fig. IV.26. Percentiles of upper arm muscle area (cm²) by age for females ranging in age from 18 to 74 years. Note: Values for females aged 18 years and older have been adjusted for bone area by subtracting 6.5 cm² from the calculated muscle area.

90

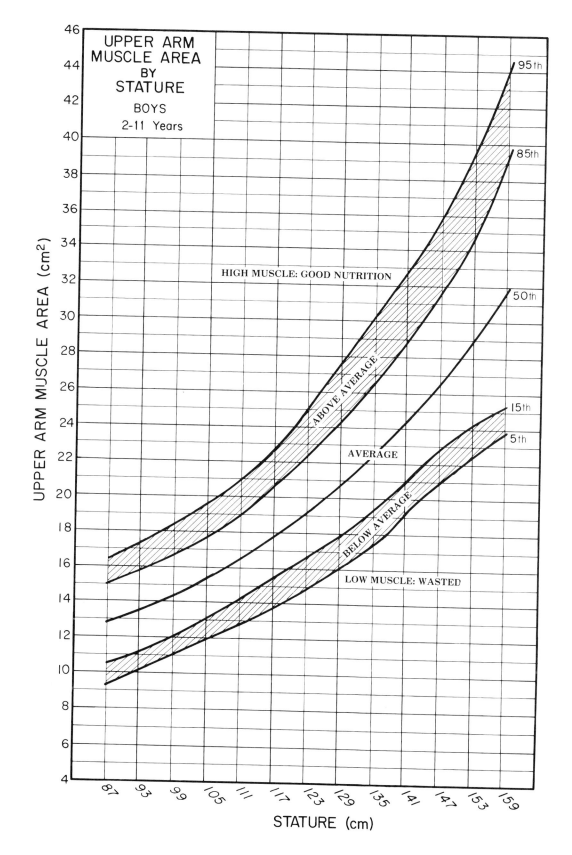

Fig. IV.27. Percentiles of upper arm muscle area (cm²) by height (cm) for boys ranging in age from 2 to 11 years.

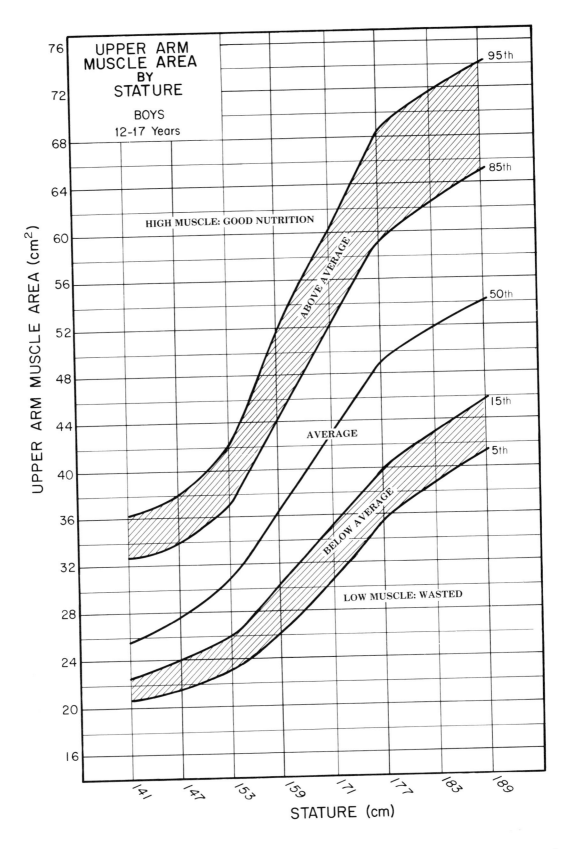

Fig. IV.28. Percentiles of upper arm muscle area (cm²) by height (cm) for boys ranging in age from 12 to 17 years.

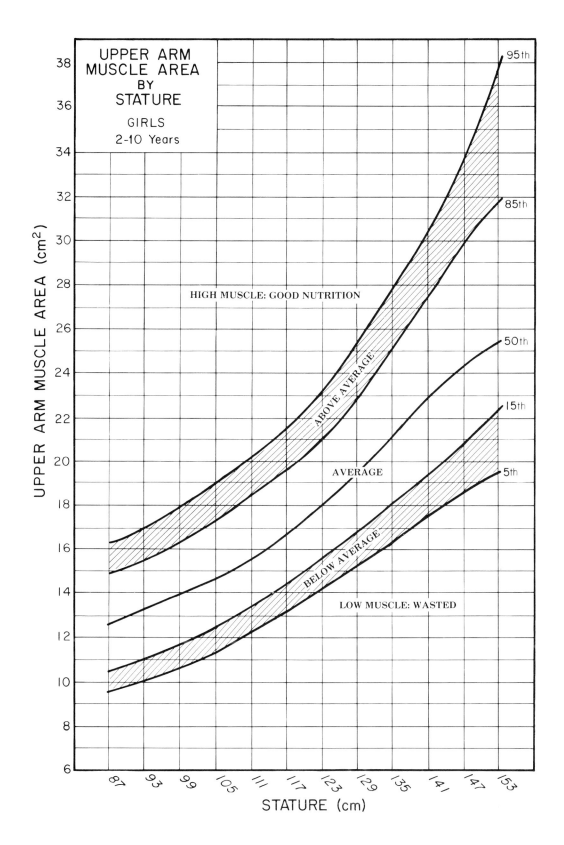

Fig. IV.29. Percentiles of upper arm muscle area (cm²) by height (cm) for girls ranging in age from 2 to 10 years.

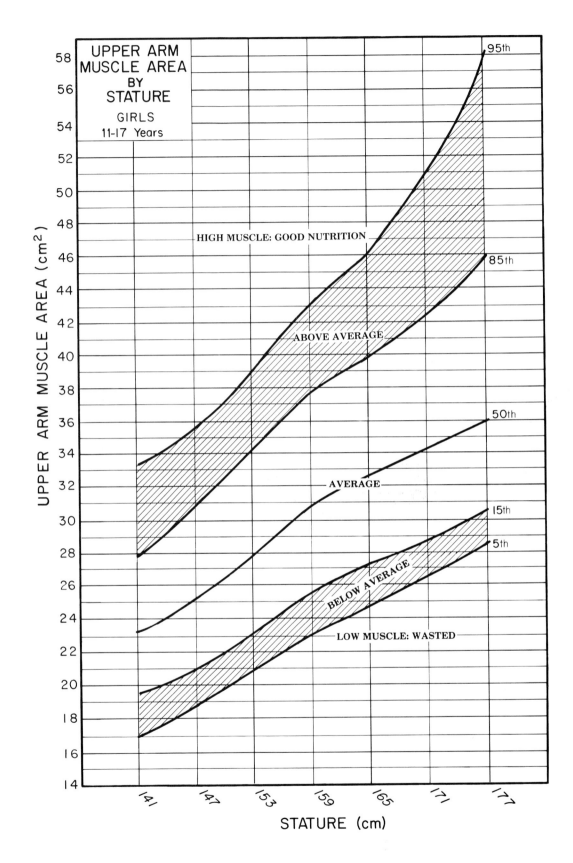

Fig. IV.30. Percentiles of upper arm muscle area (cm²) by height (cm) for girls ranging in age from 11 to 17 years.

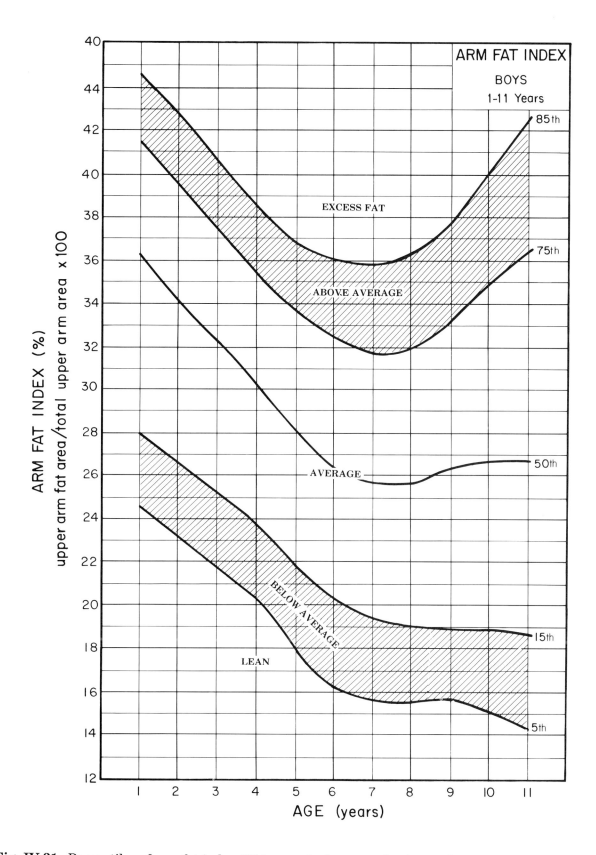

Fig. IV.31. Percentiles of arm fat index (%) by age for boys ranging in age from 1 to 11 years.

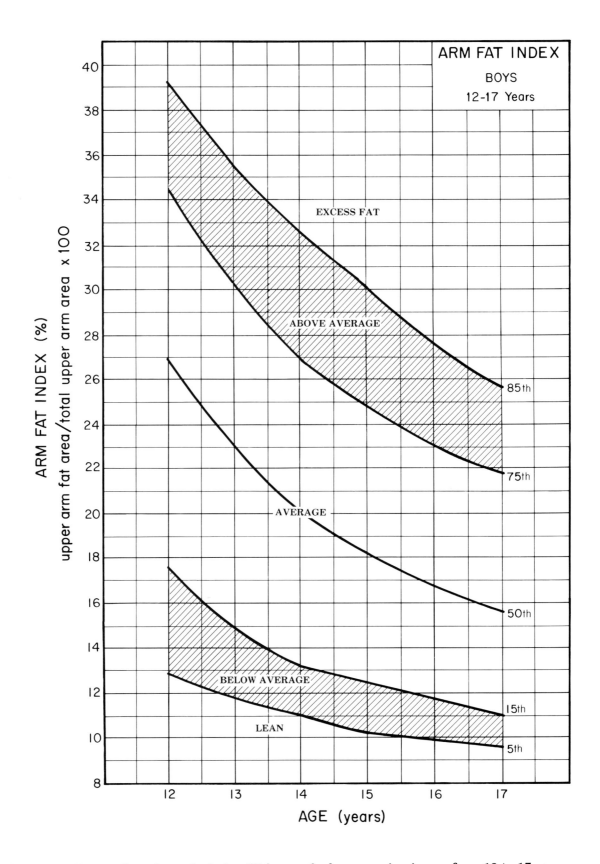

Fig. IV.32. Percentiles of arm fat index (%) by age for boys ranging in age from 12 to 17 years.

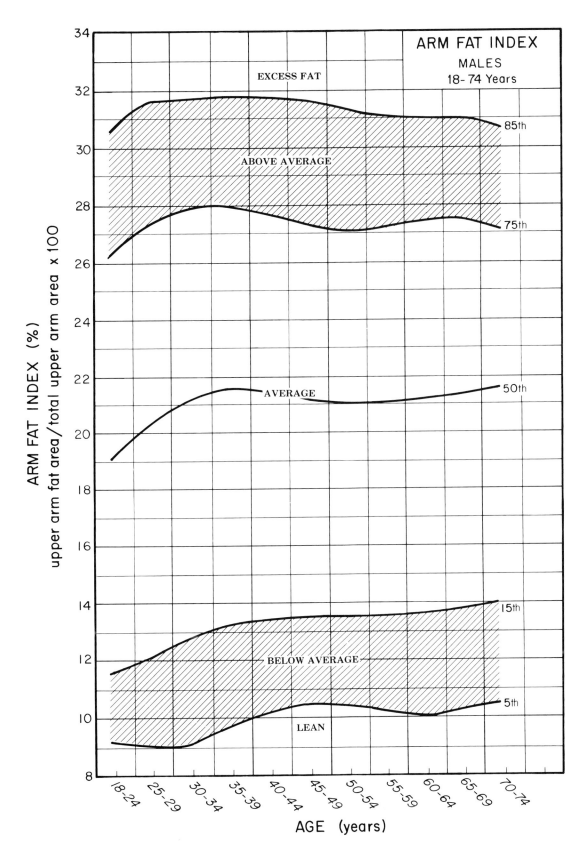

Fig. IV.33. Percentiles of arm fat index (%) by age for males ranging in age from 18 to 74 years.

97

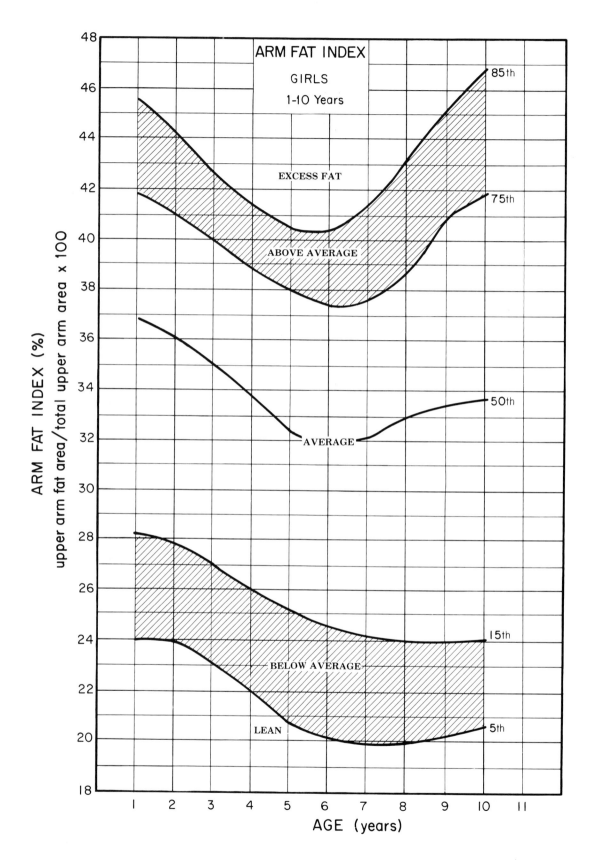

Fig.IV.34. Percentiles of arm fat index (%) by age for girls ranging in age from 1 to 10 years.

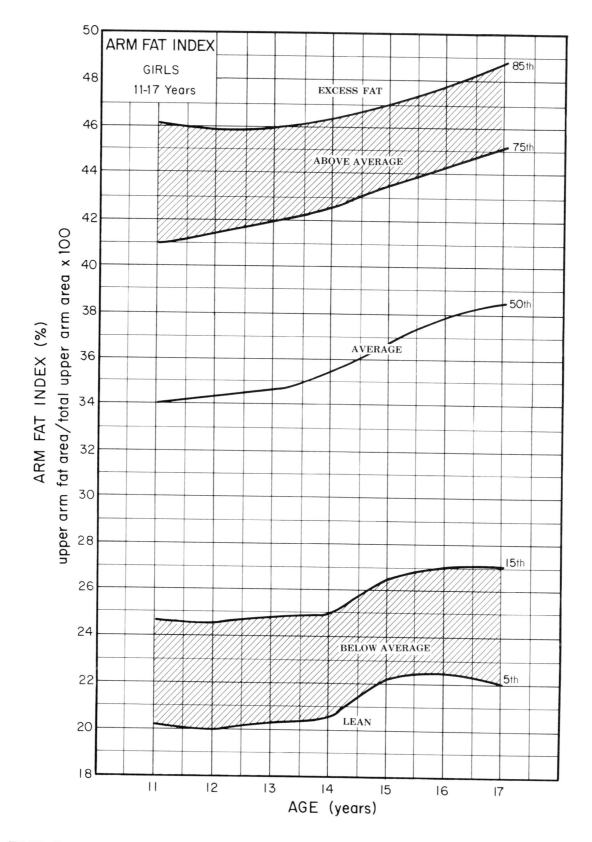

Fig. IV.35. Percentiles of arm fat index (%) by age for girls ranging in age from 11 to 17 years.

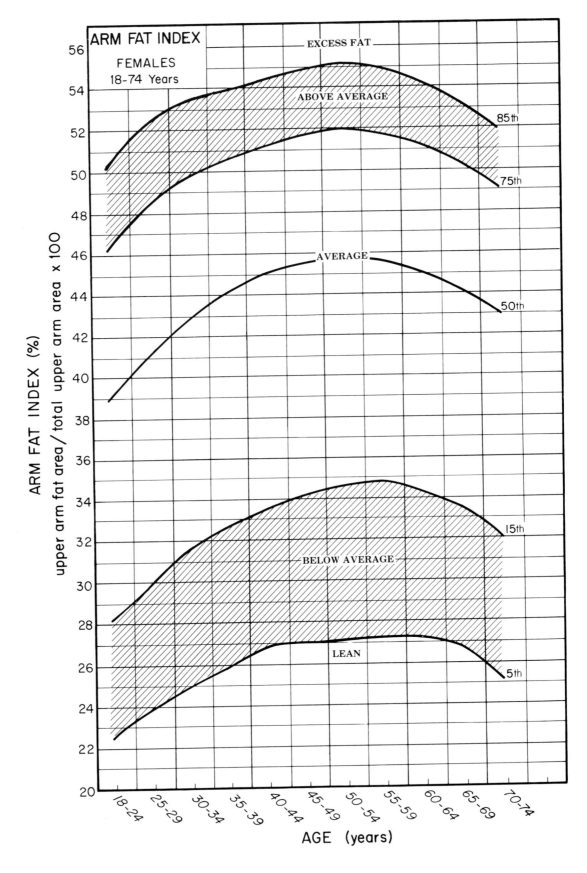

Fig. IV.36. Percentiles of arm fat index (%) by age for females ranging in age from 18 to 74 years.

100

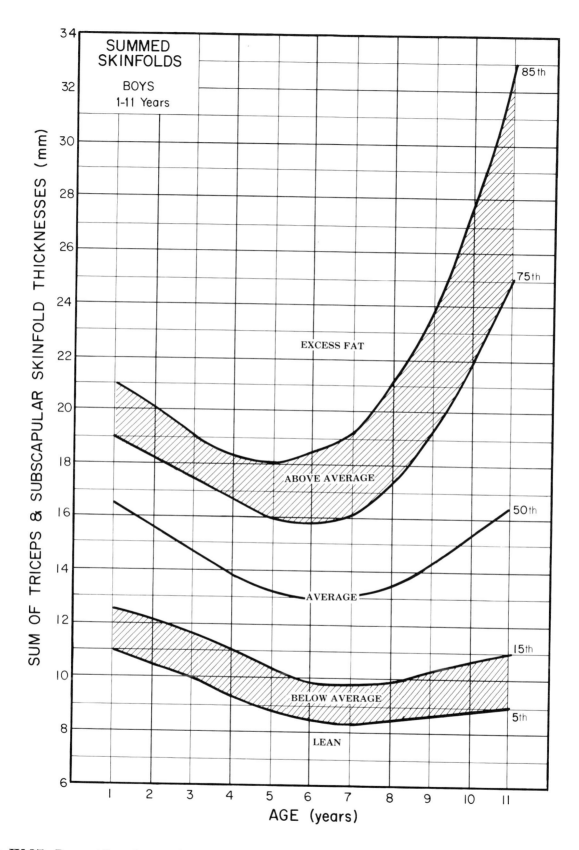

Fig. IV.37. Percentiles of sum of triceps and subscapular skinfold thicknesses by age for boys ranging in age from 1 to 11 years.

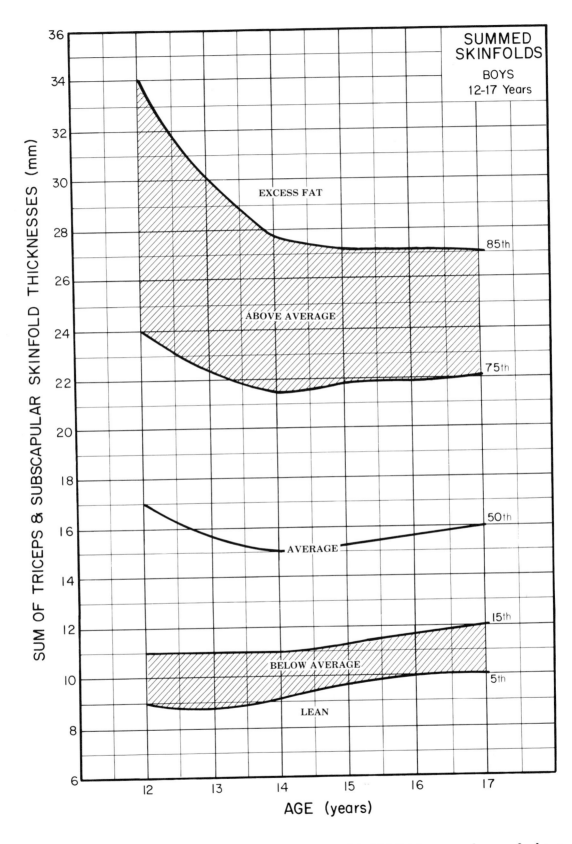

Fig. IV.38. Percentiles of sum of triceps and subscapular skinfold thicknesses by age for boys ranging in age from 12 to 17 years.

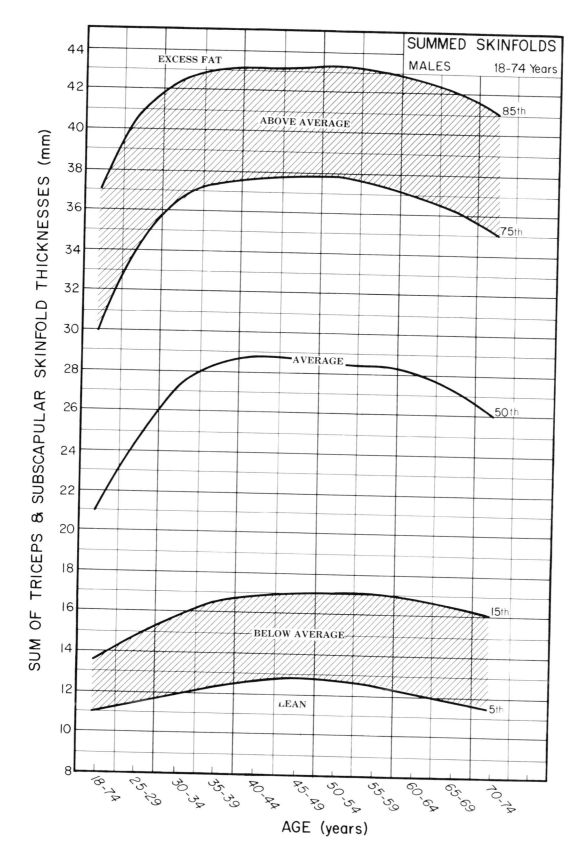

Fig. IV.39. Percentiles of sum of triceps and subscapular skinfold thicknesses by age for males ranging in age from 18 to 74 years.

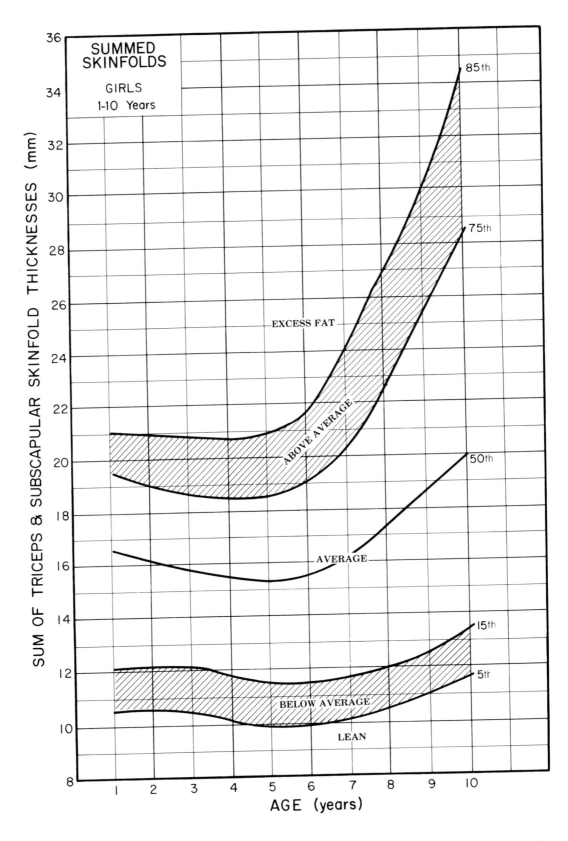

Fig. IV.40. Percentiles of sum of triceps and subscapular skinfold thicknesses by age for girls ranging in age from 1 to 10 years.

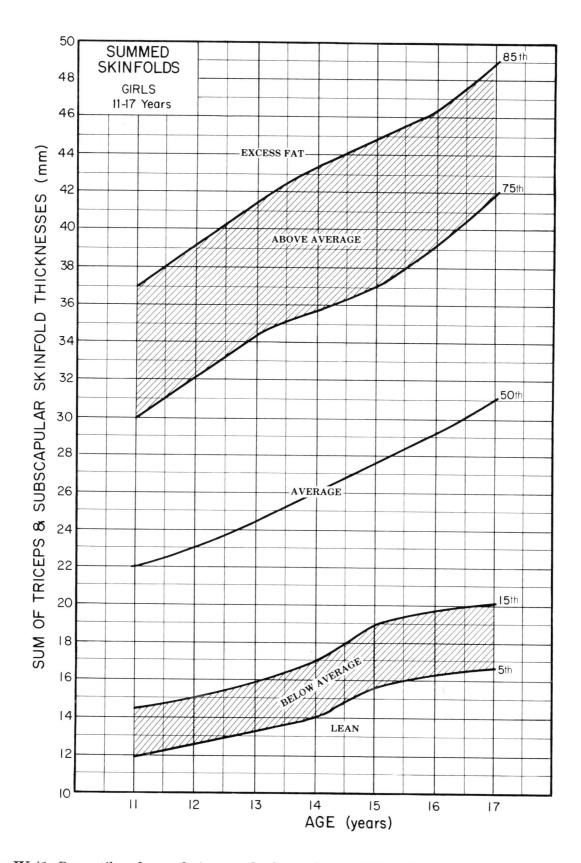

Fig. IV.41. Percentiles of sum of triceps and subscapular skinfold thicknesses by age for girls ranging in age from 11 to 17 years.

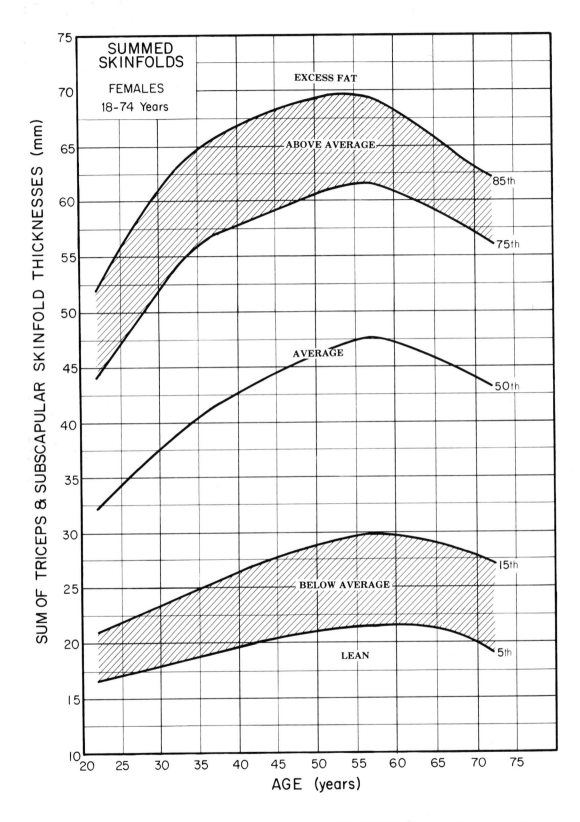

Fig. IV.42. Percentiles of sum of triceps and subscapular skinfold thicknesses by age for females ranging in age from 18 to 74 years.

106

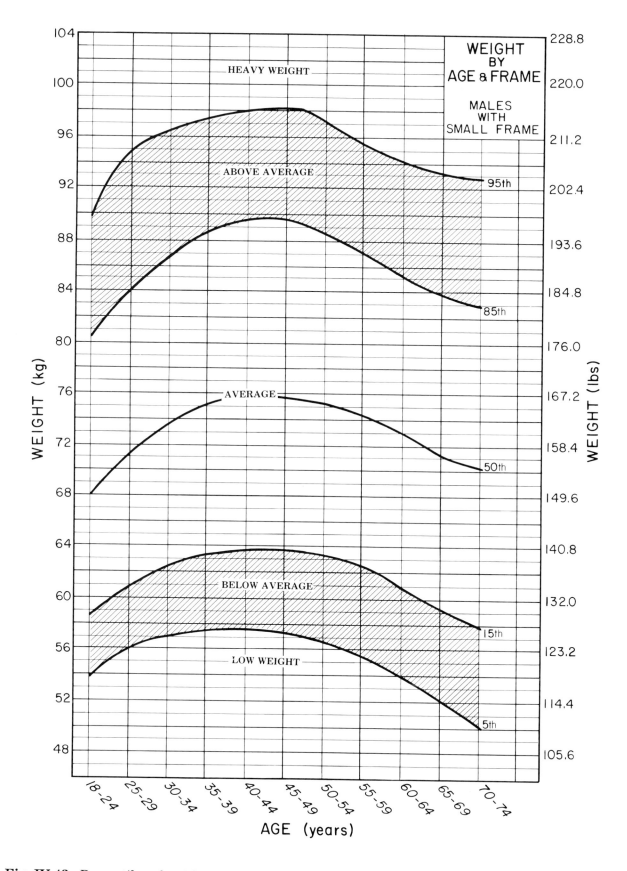

Fig. IV.43. Percentiles of weight by age for adult males with small frame.

107

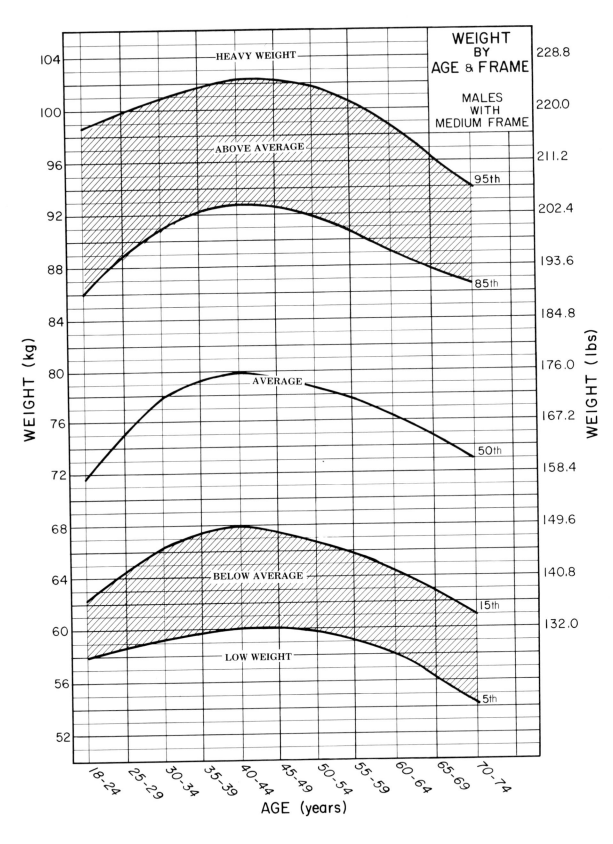

Fig. IV.44. Percentiles of weight by age for adult males with medium frame.

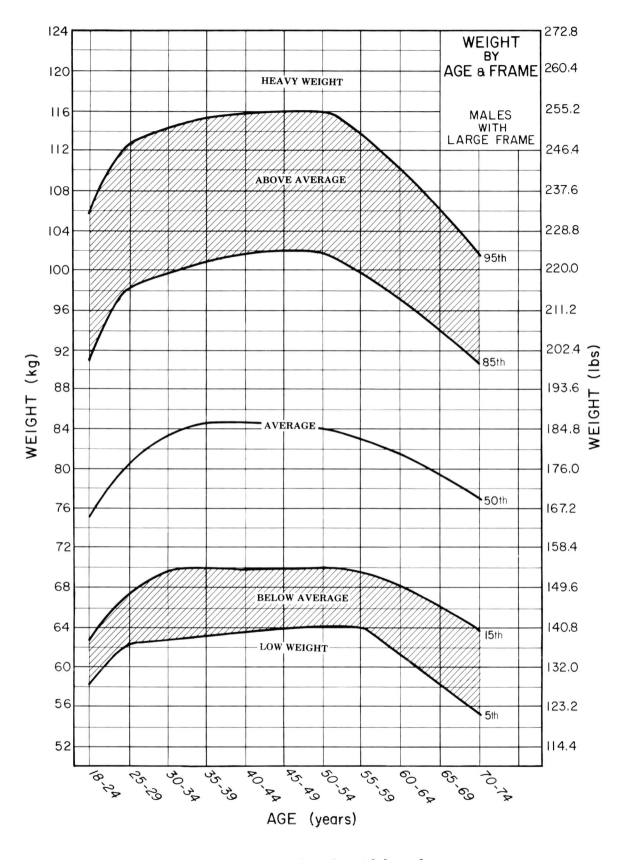

Fig. IV.45. Percentiles of weight by age for adult males with large frame.

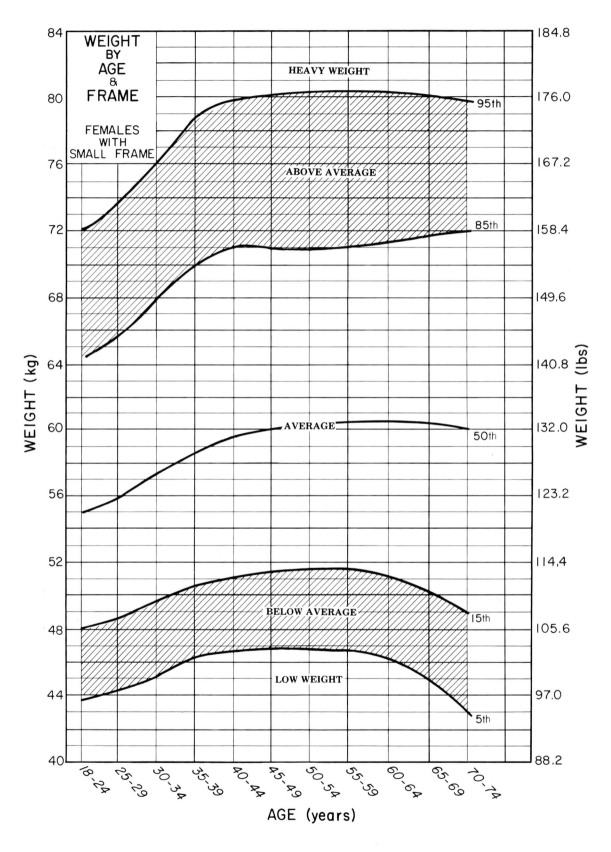

Fig. IV.46. Percentiles of weight by age for adult females with small frame.

110

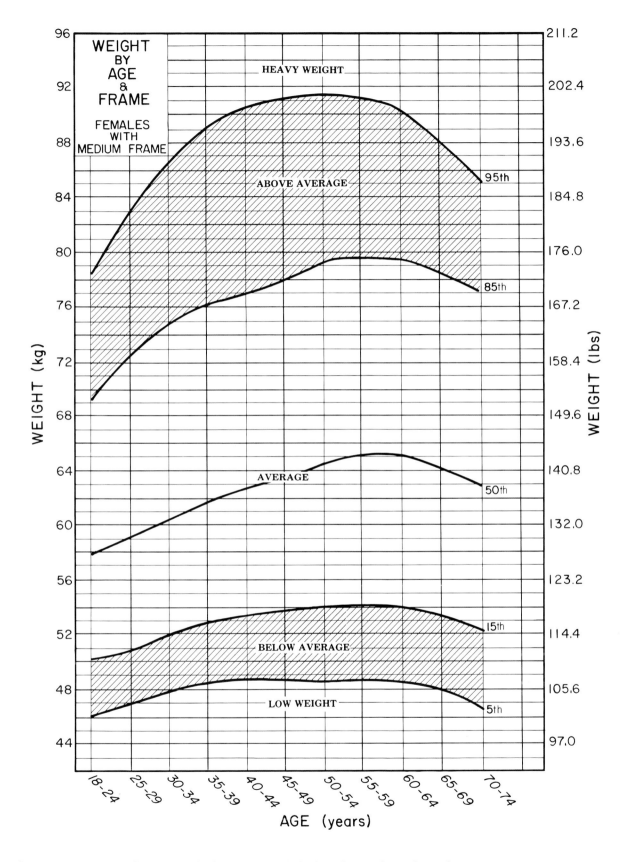

Fig. IV.47. Percentiles of weight by age for adult females with medium frame.

111

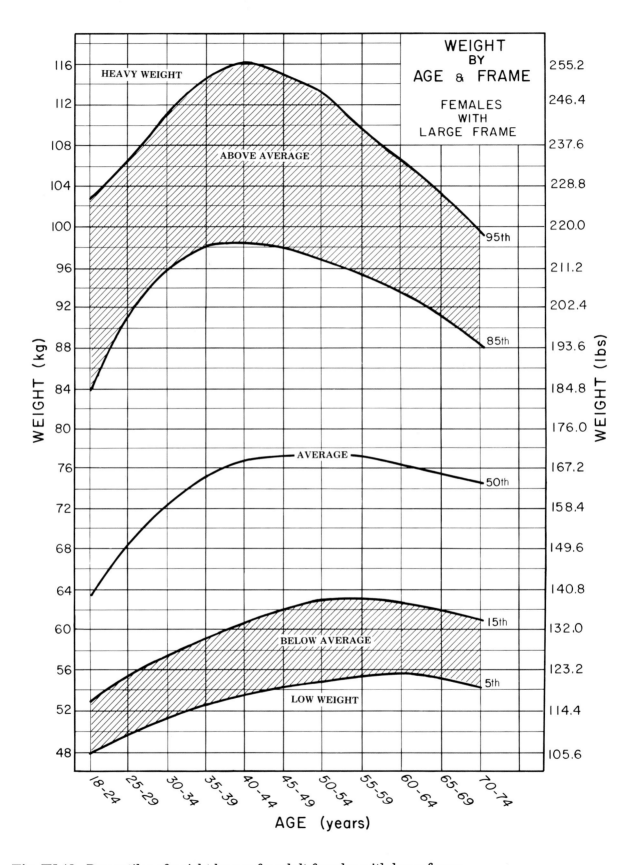

Fig. IV.48. Percentiles of weight by age for adult females with large frame.

112

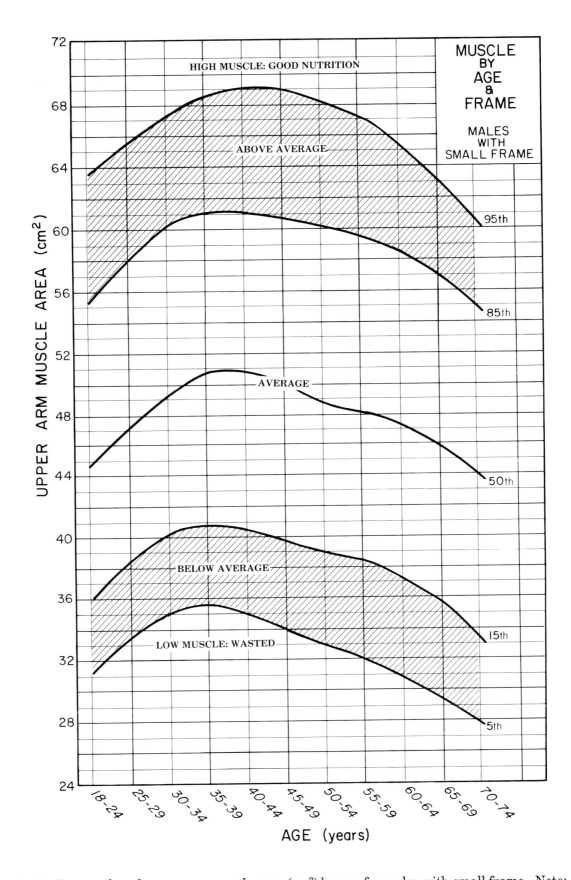

Fig. IV.49. Percentiles of upper arm muscle area (cm²) by age for males with small frame. Note: Values for males aged 18 years and older have been adjusted for bone area by subtracting 10.0 cm² from the calculated muscle area.

113

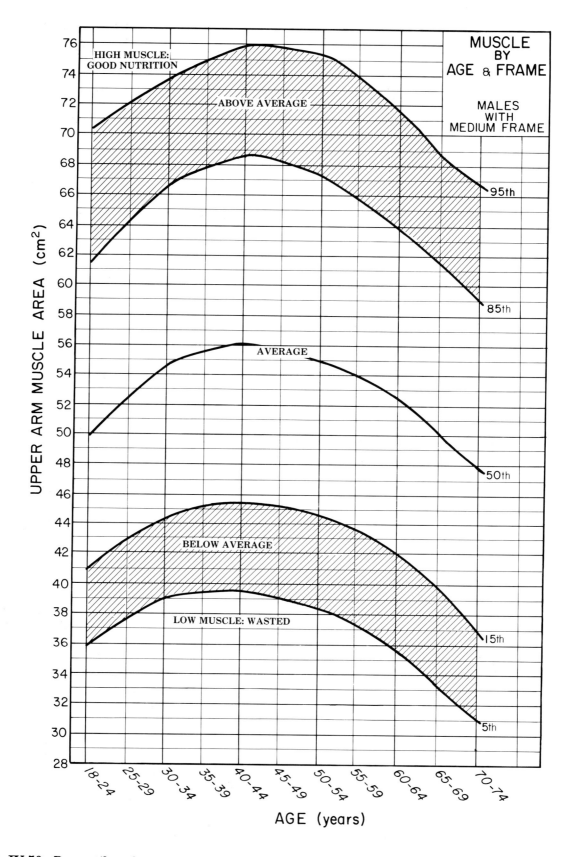

Fig. IV.50. Percentiles of upper arm muscle area (cm²) by age for males with medium frame. Note: Values for males aged 18 years and older have been adjusted for bone area by subtracting 10.0 cm² from the calculated muscle area.

114

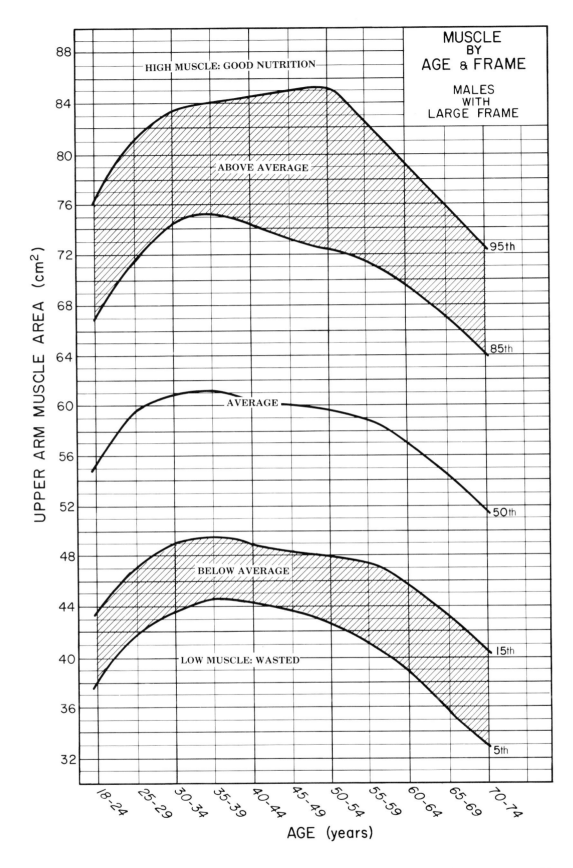

Fig. IV.51. Percentiles of upper arm muscle area (cm²) by age for males with large frame. Note: Values for males aged 18 years and older have been adjusted for bone area by subtracting 10.0 cm² from the calculated muscle area.

115

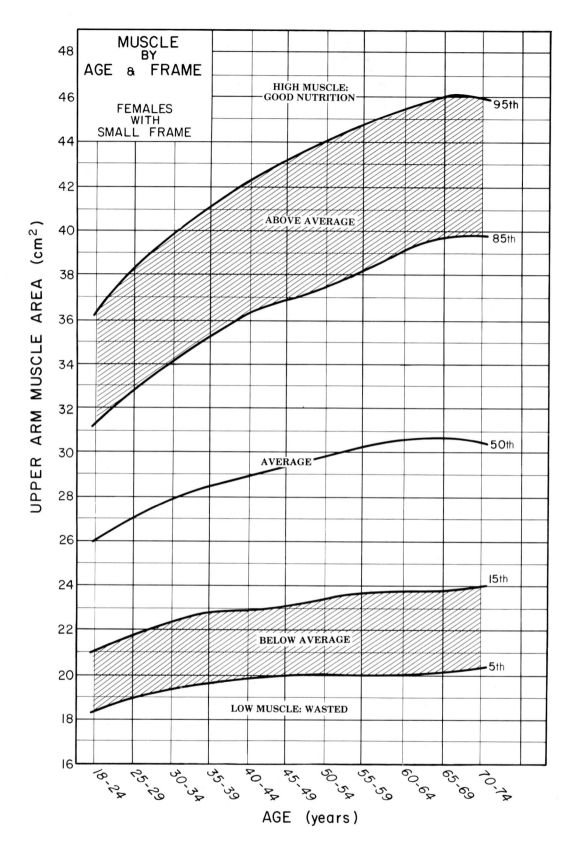

Fig. IV.52. Percentiles of upper arm muscle area (cm²) by age for females with small frame. Note: Values for males aged 18 years and older have been adjusted for bone area by subtracting 6.5 cm² from the calculated muscle area.

116

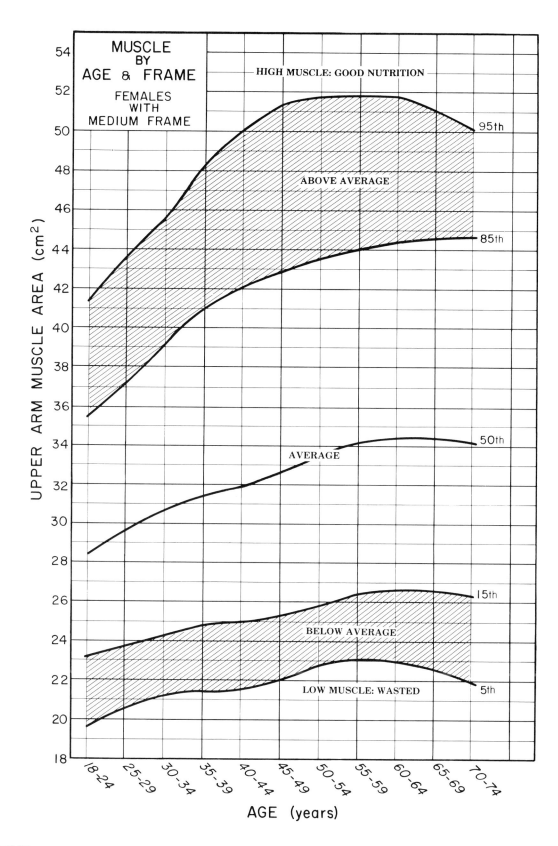

Fig. IV.53. Percentiles of upper arm muscle area (cm²) by age for females with medium frame.
Note: Values for males aged 18 years and older have been adjusted for bone area by subtracting 6.5
cm² from the calculated muscle area.

117

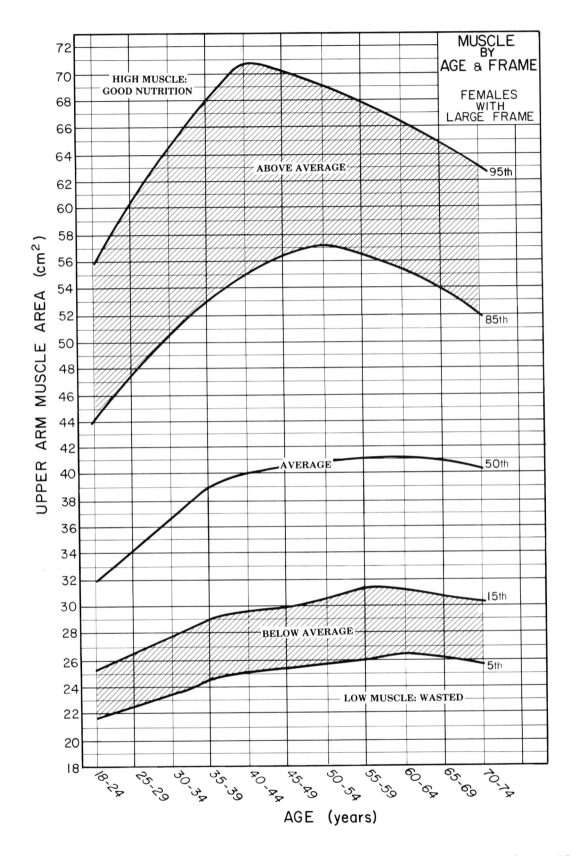

Fig. IV.54. Percentiles of upper arm muscle area (cm²) by age for females with large frame. Note: Values for males aged 18 years and older have been adjusted for bone area by subtracting 6.5 cm² from the calculated muscle area.

V
The Standard in Practice: Examples

Evaluations of Growth and Nutritional Status of Children

Adjustment of Children's Stature for Parent's Stature

Comparisons of anthropometric dimensions to a given reference permits the investigator to determine whether the child's growth is adequate or below that expected for his/her age. For example, it is usually assumed that a child whose height is below the 5th percentile is considered to be short for his age. The child could be short either because his parents are short (in which case he is probably genetically short) or because of environmental and/or pathological reasons. Therefore, evaluations of growth need to be done with reference to parental statures. For this reason, the present standards of stature are incorporated with a reference that permits adjustment of the child's stature to his or her parents' statures. Several studies addressed at parent-offspring statures have been published (1–6). Garn and associates (1–3), using samples from the Fels Longitudinal study, provided parent-specific stature tables, and Himes et al. (7) have recently updated this study and have published regression equations for the adjustment of recumbent length and stature of children ranging in age from birth to 18 years (see table V.1). The Fels Longitudinal study included 586 midparent-offspring relationships for serial measurements of recumbent length and stature of children ranging in age from birth to 18 years. An important feature of this study is that the regression equations have been incorporated into the NCHS stature data, which included the NHANES I sample used in the present standard. These data are presented in table V.1. This table provides information on age (column 1), median stature (*MdS*) (column 2 or 7), standard deviation (*SD*) (column 3 or 8), the intercept (a) (column 4 or 9), slope (b) (column 5 or 10), and error SD (column 6 or 11) of the regression equation for adjusting stature.

General Procedure

The application of the age- and sex-specific regression equations given in table V.1 can best be shown by an example.

Example. Girl aged 10 years, stature (CS) = 126 cm, mother's stature (MS) = 155 cm, father's stature (FS) = 165 cm.

The regression equation for the adjustment of stature (As) is as follows:

$$As = (\text{Standard SD} / \text{error SD}) \times \{CS - [a + (b \times MPS)] + (MdS - CS)\} ;$$

where As is the child stature adjusted for midparent height, Standard SD, error SD, a, b, and MdS correspond to the values given in table V.1, CS is the child's stature, and MPS is the midparent stature.

1. Calculate the midparent's stature (MPS) by adding the father and mother's stature and dividing the total by 2. In this case the MPS = 160 cm [MPS = (165 + 155) / 2]. When one parent's stature cannot be measured, ask the other parent whether the spouse is tall, medium, or short and using table V.2 following determine the corresponding stature to calculate the midparent stature.
2. Locate the age closest to that of the child, and for that age, use the corresponding values requested by the formula to obtain the adjustment for parent stature (As):

$$As = (5.92 / 5.51) \times \{126 - [52.69 + (0.505 \times 160)] + (138.3 - 126)\} = 5.02 \text{ cm}.$$

3. Add the parent-specific adjustment to the child's stature if the adjustment has no sign; subtract the adjustment if it has a minus sign. Thus, child's stature adjusted for midparent's stature = 126.0 + 5.02 = 131.02 cm.
4. Compare the child's parent-specific adjusted stature to the standard of stature given in table IV.1, determine in which percentile or what Z-score the child is located. In the present example, the girl's *nonadjusted* stature when compared to the standard of table IV.1 is below the 5th percentile. But the girl's adjusted stature when compared to the standard of table IV.1 is now *between the 5th and 15th percentiles.*

Interpretation.   She is as tall as other girls of similar midparent stature; probably genetically short.

The examples (examples V.1 to V.5) given in the next section have been specifically chosen to illustrate the evaluations of growth and nutritional status of children. In these examples, the child's stature is evaluated with reference to the measured height and with reference to the adjusted midparent stature. The classification into one of the five statistical anthropometric categories is done using as criterion either the Z-scores or percentile ranges where appropriate.

Note.   It should be noted that for parents who are extremely tall (midparent stature greater than 184 cm) or short (midparent stature less than 150 cm) the estimates of the parent-specific adjustments are less reliable because they are beyond the range of the sample (Fels sample) used to construct the equations. Similarly, for children who are at the extreme of the distribution (children who are extremely short or tall), the estimation of parent-specific adjustments must be considered with caution.

When applied to group data the adjusted statures of children should represent the stature of individuals with the familial variance removed. As a result, differences of statures of individuals within the distribution of adjusted statures should reflect mostly the effect of environmental factors. In this manner, the extent to which differences in growth and development between populations are due either to environmental or to familial factors can be accounted for.

Table V.1.
Medians, standard deviations, and regression equations for parent-specific adjustments of recumbent length (cm) and stature (cm) by age for boys and girls ranging in age from birth to 18 years

Age (yrs) (1)	Boys					Girls				
	Standard Regression Equation					Standard Regression Equation				
	Median (2)	SD (3)	a (4)	b (5)	error SD (6)	Median (7)	SD (8)	a (9)	b (10)	error SD (11)
Recumbent Length (cm), birth to 3 years										
Birth	50.5	2.37	35.36	0.089	2.35	49.9	1.98	44.04	0.035	1.97
0.08	54.6	2.34	35.53	0.113	2.29	53.5	2.07	42.76	0.063	2.05
0.25	61.1	2.31	37.62	0.139	2.24	59.5	2.20	41.85	0.104	2.14
0.50	67.8	2.34	40.42	0.162	2.25	65.9	2.32	40.41	0.151	2.23
0.75	72.3	2.49	41.94	0.179	2.37	70.4	2.48	37.93	0.192	2.35
1.00	76.1	2.75	42.59	0.198	2.62	74.3	2.69	36.42	0.224	2.51
1.50	82.4	3.02	44.06	0.226	2.87	80.9	2.88	38.74	0.249	2.64
2.00	87.6	3.26	42.61	0.266	3.06	86.5	3.02	40.12	0.274	2.75
2.50	92.3	3.46	41.26	0.301	3.22	91.3	3.19	40.46	0.300	2.88
3.00	96.5	3.62	41.73	0.323	3.35	95.6	3.39	40.49	0.325	3.06
Stature (cm), 2.5 to 18 years										
2.50	90.4	3.91	25.88	0.381	3.57	90.0	3.08	35.15	0.324	2.76
3.00	94.9	3.90	32.37	0.369	3.57	94.1	3.37	39.37	0.323	3.08
3.50	99.1	3.92	36.56	0.369	3.60	97.9	3.59	42.05	0.330	3.29
4.00	102.9	4.00	39.02	0.377	3.68	101.6	3.78	42.85	0.347	3.44
4.50	106.6	4.16	39.75	0.395	3.81	105.0	3.96	42.53	0.369	3.59
5.00	109.9	4.34	40.24	0.411	3.98	108.4	4.12	42.16	0.391	3.73
5.50	113.1	4.51	40.95	0.426	4.13	111.6	4.27	40.99	0.417	3.86
6.00	116.1	4.66	40.97	0.444	4.25	114.6	4.44	39.40	0.444	4.00
6.50	119.0	4.77	40.38	0.464	4.33	117.6	4.59	39.24	0.463	4.14
7.00	121.7	4.89	39.24	0.487	4.42	120.6	4.72	40.83	0.471	4.26
7.50	124.4	5.05	38.31	0.508	4.56	123.5	4.85	42.76	0.477	4.39
8.00	127.0	5.24	38.05	0.525	4.73	126.4	4.99	44.38	0.484	4.54
8.50	129.6	5.37	38.38	0.539	4.86	129.3	5.14	45.80	0.493	4.69
9.00	132.2	5.46	38.20	0.555	4.93	132.2	5.34	47.40	0.501	4.88
9.50	134.8	5.57	37.14	0.577	5.02	135.2	5.59	49.77	0.504	5.14
10.00	137.5	5.72	36.69	0.595	5.14	138.3	5.92	52.69	0.505	5.51
10.50	140.3	5.88	37.90	0.605	5.29	141.5	6.31	55.44	0.508	5.96
11.00	143.3	6.07	40.56	0.607	5.48	144.8	6.67	57.29	0.517	6.32
11.50	146.4	6.32	43.64	0.607	5.76	148.2	6.88	57.60	0.535	6.49
12.00	149.7	6.63	46.43	0.610	6.10	151.5	6.94	57.92	0.552	6.51
12.50	153.0	7.04	48.01	0.620	6.53	154.6	6.80	59.97	0.559	6.38
13.00	156.5	7.47	48.12	0.640	6.94	157.1	6.40	63.83	0.551	5.99
13.50	159.9	7.70	46.71	0.668	7.11	159.0	5.94	68.42	0.535	5.54
14.00	163.1	7.75	44.20	0.702	7.13	160.4	5.65	71.16	0.527	5.23
14.50	166.2	7.67	40.78	0.740	7.00	161.2	5.53	71.38	0.530	5.07
15.00	169.0	7.40	36.58	0.782	6.58	161.8	5.49	69.90	0.543	5.00
15.50	171.5	7.00	32.69	0.819	6.02	161.1	5.50	66.91	0.562	4.99
16.00	173.5	6.60	30.07	0.847	5.50	162.4	5.53	64.03	0.581	5.01
16.50	175.2	6.30	29.38	0.861	5.11	162.7	5.56	62.42	0.592	5.04
17.00	176.2	6.13	29.53	0.866	4.87	163.1	5.56	62.29	0.595	5.03
17.50	176.7	6.08	28.86	0.873	4.75	163.4	5.46	64.54	0.584	4.94
18.00	176.8	6.12	26.31	0.888	4.72	163.7	5.18	70.70	0.549	4.72

Source: Adapted from Himes, J. H., Roche, A. F., Thissen, D., and Moore, W. M. 1981.
Parent-specific adjustments of recumbent length and stature. Monographs in Paediatrics, vol. 13. Basel: S. Karger.

Table V.2.
Values of parental statures used in calculation of midparent stature when one
parent's stature is reported as short, medium, or tall

Parent	Short	Medium	Tall
Father	156.6	176.3	185.4
Mother	154.9	162.8	170.7

Source: Himes, J. H., Roche, A. F., Thissen, D., and Moore, W. M. 1985. Parent-specific
adjustments for evaluation of recumbent length and stature of children. Pediatrics 75:304–13.
(Reproduced by permission of Pediatrics.)

Examples: Evaluations of Growth and Nutritional Status of Children

Example V.1: 11-Year-Old Girl

Characteristics	Computation	Variable
Child's stature (CS)	N.A.	137.0cm
Father's stature	N.A.	165.0cm
Mother's stature	N.A.	155.0 cm
Midparent stature (MPS)	(165 + 155)/ 2	160.0 cm
Adjusted for midparent stature	137 + 4.61	141.6 cm
Weight	N.A.	35.0 kg
Triceps Skinfold	16/10 = 1.6 cm	16.0 mm
Subscapular Skinfold	N.A.	15.0 mm
Sum of Skinfold Thicknesses	N.A.	31.0 mm
Upper Arm Circumference	N.A.	21.0 cm
Total Upper Arm Fat Area (TUA)	$21^2/12.57$	35.1 cm²
Upper Arm Muscle Area (UMA)	$[(21.0 - 1.6) \times 3.1416]^2 /12.57$	20.3 cm²
Upper Arm Fat Area (UFA)	35.1 - 20.3	14.8 cm²
Arm Fat Index (AFI)	(14.8/35.1) x 100	42.2%

Growth and Nutritional Status Evaluation

Reference	Z-score	Category	Percentile	Category
Stature by Age	-1.35	Below Ave.	>5th but <15th	Below Ave.
Adj. midparent stature	-0.74	Average	>15th but <85th	Average
Wt. by Age	N.A	N.A.	>15th but <85th	Average
Wt. by Ht.	N.A.	N.A.	>15th but <85th	Average
UMA by Age	-1.07	Below Ave.	>5th but <15th	Below Ave
UMA by Ht.	-2.02	Below Ave.	>5th but <15th	Below Ave
Sum of Skinfolds	N.A.	N.A.	>15th but <85th	Average
Arm Fat Index	N.A.	N.A.	>15th but <85th	Average

Interpretation. Although she is below average in stature (short), her short-ness is probably of genetic origin (or related to her parents' shortness). This is evident from the fact that her adjusted height is comparable to other children with similar midparent stature. However, she is heavy for her height; this is related to her high amount of body fat indicated by the arm fat index and the low mid arm muscle area.

Example V.2: 8-Year-Old Boy

Characteristics	Computation	Variable
Child's stature (CS)	N.A.	123.0 cm
Father's stature	N.A.	187.0 cm
Mother's stature	N.A.	165.0 cm
Midparent stature (MPS)	(187 + 165)/2	176.0 cm
Adjusted for midparent stature	123 - 4.27	118.7 cm
Weight	N.A.	31.0 kg
Sitting Height	N.A.	69.0 cm
Sitting Height Index	(69/123) x 100	56.0%
Triceps Skinfold	11/10 = 1.1 cm	11.0 mm
Subscapular Skinfold	N.A.	5.0 mm
Sum of Skinfold Thicknesses	N.A.	16.0 mm
Upper Arm Circumference	N.A.	22.0 cm
Total Upper Arm Fat Area (TUA)	$22^2/12.57$	38.5 cm^2
Upper Arm Muscle Area (UMA)	$[(22.0 - 1.1) \times 3.1416]^2/12.57$	27.4 cm^2
Upper Arm Fat Area (UFA)	38.5 - 27.4	11.1 cm^2
Arm Fat Index (AFI)	(11.1/38.5) x 100	28.8%

Growth and Nutritional Status Evaluation

Reference	Z-score	Category	Percentile	Category
Stature by Age	-1.08	Below Ave.	>5th but <15	Below Ave.
Adj. midparent stature	-1.87	Short	< 5th	Short
Wt. by Age	N.A.	N.A.	>15th but <85th	Average
Wt. by Ht.	N.A.	N.A.	>95th	High Wt.
Sitting Ht. Index	0.76	Average	>95th	Large Trunk
UMA by Age	1.26	Above Ave.	>85th but <95th	Above Ave.
UMA by Ht.	2.19	Above Ave.	>85th but <95th	Above Ave.
Sum of Skinfolds	N.A.	N.A.	>15th but <85th	Average
Arm Fat Index	N.A.	N.A.	>15th but <85th	Average

Interpretation. The subject is short for his age and, considering his parents' height, he should have been taller than he is now. In other words, he seems to be below his genetic potential as far as his height is concerned. However, the subject is heavy for his age. As judged by the measurements of body composition, the excess weight is not due to an excess of fat but to the subject's high muscularity and short legs (which is indicated by the high sitting height index).

Example V.3: 13-Year-Old Girl

Characteristics	Computation	Variable
Child's stature (CS)	N.A.	165.0 cm
Father's stature	N.A.	185.0 cm
Mother's stature	N.A.	170.0 cm
Midparent stature (MPS)	(185 + 170)/2	178.0 cm
Adjusted for midparent stature	165 - 4.59	160.4 cm
Weight	N.A.	39.0 kg
Triceps Skinfold	4/10 = 0.4 cm	4.0 mm
Subscapular Skinfold	N.A.	5.0 mm
Sum of Skinfold Thicknesses	N.A.	9.0 mm
Upper Arm Circumference	N.A.	20.0 cm
Total Upper Arm Fat Area (TUA)	$20^2/12.57$	31.8 cm^2
Upper Arm Muscle Area (UMA)	$[(20.0 - 0.4) \times 3.1416]^2/12.57$	28.0 cm^2
Upper Arm Fat Area (UFA)	31.8 - 28.0	3.8 cm^2
Arm Fat Index (AFI)	$(3.8/31.8) \times 100$	11.9%

Growth and Nutritional Status Evaluation				
Reference	**Z-score**	**Category**	**Percentile**	**Category**
Stature by Age	1.00	Average	>85th but <95th	Above Ave.
Adj. midparent stature	0.20	Average	>15th but <85th	Average
Wt. by Age	N.A.	N.A.	>5th but <15th	Below Ave.
Wt. by Ht.	N.A.	N.A.	<5th	Low Wt.
UMA by Age	-0.53	Average	>15th but <85th	Average
UMA by Ht.	-0.84	Average	>15th but <85th	Average
Sum of Skinfolds	N.A.	N.A.	<5th	Lean
Arm Fat Index	N.A.	N.A.	<5th	Lean

Interpretation. Although she is tall for her age, she is not as tall as other girls with similar midparent stature. The subject's underweightness is related to her low amount of body fat. Since her muscle size is within the average range, she does not seem to be at risk of undernutrition.

Example V.4: 4-Year-Old Boy

Characteristics	Computation	Variable
Child's stature (CS)	N.A.	106.0 cm
Father's stature	N.A.	176.0 cm
Mother's stature	N.A.	163.0 cm
Midparent stature (MPS)	(176.0 + 163.0)/2	170.0 cm
Adjusted for midparent stature	106.0 + 2.93	108.9 cm
Weight	N.A.	14.0 kg
Triceps Skinfold	3.0/10 = 0.3 cm	3.0 mm
Subscapular Skinfold	N.A.	3.0 mm
Sum of Skinfold Thicknesses	N.A.	6.0 mm
Upper Arm Circumference	N.A.	12.5 cm
Total Upper Arm Fat Area (TUA)	$12.5^2/12.57$	12.4 cm^2
Upper Arm Muscle Area (UMA)	$[(12.5 - 0.3) \times 3.1416]^2/12.57$	10.6 cm^2
Upper Arm Fat Area (UFA)	12.4 - 10.6	1.8 cm^2
Arm Fat Index (AFI)	(1.8/12.4) x 100	14.5%

Growth and Nutritional Status Evaluation				
Reference	**Z-score**	**Category**	**Percentile**	**Category**
Stature by Age	0.00	Average	>15th but <85th	Average
Adj. midparent stature	0.02	Average	>15th but <85th	Average
Wt. by Age	N.A.	N.A.	<5th	Low Wt.
Wt. by Ht.	N.A.	N.A.	<5th	Low Wt.
UMA by Age	-2.11	Wasted	<5th	Wasted
UMA by Ht.	-1.64	Wasted	<5th	Wasted
Sum of Skinfolds	N.A.	N.A.	<5th	Lean
Arm Fat Index	N.A.	N.A.	<5th	Lean

Interpretation. The subject is obviously underweight and emaciated as indicated by the drastic reduction in upper arm muscle area and subcutaneous fat. The subject is clearly at severe risk of malnutrition. Since in terms of stature he approaches the average, this problem is probably of recent origin and, unless the factors leading to this condition are modified, the subject's growth will be stunted.

Example V.5: 6-Year-Old Girl

Characteristics	Computation	Variable
Child's stature (CS)	N.A.	108.0 cm
Father's stature	N.A.	178.0 cm
Mother's stature	N.A.	165.0 cm
Midparent stature (MPS)	(178.0 + 165.0)/2	172.0 cm
Adjusted for midparent stature	108.0 - 2.02	106.0 cm
Weight	N.A.	19.0 kg
Triceps Skinfold	3.0/10 = 0.3 cm	3.0 mm
Subscapular Skinfold	N.A.	3.0 mm
Sum of Skinfold Thicknesses	N.A.	6.0 mm
Upper Arm Circumference	N.A.	13.0 cm
Total Upper Arm Fat Area (TUA)	$13.0^2/12.57$	13.5 cm²
Upper Arm Muscle Area (UMA)	$[(13.0 - 0.3) \times 3.1416]^2/12.57$	11.6 cm²
Upper Arm Fat Area (UFA)	13.5 - 11.6	1.9 cm²
Arm Fat Index (AFI)	(1.9/13.5) x 100	14.0%

Growth and Nutritional Status Evaluation

Reference	Z-score	Category	Percentile	Category
Stature by Age	-1.94	Short	<5th	Short
Adj. midparent stature	-2.02	Short	<5th	Short
Wt. by Age	N.A.	N.A.	>15th but <85th	Average
Wt. by Ht.	N.A.	N.A.	>15th but <85th	Average
UMA by Age	-1.64	Wasted	<5th	Wasted
UMA by Ht.	-1.33	Low Musc.	>5th but <15th	Low Musc.
Sum of skinfolds	N.A.	N.A.	<5th	Lean
Arm Fat Index	N.A.	N.A.	<5th	Lean

Interpretation. Despite the fact that the subject's weight is within the average range, she exhibits a symmetrical reduction of both upper arm muscle area and subcutaneous fat. Furthermore, she is clearly shorter than her peers of similar age and similar midparent height. This evidence suggests that this child has been suffering from severe chronic malnutrition.

Examples: Evaluations of Nutritional Status of Adults

Example V.6: 70-Year-Old Male

Characteristics	Computation	Variable
Elbow Breadth from Frameter	8.0 x 10 = 80 mm	8.0 cm
Stature	N.A.	160.0 cm
Weight	N.A.	72.0 kg
Frame Size from Frame Index 1	N.A.	Large
Frame Size from Frame Index 2	(80/160) x 100 = 50.0	Large
Triceps Skinfolds	20/10 = 2.0 cm	20.0 mm
Subscapular Skinfold	N.A.	23.0 mm
Sum of Skinfold Thicknesses	N.A.	43.0 mm
Density from table II.2	$D = 1.1527 - (0.0793 \times \log 43.0)$	1.0232 gm/cc
Percent Fat Weight	$\%fat = [(4.95/1.0232) - 4.50] \times 100$	33.8%
Upper Arm Circumference	N.A.	32.0 cm
Total Upper Arm Area (TUA)	$32.0^2/12.57$	81.46 cm^2
Upper Arm Muscle Area (UMA)	$[(30.0 - 2.0) \times 3.1416]^2/12.57$	52.61 cm^2
Upper Arm Fat Area (UFA)	81.46 - 52.61	28.85 cm^2
Bone-Free Muscle Area (UMAc)	52.61 - 10.0	42.61
Arm Fat Index (AFI)	(28.85/81.46) x 100	35.42%

Nutritional Status Evaluation

Reference	Z-score	Category	Percentile	Category
Wt. by Age	N.A.	N.A.	>15th but <85th	Average
Wt. by Height	N.A.	N.A.	>15th but <85th	Average
Wt. by Age/Large Frame	N.A.	N.A.	>85th but <95th	High Wt.
UMA by Age	-0.46	Average	>15th but <85th	Average
UMA by Age/Large Frame	-0.74	Average	>15th but <85th	Average
Sum of Skinfolds	N.A.	N.A.	>85th	Excess Fat
Arm Fat Index	N.A.	N.A.	>85th	Excess Fat
Percent Fat Weight	N.A.	N.A.	N.A.	Excess Fat

Interpretation. The subject is heavy for his age when compared to others of similar frame size. This high weight is associated with an excess of fat. Although the subject's muscle area is within the normal range, he is clearly at risk for obesity.

Example V.7: 36-Year-Old Female

Characteristics	Computation	Variable
Elbow Breadth from Frameter	7.2 x 10 = 72 mm	7.2 cm
Stature	N.A.	173.0 cm
Weight	N.A.	83.0 kg
Frame Size from Frameter	N.A.	Large
Frame Size from Frame Index 1	N.A.	Large
Triceps Skinfolds	25/10 = 2.5 cm	25.0 mm
Subscapular Skinfold	N.A.	42.0 mm
Sum of Skinfold Thicknesses	N.A.	67.0 mm
Density from table II.2	$D = 1.1356 - (0.0680 \times \log 67.0)$	1.0114 gm/cc
Percent Fat Weight	$\%fat = [(4.95/1.0114) - 4.50] \times 100$	39.4%
Upper Arm Circumference	N.A.	32.0 cm
Total Upper Arm Area (TUA)	$32.0^2/12.57$	81.46 cm^2
Upper Arm Muscle Area (UMA)	$[(32.0 - 2.5) \times 3.1416]^2/12.57$	46.38 cm^2
Upper Arm Fat Area (UFA)	81.46 - 46.38	40.08 cm^2
Bone-Free Muscle Area (UMAc)	46.38 - 6.5	39.88 cm^2
Arm Fat Index (AFI)	$(40.08/81.46) \times 100$	56.90%

Nutritional Status Evaluation

Reference	Z-score	Category	Percentile	Category
Wt. by Age	N.A.	N.A.	>85th	High Wt.
Wt. by Height	N.A.	N.A.	>15th but <85th	Average
Wt. by Age/Large Frame	N.A.	N.A.	>85th but <95th	High Wt.
UMA by Age	0.49	Average	>15th but <85th	Average
UMA by Age/Large Frame	-0.11	Average	>15th but <85th	Average
Sum of Skinfolds	N.A.	N.A.	>85th	Excess Fat
Arm Fat Index	N.A.	N.A.	>85th	Excess Fat
Percent Fat Weight	N.A.	N.A.	N.A.	Excess Fat

Interpretation. The subject is heavy for her age and for her height and frame size. The high weight is associated with an excess of body fat.

Example V.8: 20-Year-Old Female

Characteristics	Computation	Variable
Elbow Breadth from Frameter	5.6 x 10 = 56 mm	5.6 cm
Stature	N.A.	166.0 cm
Weight	N.A.	49.5 kg Frame
Size from Frameter	N.A.	Small Frame
Size from Frame Index 1	N.A.	Small
Triceps Skinfolds	5.0/10 = 0.5 cm	5.0 mm
Subscapular Skinfold	N.A.	5.0 mm Sum
of Skinfold Thicknesses	N.A.	10.0 mm
Density from table II. 2	$D = 1.1582 - (0.0813 \times \log 10.0)$	1.0769 gm/cc
Percent Fat Weight	%fat = [(4.95/1.0769) - 4.50] x 100	9.7 %
Upper Arm Circumference	N.A.	23.0 cm
Total Upper Arm Area (TUA)	$23.0^2/12.57$	42.08 cm^2
Upper Arm Muscle Area (UMA)	$[(23.0 - 0.5) \times 3.1416]^2/12.57$	36.53 cm^2
Upper Arm Fat Area (UFA)	42.08 - 36.53	5.6 cm^2
Bone-Free Muscle Area (UMAc)	36.5 - 6.5	30.0 cm^2
Arm Fat Index (AFI)	(5.6/42.1) x 100	13.2%

Nutritional Status Evaluation

Reference	Z-score	Category	Percentile	Category
Wt. by Age	N.A.	N.A.	>5th but <15th	Below Ave.
Wt. by Height	N.A.	N.A.	<5th but <15th	Below Ave.
Wt.by Age/Small Frame	-0.72	Average	>10th but <75th	Average
UMA by Age	0.02	Average	>15th but <85th	Average
UMA by Age/Small Frame	0.61	Average	>15th but <85th	Average
Sum of Skinfolds	N.A.	N.A.	<5th	Lean
Arm Fat Index	N.A.	N.A.	<5th	Lean
Percent Fat Weight	N.A.	N.A.	N.A.	Lean

Interpretation.   The subject is lean, but as shown by her upper arm muscle area, which is within the average range, she is not undernourished. Her low weight reflects her leanness.

Example V.9: 24-Year-Old Male

Characteristics	Computation	Variable
Elbow Breadth from Frameter	7.3 x 10 = 73 mm	7.3 cm
Stature	N.A.	178.0 cm
Weight	N.A.	88.0 kg
Frame Size from Frameter	N.A.	Medium
Frame Size from Frameter Index 1	N.A.	Medium
Frame Size from Frame Index 2	(73/178) x 100 = 41.0	Medium
Triceps Skinfolds	9.0/10 = 0.9 cm	9.0 mm
Subscapular Skinfold	N.A.	10.0 mm
Sum of Skinfold Thicknesses	N.A.	19.0 mm
Density from table II. 2	D = 1.1525 - (0.0687 x log 19.0)	1.0646 gm/cc
Percent Fat Weight	%fat = [(4.95/1.0646) - 4.50] x 100	15.0 %
Upper Arm Circumference	N.A.	35.0 cm
Total Upper Arm Area (TUA)	$35.0^2/12.57$	97.5 cm²
Upper Arm Muscle Area (UMA)	$[(35.0 - 0.9) \times 3.1416]^2/12.57$	36.53 cm²
Upper Arm Fat Area (UFA)	97.5 - 82.4	13.3 cm²
Bone-Free Muscle Area (UMAc)	82.4 - 10.0	72.4 cm²
Arm Fat Index (AFI)	(13.3/97.5) x 100	13.6%

Nutritional Status Evaluation

Reference	Z-score	Category	Percentile	Category
Wt. by Age	N.A.	N.A.	>85th but <95th	Heavy Wt.
Wt. by Height	N.A.	N.A.	>15th but <15th	Average
Wt. by Age/Medium Frame	N.A.	N.A.	>85th but <95th	Heavy Wt.
UMA by Age	1.87	High Muscle	>95th	High Muscle
UMA by Age/Medium Frame	1.97	High Muscle	>95th	High Muscle
Sum of Skinfolds	N.A.	N.A.	>10th but <75th	Average
Arm Fat Index	N.A.	N.A.	>10th but <75th	Average
Percent Fat Weight	N.A.	N.A.	N.A.	Average

Interpretation. The subject is clearly heavy for his height, age, and frame size. However, his excess weight is mostly due to his high muscularity since, in terms of fatness measurements, he is in the average range.

Literature Cited

Chapter I

1. Stuart, H. C., and Stevenson, S. S. 1969. Growth and development. In: Textbook of Pediatrics, 9th ed., ed. W. E. Nelson. Philadelphia: W. B. Saunders.

2. Hamill, P. V., Drizd, T. A., Johnson, C. L., Reed, R. B., and Roche, A. F. 1977. NCHS growth curves for children, birth–18 years, United States. Vital and Health Statistics, series 11, no. 165. Hyattsville, Md.: National Center for Health Statistics. DHEW Publication no. (PHS) 78-1650.

3. Tanner, J. M., and Davies, P. S. 1985. Clinical longitudinal standards of height and height velocity for North American children. J. Pedia. 107: 317–29.

4. Waterlow, J. C., Buzina, R., Keller, W., Lane, J. M., and Nichamon, M. Z. 1977. The presentation and use of height and weight data for comparing the nutritional status of groups of children under the age of 10 years. Bulletin of the World Health Organization 55 (4): 489–98.

5. Rivers, J. P. W. 1988. The nutritional biology of famine. In: Famine, ed. G. A. Harrison. Oxford: Oxford University Press.

6. Martorell, R. 1985. Child growth retardation: a discussion of its causes and its relationship to health. In: Nutritional Adaptation in Man, ed. K. L. Blaxter and J. C. Waterlow. London: John Libbey.

7. Dibley, M. J., Staehling, N., Nieburg, P., and Trowbridge, F. L. 1985. Pitfalls in the interpretation of weight-for-height. XII International Congress of Nutrition, Brighton, U.K. (abstr.).

8. Keller, W., and Filmore, C. M. 1983. Prevalence of protein-energy malnutrition. World Health Statistics Quarterly 36:129–67.

9. Monteiro, C. A. 1985. A critical assessment of recently proposed changes in anthropometric evaluation of nutritional status of children. XII International Congress of Nutrition, Brighton, U.K. (abstr.).

10. Trowbridge, F. L. 1979. Clinical and biochemical characteristics associated with anthropometric nutritional categories. Am. J. Clin. Nutr. 32:758–66.

11. Buckler, J. M. H. 1979. A reference manual of growth and development. Oxford, London: Blackwell Scientific Publications.

12. Tanner, J. M., Whitehouse, R. H., and Takaishi, M. 1965. Standards from birth to maturity for height, weight, height velocity, and weight velocity: British children. Arch. Dis. Child. 41: 454–64.

13. Johnson, C. L., Fulwood, R., Abraham, S., and Bryner, J. D. 1981. Basic data on anthropometric measurements and angular measure-

ments of the hip and knee joints for selected age groups 1–74 years of age: United States, 1971–1975. Vital and Health Statistics, series 11, no. 219. Hyattsville, Md.: National Center for Health Statistics. DHEW Publication no. (PHS) 81-1669.

14. Schell, L. M., and Johnston, F. E. 1978. Physical growth and development of American Indian and Eskimo children and youth. In: Handbook of North American Indians, ed. W. C. Sturtevant. Washington: Smithsonian Institution, U. S. Government Printing Office.

15. Stinson, S. 1985. Sex differences in environmental sensitivity during growth and development. Yearbook of Physical Anthropology 28:123–47.

16. Johnston, F. E., and Schell, L. 1979. Anthropometric variations of Native American children and adults. In: The First Americans: Origins, Affinities and Adaptations, ed. W. S. Laughlin and A. B. Harper. New York: Gustav Fisher.

17. Buschang, P. H., Malina, R. M., and Little, B. B. 1986. Linear growth of Zapotec school children: growth status and yearly velocity for leg length and sitting height. Ann. Hum. Biol. 13:225–34.

18. Metropolitan Life Insurance Co. 1959. New weight standards for men and women. Stat. Bull. 140:1–4.

19. Metropolitan Life Insurance Co. 1983. Metropolitan height and weight tables. Stat. Bull. 64:1–9.

20. Welham, W. C., and Behnke, A. R. 1942. The specific gravity of healthy man: body weight, volume and other physical characteristics of exceptional athletes and of naval personnel. JAMA 118:498–501.

21. Abraham, S., Carroll, M. D., Najjar, M. F., and Fulwood, R. 1983. Obese and overweight adults in the United States. Vital and Health Statistics, series 11, no. 230. Hyattsville, Md.: National Center for Health Statistics. DHHS Publication no. (PHS) 83-1680.

22. Hubert, H. B., Feinleib, M., and McNamara, P. M. 1983. Obesity as an independent risk factor for cardiovascular disease: a 26-year follow up of participants in the Framingham Heart Study. Circulation 67:968–77.

23. Jensen, T. G. 1984. Determination of nutritional status in critical care. J. Am. Diet. Assoc. 84:1345–48.

24. Simopoulos, A. P., and van Itallie, T. B. 1984. Body weight, health, and longevity. Ann. Int. Med. 100:285–95.

25. Adibi, S. A. 1976. Metabolism of branched-chain amino acids in altered nutrition. Metabolism 25:1287–1302.

26. Furst, P., Bergstrom, J., Vinnars, E., Schildt, B., and Holstrom, B. 1978. Intracellular amino acids and energy metabolism in catabolic patients with regard to muscle tissue. In: Advances in Parenteral Nutrition, ed. I. Johnston, pp. 85–104. Lancaster: M.T.P. Press.

27. Young, G. A., and Hill, G. L. 1978. Assessment of protein-calorie malnutrition in surgical patients from plasma proteins and anthropometric measurements. Am. J. Clin. Nutr. 31:429–35.

28. Young, G. A., and Hill, G. L. 1981. Evaluation of protein-energy

malnutrition in surgical patients from plasma valine and other amino acids, proteins, and anthropometric measurements. Am. J. Clin. Nutr. 34:166–72.

29.   Heymsfield, S. B., McManus, C., Smith, J., Stevens, V., and Nixon, D. W. 1982. Anthropometric measurement of muscle mass: revised equations for calculating bone-free arm muscle area. Am. J. Clin. Nutr. 36:680–90.

30.   Trowbridge, F. L., Hiner, C. D., and Robertson, A. D. 1982. Arm muscle indicators and creatinine excretion in children. Am. J. Clin. Nutr. 36:691–96.

Chapter II

1.   Abraham, S., Carroll, M. D., Najjar, M. F., and Fulwood, R. 1983. Obese and overweight adults in the United States. Vital and Health Statistics, series 11, no. 230. Hyattsville, Md.: National Center for Health Statistics. DHHS Publication no. (PHS) 83-1680.

2.   Frisancho, A. R. 1984. New standards of weight and body composition by frame size and height for assessment of nutritional status of adults and the elderly. Am. J. Clin. Nutr. 40:808–19.

3.   Lohman, T. G., Roche, A. F., and Martorell, R. (eds). 1988. Anthropometric Standardization Reference Manual. Champaign, Ill.: Human Kinetics Books.

4.   Chumlea, W. C. 1988. Methods of nutritional anthropometric assessment for special groups. In: Anthropometric Standardization Reference Manual, ed. T. G. Lohman, A. F. Roche, and R. Martorell. Champaign, Ill.: Human Kinetics Books.

5.   Simopoulos, A. P., and van Itallie, T. B. 1984. Body weight, health, and longevity. Ann. Int. Med. 100:285–95.

6.   Katch, V. L., and Freedson, P. S. 1982. Body size and shape: derivation of the HAT frame size model. Am. J. Clin. Nutr. 36: 669–75.

7.   Katch, V. L., Freedson, P. S., Katch, F. I., and Smith, L. 1982. Body frame size: validity of self-appraisal. Am. J. Clin. Nutr. 36:676–79.

8.   Best, W. R., and Kuhl, W. J. 1953. Estimation of active protoplasmic mass by physical and roentgenological anthropometry. Medical Nutrition Laboratory Report no. 114, Surgeon General's Department, U.S. Army.

9.   Baker, P. T., Frisancho, A. R., and Thomas, R. B. 1965. A preliminary analysis of human growth in the Peruvian Andes. In: Human Adaptability to Environments and Physical Fitness, ed. M. S. Malhotra, pp. 259–69. Defense Institute of Physiology and Allied Sciences, Madras-3, Research and Development Organization, Ministry of Defense, Government of India.

10.   Baker, P. T., Hunt, E. E., Jr., and Sen, T. 1958. The growth and interrelations of skinfolds and brachial tissues in man. Am. J. Phys. Anthropol. 16:39–58.

11. Frisancho, A. R., and Garn, S. M. 1971. Skinfold thickness and muscle size: implications for developmental status and nutritional evaluation of children from Honduras. Am. J. Clin. Nutr. 24:541–46.

12. Amador, M., Gonzales, M. E., Cordova, L., and Perez, N. 1982. Diagnosing and misdiagnosing malnutrition. Acta Paediatrica Academiae Scientiarum Hungaricae 23:391–401.

13. Anderson, M. A. 1975. Use of height-arm circumference measurement for nutritional selectivity in Sri Lanka school feeding. Am. J. Clin. Nutr. 28:775–81.

14. Arnhold, R. 1969. The QUAC stick: a field measure used by the Quaker service team, Nigeria. J. Trop. Pediatr. 15:241–47.

15. Frisancho, A. R. 1974. Triceps skinfold and upper arm muscle size norms for assessment of nutritional status. Am. J. Clin. Nutr. 27:1052–57.

16. Gonzales, M. E., and Rodriguez, C. 1983. Estudio de algunos indicadores anthropometricos y funcionales en varones de 11–20 años. Revista Cubana Pediatria 5:644–60.

17. Gurney, T. M., and Jelliffe, D. B. 1973. Arm of muscle circumference and cross-sectional muscle and fat areas. Am. J. Clin. Nutr. 26:912–15.

18. Pena, M., Barta, L., Regoly-Merei, A., and Tichy, M. 1979. Anthropometric considerations regarding obese children. Acta Sci. Hung. 20:333–36.

19. Furst, P., Bergstrom, J., Vinnars, E., Schildt, B., and Holstrom, B. 1978. Intracellular amino acids and energy metabolism in catabolic patients with regard to muscle tissue. In: Advances in Parenteral Nutrition, ed. I. Johnston, pp. 85–104. Lancaster: M.T.P. Press.

20. Heymsfield, S. B., McManus, C., Smith, J., Stevens, V., and Nixon, D. W. 1982. Anthropometric measurement of muscle mass: revised equations for calculating bone-free arm muscle area. Am. J. Clin. Nutr. 36:680–90.

21. Forbes, G. B., Brown, M. R., and Griffiths, H. J. L. 1988. Arm muscle plus bone area: anthropometry and CAT scan compared. Am. J. Clin. Nutr. 47:929–31.

22. Katch, F. I., and Spiak, D. L. 1984. Validity of the Mellits and Cheek method for body-fat estimation in relation to menstrual cycle status in athletes and non-athletes below 22 percent fat. Ann. Hum. Biol. 11:389–94.

23. Katch, F. I., Behnke, A. R., and Katch, V. L. 1979. Estimation of body fat from skinfolds and surface area. Hum. Biol. 51:411–24.

24. Norgan, N. G., and Ferro-Luzzi, A. 1985. The estimation of body density in men: are general equations general? Ann. of Hum. Biol. 12:1–15.

25. Katch, V. L., Michael, E. D., Jr., and Amuchie, F. A. 1973. The use of body weight and girth measurements in predicting segmental leg volume of females. Hum. Biol. 45:293–303.

26. Frerichs, R. R., Harsha, D. W., and Berenson, G. S. 1979. Equations

for estimating percentage of body fat in children 10–14 years old. Pediat. Res. 13:170–74.

27.   Lewis, S., Haskell, W. L., Klein, H., Halpern, J., and Wood, P. D. 1975. Prediction of body composition in habitually active middle-aged men. J. Appl. Physiol. 39:221–25.

28.   Lohman, T. G. 1981. Skinfolds and body density and their relation to body fatness: a review. Hum. Biol. 53:181–225.

29.   Seltzer, C. C., Goldman, R. F., and Mayer, J. 1970. The triceps skinfold and girth assessment for predicting alterations in body composition. J. Appl. Physiol. 29:313–17.

30.   Wilmore, J. H., Girandola, R. N., and Moody, D. L. 1970. Validity of skinfold and girth assessment for predicting alterations in body composition. J. Appl. Physiol. 29:313–17.

31.   Durnin, J. V. G. A., and Womersley, J. 1974. Body fat assessed from total body density and its estimation from skinfold thickness: measurements on 481 men and women aged from 16 to 72 years. Brit. J. Nutr. 32:77–97.

32.   Siri, W. E. 1956. Body composition from fluid spaces and density: analysis of methods. University of Calif., Berkeley, Donner Lab Med. Phys. Rept. (UCRL-3349).

33.   Metropolitan Life Insurance Co. 1959. New weight standards for men and women. Stat. Bull. 140:1–4.

34.   Metropolitan Life Insurance Co. 1983. Metropolitan height and weight tables. Stat. Bull. 64:1–9.

35.   Himes, J. H., and Bouchard, C. 1985. Do the new Metropolitan Life Insurance weight-height tables correctly assess body frame and body fat relationships? Am. J. Public Health 75:1076–79.

36.   Grant, J. P. 1980. Handbook of Total Parenteral Nutrition. Philadelphia: Saunders.

37.   Garn, S. M., Pesick, S. D., and Hawthorne, V. M. 1983. The bony chest breadth as a frame size standard in nutritional assessment. Am. J. Clin. Nutr. 37:315–18.

38.   Frisancho, A. R., and Flegel, P. N. 1983. Elbow breadth as a measure of frame size for U.S. males and females. Am. J. Clin. Nutr. 37:311–14.

39.   Frisancho, A. R. 1981. New norms of upper limb fat and muscle areas for assessment of nutritional status. Am. J. Clin. Nutr. 34:2540–45.

40.   Rookus, M. A., Burema, J., Deurenberg, P., and Van Der Wiel-Wetzels, W. 1985. The impact of adjustment of a weight-height index (W/H2) for frame size on the prediction of body fatness. British J. Nutr. 54:335–42.

41.   Mueller, W. H., and Martorell, R. 1988. Reliability and accuracy of measurement. In: Anthropometric Standardization Reference Manual, ed. T. G. Lohman, A. F. Roche, and R. Martorell. Champaign, Ill.: Human Kinetics Books.

42.   Hill, G. L., Blackett, R. L., Pickford, I., Burkinshaw, L., Young, G. A.,

Warren, J. V., Schorah, C. J., and Morgan, D. B. 1977. Malnutrition in surgical patients. Lancet 1:689.

43.   Hall, J. C., O'Quigley, J., Giles, G. R., Appleton, N., and Stocks, H. 1980. Upper limb anthropometry: the value of measurement variance studies. Am. J. Clin. Nutr. 33:1846–51.

44.   Zerfas, A. J. 1985. Checking Continuous Measures: Manual for Anthropometry. Division of Epidemiology, School of Public Health, University of California, Los Angeles.

Chapter III

1.   Gomez, F., Galvan, R. R., Frenk, S., Munoz, J. C., Chavez, R., and Vasquez, J. 1956. Mortality in second and third degree malnutrition. J. Trop. Pediatr. 2:77–83.

2.   Waterlow, J. C., Buzina, R., Keller, W., Lane, J. M., and Nichamon, M. Z. 1977. The presentation and use of height and weight data for comparing the nutritional status of groups of children under the age of 10 years. Bulletin of the World Health Organization 55 (4): 489–98.

3.   Hubert, H. B., Feinleib, M., and McNamara, P. M. 1983. Obesity as an independent risk factor for cardiovascular disease: a 26-year follow up of participants in the Framingham Heart Study. Circulation 67:968–77.

4.   Simopoulos, A. P., and van Itallie, T. B. 1984. Body weight, health, and longevity. Ann. Int. Med. 100:285–95.

5.   Garn, S. M., Sullivan, T. V., and Hawthorne, V. M. 1988. Effects of skinfold levels on lipids and blood pressure in younger and older adults. J. Geront. 43 (6): 170–74.

6.   Harlan, W. R., Hull, A. L., Schmouder, R. P., Thompson, F. E., Larkin, F. A., and Landis, J. R. 1983. Dietary intake and cardiovascular risk factors. Part I: Blood pressure correlates. Vital and Health Statistics, series 11, no. 226. Hyattsville, Md.: National Center for Health Statistics. DHHS Publication no. (PHS) 83-1676.

7.   Heymsfield, S. B., McManus, C., Smith, J., Stevens, V., and Nixon, D. W. 1982. Anthropometric measurement of muscle mass: revised equations for calculating bone-free arm muscle area. Am. J. Clin. Nutr. 36:680–90.

Chapter IV

1.   Abraham, S., Carroll, M. D., Najjar, M. F., and Fulwood, R. 1983. Obese and overweight adults in the United States. Vital and Health Statistics, series 11, no. 230. Hyattsville, Md.: National Center for Health Statistics. DHHS Publication no. (PHS) 83-1680.

2.   Abraham, S., Johnson, C. L., and Najjar, M. F. 1979. Weight by height and age for adults 18–74 years: United States, 1971–1974. Vital and Health Statistics, series 11, no. 208. Hyattsville, Md.: Na-

tional Center for Health Statistics. DHEW publication no. (PHS) 79-1656.

3. Frisancho, A. R. 1984. New standards of weight and body composition by frame size and height for assessment of nutritional status of adults and the elderly. Am. J. Clin. Nutr. 40:808–19.

Chapter V

1. Garn, S. M. 1965. The applicability of North America growth standards in developing countries. Can. Med. Ass. J. 93:914–19.
2. Garn, S. M. 1966. Body size and its implications. In: Review of Child Development Research, vol. 2, ed. L. W. Hoffman and M. L. Hoffman, pp. 529–61. New York: Russell Sage Foundation.
3. Garn, S. M., and Rohmann, C. G. 1966. Interaction of nutrition and genetics in the timing of growth and development. Pediat. Clins. N. Am. 13:353–79.
4. Tanner, J. M., Goldstein, H., Graffar, M., Asiel, M., Karlberg, P., Prader, A., and Sempe, R. 1968. Standards for children's height at ages 3 to 9 adjusted for height of parents. Int. Pediatrics Congr., Mexico City.
5. Tanner, J. M., Goldstein, H., and Whitehouse, R. H. 1970. Standards for children's height at ages 2–9 years allowing for height of parents. Archs. Dis. Childh. 45:755–62.
6. Wingerd, J., Solomon, I. L., and Schoen, E. J. 1973. Parent-specific height standards for preadolescent children of three racial groups, with method for rapid determination. Pediatrics 52:555–66.
7. Himes, J. H., Roche, A. F., and Thissen, D. 1981. Parent-Specific Adjustments for Assessment of Recumbent Length and Stature. In: Monographs in Pediatrics, vol. 13, ed. F. Falkner, N. Kretchmer, and E. Rossi. New York: Karger.

APPENDICES

Appendix A
Anthropometric Tables for Blacks

Based on a cross-sectional sample of 6,954 subjects aged 1 to 74 years derived from the first and second National Health and Nutrition Examination Surveys (NHANES I and II) of the United States conducted during 1971–74 and 1976–80.

Means, standard deviations, and percentiles of stature (cm) by age (yrs) for Black males and females of 1 to 74 years

Age (yrs)	N	Mean	SD	Percentiles								
				5	10	15	25	50	75	85	90	95
Males												
1.0–1.9	77	82.3	5.4	74.3	76.1	77.5	79.0	81.7	86.0	87.2	89.5	94.0
2.0–2.9	139	90.7	4.7	83.5	84.8	85.8	87.2	90.1	94.2	96.0	96.8	98.0
3.0–3.9	151	99.1	5.4	90.2	93.0	94.3	95.8	98.3	102.5	104.5	106.7	108.4
4.0–4.9	151	107.1	5.7	98.1	99.6	101.3	103.5	107.7	110.7	112.4	113.7	116.7
5.0–5.9	122	114.3	5.5	106.5	107.5	108.7	110.8	113.7	118.0	120.2	122.0	123.5
6.0–6.9	60	119.7	5.5	109.3	113.0	115.6	116.3	119.7	122.9	124.7	125.8	127.6
7.0–7.9	67	125.1	6.1	114.7	117.2	119.9	121.0	125.5	128.3	130.1	132.8	133.5
8.0–8.9	49	131.8	6.3	123.7	124.4	125.1	127.4	131.4	135.4	138.4	140.7	143.9
9.0–9.9	74	135.9	5.7	126.1	129.3	129.8	131.0	135.7	139.5	142.0	143.7	144.7
10.0–10.9	60	141.4	7.8	127.5	131.0	132.2	136.1	141.5	147.5	149.8	151.3	154.4
11.0–11.9	71	147.3	7.8	132.4	135.8	140.0	143.1	148.0	153.2	154.3	155.5	158.9
12.0–12.9	71	151.3	9.4	137.3	138.8	140.4	144.4	150.5	158.2	161.3	162.4	167.8
13.0–13.9	74	159.1	9.1	144.2	148.9	150.6	153.1	159.1	165.6	167.3	168.8	173.2
14.0–14.9	68	165.8	9.3	151.2	154.9	156.3	157.9	165.5	171.5	175.2	179.6	181.8
15.0–15.9	65	170.6	6.0	162.2	163.4	164.0	165.9	170.2	175.4	177.6	178.1	180.7
16.0–16.9	66	173.7	6.8	164.2	165.6	166.7	168.9	172.6	177.6	181.5	183.1	184.5
17.0–17.9	63	175.5	6.9	165.1	167.3	168.8	170.4	174.5	180.6	183.9	185.1	187.2
18.0–24.9	254	175.8	7.0	164.1	167.2	168.6	171.1	176.5	180.7	183.3	184.3	186.3
25.0–29.9	161	175.7	7.4	163.8	166.2	168.0	170.6	176.2	181.2	183.3	184.6	186.5
30.0–34.9	121	175.9	6.4	165.6	168.1	169.2	171.5	176.5	179.8	183.1	183.8	186.4
35.0–39.9	88	175.4	7.3	164.2	165.6	167.7	171.1	175.1	179.7	182.2	184.3	189.8
40.0–44.9	89	174.8	6.2	164.0	167.1	169.0	171.3	174.6	178.4	181.2	183.7	184.8
45.0–49.9	113	175.3	8.0	164.1	166.1	167.6	170.3	174.5	181.1	184.2	185.2	187.6
50.0–54.9	105	173.7	6.1	163.5	166.8	167.7	169.3	172.8	178.3	180.5	181.1	182.8
55.0–59.9	105	173.5	6.7	162.7	164.9	165.6	168.3	174.0	178.4	180.2	181.6	184.4
60.0–64.9	126	174.1	6.5	164.1	166.3	167.0	169.6	173.8	178.1	181.6	183.1	185.4
65.0–69.9	254	170.8	6.3	159.4	162.5	164.7	166.7	170.9	175.6	177.5	178.7	180.4
70.0–74.9	186	170.9	6.9	159.6	162.4	163.7	166.5	171.5	175.0	177.0	179.0	182.1
Females												
1.0–1.9	56	81.0	4.0	73.9	75.7	77.4	78.3	81.2	83.0	84.3	87.0	87.4
2.0–2.9	118	90.0	5.1	81.5	84.6	85.1	86.5	89.8	93.2	95.0	96.7	97.9
3.0–3.9	126	98.6	4.7	92.3	93.1	94.2	95.3	98.5	101.0	102.7	103.7	105.7
4.0–4.9	147	106.6	5.1	98.4	100.0	101.3	103.1	106.6	109.8	111.9	113.9	115.0
5.0–5.9	163	113.5	5.7	103.8	105.6	107.7	110.3	113.9	117.2	119.0	120.2	122.8
6.0–6.9	72	120.3	4.7	113.2	114.6	115.2	117.0	119.7	124.0	125.3	126.4	128.7
7.0–7.9	81	125.7	6.4	115.8	118.3	119.3	121.9	126.3	130.1	132.5	134.4	135.0
8.0–8.9	54	130.7	6.8	121.3	122.1	123.8	125.7	130.5	134.5	137.9	140.1	141.3
9.0–9.9	71	137.0	6.9	127.4	128.7	129.3	131.7	136.6	141.8	143.9	144.1	148.2
10.0–10.9	62	144.1	8.3	127.9	135.4	136.5	139.2	144.7	148.0	150.9	155.0	159.1
11.0–11.9	67	149.3	7.5	135.7	139.8	140.5	144.5	149.1	154.8	155.7	158.2	161.8
12.0–12.9	72	154.5	7.3	143.2	144.7	146.7	149.4	153.9	159.8	162.0	162.7	166.1
13.0–13.9	82	159.2	5.2	151.8	152.9	153.7	155.0	159.2	162.3	164.1	165.3	168.8
14.0–14.9	79	160.2	5.7	152.4	153.6	154.7	156.3	160.1	163.5	165.8	167.8	170.5
15.0–15.9	73	163.0	7.0	149.7	154.2	156.4	159.0	162.7	167.1	168.1	170.4	176.5
16.0–16.9	54	162.8	7.5	149.2	151.9	156.6	158.3	163.4	167.3	170.8	173.0	174.7
17.0–17.9	68	162.0	5.3	154.0	155.1	156.9	158.8	161.8	165.3	167.0	169.0	169.4
18.0–24.9	474	162.6	6.5	152.6	154.8	156.2	158.4	162.5	166.5	168.8	170.7	173.6
25.0–29.9	279	162.9	5.9	154.3	155.8	157.2	158.6	163.2	166.8	169.2	170.4	172.3
30.0–34.9	237	162.6	6.2	152.4	154.9	156.1	158.5	162.6	166.5	168.8	171.1	173.1
35.0–39.9	239	163.2	6.3	153.0	155.9	157.3	159.5	163.0	167.3	169.5	171.2	175.6
40.0–44.9	232	163.4	6.4	151.6	154.5	156.9	159.7	163.8	167.3	170.1	171.2	174.6
45.0–49.9	126	161.7	6.7	151.8	153.2	154.4	157.5	160.9	166.5	168.8	170.2	171.7
50.0–54.9	136	162.1	6.3	151.8	154.3	155.0	157.6	162.0	166.8	169.3	170.3	172.3
55.0–59.9	124	160.8	7.0	149.0	150.8	153.2	156.0	161.1	165.2	168.5	169.9	172.5
60.0–64.9	153	160.1	6.7	149.0	151.9	153.4	155.7	160.4	164.3	167.0	168.3	171.0
65.0–69.9	281	159.1	5.9	149.1	151.5	153.1	155.7	158.8	162.7	165.0	166.5	168.0
70.0–74.9	198	158.4	5.8	147.9	151.1	152.9	155.1	157.9	162.1	164.6	166.1	169.6

Means, standard deviations, and percentiles of weight (kg) by age (yrs) for Black males and females of 1 to 74 years

Age (yrs)	N	Mean	SD	Percentiles								
				5	10	15	25	50	75	85	90	95
Males												
1.0–1.9	157	11.8	1.6	9.6	9.9	10.2	10.7	11.6	12.6	13.4	14.4	15.0
2.0–2.9	142	13.5	1.8	11.1	11.3	11.7	12.1	13.4	14.5	15.6	15.9	16.6
3.0–3.9	151	15.7	2.4	12.6	13.1	13.4	14.1	15.4	16.8	17.6	18.6	19.8
4.0–4.9	151	17.9	2.4	13.7	14.7	15.4	16.2	17.9	19.5	20.2	20.8	21.7
5.0–5.9	122	20.5	3.2	16.6	17.1	17.6	18.4	19.8	21.8	23.3	24.6	25.8
6.0–6.9	60	23.0	3.7	18.7	19.4	20.1	20.4	22.2	24.1	25.6	27.3	29.6
7.0–7.9	67	24.7	4.4	18.9	19.6	20.3	21.3	24.4	26.6	28.2	31.2	32.5
8.0–8.9	49	28.1	4.6	22.6	23.5	24.1	25.1	26.8	30.0	31.8	37.1	38.4
9.0–9.9	74	30.4	5.6	23.5	24.0	25.7	26.5	28.9	33.6	34.9	38.2	39.5
10.0–10.9	60	35.3	7.9	25.1	26.5	27.6	29.5	33.3	39.5	42.0	44.4	53.9
11.0–11.9	71	38.9	9.7	28.7	30.4	31.4	33.9	36.5	41.0	45.0	48.6	57.1
12.0–12.9	71	43.4	14.7	30.3	32.0	33.0	35.0	39.7	46.1	51.7	58.8	73.7
13.0–13.9	74	47.2	9.4	34.1	37.1	38.3	39.9	44.7	52.4	56.5	61.3	66.0
14.0–14.9	68	54.2	9.8	38.8	41.6	44.8	46.5	53.0	60.7	65.4	67.8	71.0
15.0–15.9	65	62.1	10.9	49.1	50.9	51.3	55.8	59.6	68.1	72.0	76.0	87.2
16.0–16.9	66	66.2	9.9	54.0	55.1	56.9	59.4	63.8	71.7	77.1	81.6	88.7
17.0–17.9	63	65.6	11.7	50.2	52.7	54.2	57.3	64.9	71.2	74.7	82.3	89.9
18.0–24.9	255	72.8	15.5	56.1	59.3	60.9	63.0	69.5	78.2	83.2	90.1	102.8
25.0–29.9	162	76.4	17.6	58.3	60.7	63.4	66.0	71.2	82.4	90.1	94.2	106.3
30.0–34.9	121	80.5	17.9	59.3	64.8	66.9	69.6	76.2	88.7	93.7	99.3	106.7
35.0–39.9	88	81.2	15.9	59.6	60.9	63.2	66.2	83.0	89.3	97.3	100.6	113.3
40.0–44.9	90	79.7	15.3	58.3	60.8	62.0	68.1	78.9	90.3	96.2	98.4	104.4
45.0–49.9	113	81.0	15.9	59.9	62.6	65.4	69.8	78.4	91.7	98.3	101.3	110.3
50.0–54.9	105	79.6	15.8	58.3	61.7	63.2	66.8	77.7	90.5	100.7	105.1	107.0
55.0–59.9	105	79.4	17.0	56.8	60.9	64.0	67.1	76.9	85.7	96.7	102.3	111.8
60.0–64.9	126	77.5	14.5	56.6	60.9	62.9	68.4	76.4	85.4	89.6	94.8	108.2
65.0–69.9	254	73.5	14.5	53.5	56.6	58.5	62.9	71.1	83.3	90.8	94.9	100.6
70.0–74.9	186	72.1	14.9	54.2	56.1	57.3	60.2	70.0	80.8	87.0	90.6	100.9
Females												
1.0–1.9	134	10.9	1.5	8.6	9.1	9.6	10.0	10.8	11.7	12.3	12.8	13.5
2.0–2.9	119	13.0	1.8	10.3	10.7	11.2	11.9	12.8	13.9	14.5	15.2	16.2
3.0–3.9	128	15.0	2.2	11.8	12.6	13.0	13.7	14.7	16.1	17.2	17.6	18.5
4.0–4.9	147	17.7	3.0	13.7	14.3	15.0	16.0	17.2	19.2	20.8	21.2	22.4
5.0–5.9	163	20.0	3.8	15.0	16.1	16.7	17.5	19.5	21.9	23.5	24.9	26.0
6.0–6.9	72	22.4	3.7	18.1	18.8	19.3	19.7	21.4	24.1	25.5	26.3	27.6
7.0–7.9	81	25.0	4.2	19.3	20.3	21.1	22.0	24.8	26.9	28.8	29.9	31.3
8.0–8.9	54	27.6	5.1	21.9	22.4	22.7	23.6	26.4	29.9	33.4	34.4	37.2
9.0–9.9	71	31.5	6.4	23.7	24.4	25.7	26.3	30.3	35.5	39.3	41.6	43.4
10.0–10.9	62	38.3	10.8	24.7	27.7	29.0	31.3	35.3	43.4	49.3	54.8	61.1
11.0–11.9	67	43.5	12.9	29.7	31.4	32.3	34.9	40.1	46.9	54.5	59.1	72.3
12.0–12.9	72	48.3	13.2	31.1	32.7	33.4	38.3	47.5	56.5	61.7	64.1	69.3
13.0–13.9	82	52.9	10.6	39.3	40.3	44.3	46.1	50.7	58.8	62.9	67.9	78.5
14.0–14.9	79	54.8	13.5	39.2	40.8	42.6	45.8	50.6	60.6	68.4	74.4	85.0
15.0–15.9	73	58.3	13.9	44.4	46.6	47.8	49.0	54.0	60.6	67.7	79.4	91.1
16.0–16.9	54	62.4	14.1	46.8	48.3	51.4	53.9	57.0	67.3	73.8	84.6	92.3
17.0–17.9	68	59.9	13.9	41.6	45.8	47.8	51.4	56.7	64.3	69.4	84.0	89.1
18.0–24.9	474	63.2	15.1	45.8	48.5	50.3	52.8	60.2	70.0	76.9	82.3	92.9
25.0–29.9	279	67.8	15.7	48.5	50.1	52.5	56.3	64.2	76.9	85.7	90.6	102.3
30.0–34.9	237	72.1	19.1	46.6	50.3	54.2	59.6	69.3	81.1	86.8	95.6	105.7
35.0–39.9	239	75.6	18.9	50.2	53.1	56.6	61.8	71.5	86.4	95.5	103.1	112.6
40.0–44.9	232	75.9	18.5	50.7	55.3	58.7	63.5	73.5	85.3	93.9	100.1	106.5
45.0–49.9	126	75.4	20.8	50.1	53.6	56.9	60.8	73.1	81.2	89.5	98.7	111.0
50.0–54.9	136	77.6	18.1	51.6	56.8	60.7	64.4	74.8	86.5	95.0	101.9	113.3
55.0–59.9	124	78.7	22.4	52.0	56.7	60.2	65.3	73.9	86.6	95.6	104.0	134.3
60.0–64.9	153	74.1	16.1	51.9	55.8	57.4	63.3	71.7	83.0	90.7	95.8	102.4
65.0–69.9	282	71.8	14.8	48.8	53.5	57.8	61.9	70.5	81.1	87.3	90.7	98.4
70.0–74.9	198	69.5	15.8	46.6	50.2	52.6	60.2	67.4	77.2	84.5	89.7	99.1

Means, standard deviations, and percentiles of weight (kg) by height (cm) for Black males of 2 to 74 years

Height (cm)	N	Mean	SD	Percentiles								
				5	10	15	25	50	75	85	90	95
Boys: 2 to 11 years												
84–086	25	12.3	1.2	10.9	11.1	11.1	11.3	11.9	13.0	13.6	13.7	14.4
87–089	40	12.8	1.0	11.3	11.6	11.6	12.0	12.7	13.5	13.9	14.2	14.7
90–092	38	13.5	1.3	11.6	12.0	12.3	12.7	13.3	14.4	14.9	15.9	16.1
93–095	49	14.3	1.2	12.3	13.0	13.3	13.5	14.2	15.0	15.6	15.8	16.6
96–098	69	15.1	1.6	13.4	13.6	13.7	14.1	14.9	15.6	16.0	16.8	17.3
99–101	45	15.9	1.2	13.5	14.5	14.7	15.3	15.9	16.6	17.1	17.2	18.0
102–104	50	16.7	1.5	14.4	15.0	15.4	15.9	16.6	17.5	17.8	18.0	18.9
105–107	52	17.5	1.3	15.4	15.9	16.1	16.4	17.5	18.4	19.0	19.4	19.8
108–110	60	18.8	1.3	17.0	17.2	17.6	17.8	18.8	19.6	20.0	20.2	20.5
111–113	59	19.8	2.0	16.2	17.6	18.1	18.6	19.4	20.8	21.5	22.6	24.9
114–116	48	21.1	2.7	18.8	19.0	19.0	19.5	20.5	21.7	22.2	22.9	23.6
117–119	40	21.3	1.8	18.8	19.3	19.4	20.2	21.0	22.2	23.4	24.0	24.3
120–122	43	22.9	2.6	19.8	20.2	20.8	21.2	22.4	23.8	25.4	25.6	26.4
123–125	37	25.5	3.1	22.0	23.1	23.3	23.5	24.6	26.5	27.2	28.3	32.5
126–128	39	26.0	2.7	22.6	23.6	23.7	24.3	25.4	26.5	29.3	31.8	31.9
129–131	39	27.0	2.4	22.7	23.6	24.3	25.1	26.9	28.7	29.4	30.0	30.6
132–134	31	28.8	3.6	24.9	25.4	25.7	26.6	28.0	30.5	31.2	32.4	34.6
135–137	32	30.3	4.0	25.4	26.5	26.8	27.6	29.5	32.1	33.7	34.5	39.0
138–140	25	33.1	5.2	28.7	28.8	29.4	30.5	32.2	33.8	37.0	37.1	39.9
141–143	32	34.7	4.4	30.0	30.5	31.1	31.6	33.6	35.3	38.2	39.1	46.9
144–146	23	36.7	2.8	33.4	33.7	33.9	35.1	35.9	39.0	39.7	39.9	40.0
147–149	23	41.0	7.0	33.9	34.3	34.9	36.2	38.6	44.4	47.2	47.3	58.2
Boys: 12 to 17 years												
150–152	19	41.2	4.9	36.2	36.5	37.2	38.3	39.3	42.5	48.6	49.3	54.5
153–155	22	43.7	5.5	38.8	39.1	39.2	39.7	42.2	44.4	46.5	51.7	51.9
156–158	24	47.5	8.9	40.6	40.6	40.7	42.2	43.8	49.1	54.2	59.9	64.6
159–161	28	47.9	5.6	40.3	41.6	42.8	44.7	45.9	49.8	52.5	56.1	60.9
162–164	34	55.9	8.3	44.2	45.5	48.3	51.1	56.7	58.8	59.5	63.3	69.2
165–167	52	56.8	8.1	46.7	49.7	50.3	50.9	55.1	60.7	62.9	66.0	69.6
168–170	42	62.6	13.2	50.0	51.3	51.6	54.3	59.4	66.2	69.8	74.2	89.9
171–173	41	62.1	6.9	51.0	54.2	55.3	56.9	62.1	67.9	69.6	71.4	73.7
174–176	34	67.3	12.0	51.8	54.0	56.5	60.3	64.4	72.0	82.3	87.9	90.8
177–179	29	66.8	7.3	54.8	55.0	59.6	60.9	67.9	71.8	74.7	75.5	78.7
Males: 18 to 74 years												
156–158	21	64.1	12.3	48.6	51.4	53.0	54.7	64.5	69.6	74.7	77.3	88.2
159–161	39	64.2	14.2	49.1	52.4	53.6	56.3	63.8	68.3	71.3	76.9	88.0
162–164	92	67.3	10.9	50.2	55.1	57.0	59.8	65.9	73.8	78.4	82.8	90.0
165–167	156	70.6	13.6	53.3	55.2	58.1	61.0	68.8	76.9	83.9	88.0	92.4
168–170	221	71.6	12.2	54.0	56.6	58.7	61.9	70.6	78.2	84.4	87.9	92.9
171–173	256	74.6	14.9	56.4	59.6	61.0	64.8	71.1	83.0	87.9	93.0	100.5
174–176	268	77.9	15.2	58.4	61.1	63.7	66.9	75.4	85.4	92.3	97.3	105.9
177–179	217	79.7	16.0	60.9	62.6	64.8	68.0	78.2	88.6	94.5	100.2	107.8
180–182	155	84.1	16.6	62.5	65.0	67.3	72.6	82.5	92.8	99.9	105.9	111.8
183–185	103	84.0	16.0	62.5	67.3	68.9	72.7	80.5	94.5	101.6	106.9	111.8
186–188	39	90.2	19.1	64.9	70.0	70.4	76.0	88.0	97.5	109.8	118.2	127.3

Appendix A: Table 4.

Means, standard deviations, and percentiles of weight (kg) by height (cm) for Black females of 2 to 74 years

Height (cm)	N	Mean	SD	Percentiles								
				5	10	15	25	50	75	85	90	95
Girls: 2 to 10 years												
84–086	23	11.9	1.0	10.5	10.7	10.7	10.8	12.1	12.7	12.7	12.9	13.6
87–089	29	12.6	1.8	10.1	10.4	11.2	11.4	12.4	13.5	13.8	14.6	15.1
90–092	32	13.1	1.1	11.3	11.6	11.7	12.1	13.5	13.8	14.1	14.4	14.9
93–095	50	13.7	1.1	11.8	12.0	12.8	13.1	13.7	14.5	14.9	14.9	15.3
96–098	50	14.7	1.4	12.9	13.1	13.5	13.7	14.7	15.4	16.1	16.8	17.0
99–101	55	15.6	1.9	12.6	13.8	13.9	14.3	15.6	17.1	17.6	17.6	18.6
102–104	55	16.2	1.9	13.5	14.2	14.3	14.6	16.2	17.0	18.3	18.8	20.4
105–107	52	16.9	1.4	15.0	15.0	15.5	16.1	16.9	17.7	18.1	18.7	19.2
108–110	57	18.5	1.8	16.1	16.6	16.9	17.2	18.3	19.7	20.5	21.1	21.7
111–113	55	19.4	2.2	16.8	17.1	17.2	17.8	19.2	20.5	21.2	21.7	23.5
114–116	62	20.5	2.3	17.8	18.3	18.7	19.0	20.2	21.8	22.4	23.7	24.9
117–119	55	22.3	3.5	18.8	19.3	19.5	20.0	21.3	23.4	24.8	25.3	27.0
120–122	41	22.7	2.3	20.2	20.3	20.8	21.4	22.3	23.3	23.9	25.7	27.0
123–125	44	24.8	2.7	21.3	22.3	22.3	22.8	24.4	25.6	26.4	27.1	29.0
126–128	45	25.3	2.9	21.2	22.7	23.0	23.5	24.8	26.3	27.1	28.5	29.4
129–131	30	27.0	3.2	23.0	23.6	24.4	25.2	25.8	28.1	29.9	31.3	34.4
132–134	33	29.0	3.6	25.4	25.9	26.2	26.8	27.7	29.8	32.5	33.3	39.1
135–137	28	32.9	6.5	24.7	25.2	28.5	28.8	31.0	34.1	41.6	44.9	46.5
138–140	22	32.5	3.4	28.3	28.8	29.0	30.3	32.5	34.4	34.6	36.6	38.8
141–143	20	35.5	6.0	28.7	29.6	29.8	31.1	33.4	36.5	41.7	43.4	47.6
144–146	20	38.7	7.9	30.4	30.7	31.0	31.9	36.2	42.9	43.8	44.2	45.3
Girls: 11 to 17 years												
147–149	29	44.5	14.3	32.7	33.8	34.3	36.3	40.4	49.4	54.3	56.4	59.2
150–152	39	48.9	11.4	33.4	35.3	38.0	41.0	46.4	55.3	61.1	66.4	78.8
153–155	55	51.0	10.8	38.6	39.3	40.1	45.4	49.4	54.1	56.6	62.5	78.7
156–158	74	52.8	12.8	39.3	39.8	40.8	45.0	49.0	56.7	63.4	72.3	84.6
159–161	87	56.0	12.8	41.6	44.3	45.8	48.2	53.3	59.4	62.9	71.4	86.0
162–164	68	59.6	12.2	46.4	47.5	48.6	50.5	56.9	64.3	69.4	76.4	82.6
165–167	58	59.7	11.2	46.5	48.9	50.3	52.8	57.9	61.5	67.7	73.3	91.1
168–170	22	63.3	13.8	48.0	49.6	50.6	54.8	58.2	68.4	73.4	78.5	92.3
Females: 18 to 74 years												
144–146	24	58.1	15.9	42.2	44.3	44.9	46.0	50.3	66.6	82.0	82.5	85.0
147–149	71	63.9	14.7	40.8	45.0	48.8	53.1	62.7	71.5	77.8	81.5	90.3
150–152	113	65.4	13.6	44.3	48.9	51.3	54.9	65.4	73.5	78.3	80.2	86.6
153–155	222	68.3	15.7	46.8	49.9	52.0	56.9	67.3	77.1	83.2	88.1	97.1
156–158	414	69.3	18.1	46.9	49.8	51.8	57.1	66.6	77.8	86.1	90.8	101.5
159–161	441	69.5	17.0	47.2	50.2	53.8	57.9	66.6	78.0	86.2	90.7	98.9
162–164	437	72.5	17.2	49.2	52.2	55.3	60.3	69.7	82.8	89.5	94.9	102.3
165–167	348	73.2	18.5	50.8	53.2	56.3	60.4	70.0	81.6	91.1	95.9	108.4
168–170	220	76.5	18.8	51.9	55.3	57.8	60.7	74.2	87.9	96.0	101.6	108.8
171–173	101	78.0	18.4	55.7	58.5	60.5	64.2	75.4	85.7	93.9	99.8	113.1
174–176	53	80.7	22.4	56.8	60.9	62.8	66.7	75.6	87.5	95.5	98.2	112.7

Means, standard deviations, and percentiles of Body mass index (w/s^2) by age (yrs) for Black males and females of 1 to 74 years

Age (yrs)	N	Mean	SD	Percentiles								
				5	10	15	25	50	75	85	90	95
Males												
1.0–1.9	77	17.4	1.8	14.8	15.4	15.8	16.4	17.3	18.2	19.0	19.4	20.2
2.0–2.9	139	16.4	1.4	14.5	14.8	15.0	15.4	16.2	17.2	17.9	18.6	19.0
3.0–3.9	151	15.9	1.4	13.9	14.6	14.8	15.1	15.7	16.5	16.9	17.2	18.1
4.0–4.9	151	15.5	1.3	13.6	13.9	14.3	14.8	15.5	16.3	16.8	17.0	17.4
5.0–5.9	122	15.6	1.6	13.8	14.0	14.3	14.7	15.6	16.3	16.7	17.1	17.6
6.0–6.9	60	16.1	2.2	13.9	14.3	14.4	14.9	15.3	16.4	17.4	18.1	20.1
7.0–7.9	67	15.7	1.9	13.7	13.9	14.1	14.6	15.3	16.3	17.0	17.4	19.6
8.0–8.9	49	16.1	1.7	13.8	14.3	14.4	14.8	15.7	17.4	18.0	18.7	19.3
9.0–9.9	74	16.4	2.1	13.7	14.1	14.6	15.2	16.0	17.1	18.0	18.6	20.6
10.0–10.9	60	17.5	2.8	14.9	15.1	15.2	15.8	16.8	18.0	19.3	20.1	22.7
11.0–11.9	71	17.7	3.0	14.8	15.3	15.7	16.3	16.9	18.0	19.7	21.7	24.3
12.0–12.9	71	18.6	4.1	15.4	15.7	15.9	16.5	17.4	18.8	21.7	23.2	25.1
13.0–13.9	74	18.5	2.4	15.6	16.3	16.4	16.7	17.7	19.7	21.4	21.9	23.7
14.0–14.9	68	19.6	2.6	16.5	16.8	17.2	17.9	18.9	21.3	21.8	22.7	23.8
15.0–15.9	65	21.3	3.2	17.4	17.7	18.0	19.1	20.9	22.4	23.9	24.8	26.4
16.0–16.9	66	21.9	3.0	18.9	19.0	19.3	19.6	21.2	23.1	24.5	25.5	27.3
17.0–17.9	63	21.3	3.2	16.8	18.0	18.2	19.3	20.7	22.7	24.0	25.7	27.4
18.0–24.9	254	23.5	4.6	19.0	19.4	19.9	20.6	22.5	25.0	26.6	27.8	31.6
25.0–29.9	161	24.7	5.5	19.1	19.7	20.2	21.0	23.8	26.7	28.1	29.9	34.3
30.0–34.9	121	26.0	5.5	19.6	20.7	21.4	22.8	25.1	28.1	29.4	30.7	34.7
35.0–39.9	88	26.4	4.9	19.3	20.5	21.6	23.0	26.4	28.9	30.7	32.1	34.1
40.0–44.9	89	26.2	4.7	18.9	20.1	21.5	22.6	26.2	29.2	31.0	32.0	32.9
45.0–49.9	113	26.4	5.0	20.1	21.4	21.7	22.8	25.3	29.2	32.5	33.3	35.0
50.0–54.9	105	26.3	4.7	19.3	20.0	21.1	22.4	26.0	29.6	32.0	32.6	34.6
55.0–59.9	105	26.3	5.1	19.7	21.0	22.0	22.6	25.8	28.2	31.3	33.0	35.3
60.0–64.9	126	25.5	4.2	19.3	20.2	21.1	22.1	25.4	27.8	30.1	31.4	33.7
65.0–69.9	254	25.1	4.6	18.9	20.1	20.7	21.6	24.4	28.3	30.4	31.8	33.7
70.0–74.9	186	24.6	4.4	18.6	19.4	20.2	21.5	24.0	27.2	28.9	30.3	33.4
Females												
1.0–1.9	56	16.8	1.4	14.6	15.2	15.4	15.8	16.5	17.6	18.2	18.5	19.6
2.0–2.9	118	16.1	1.8	13.7	14.1	14.6	14.9	16.1	17.0	17.5	18.1	18.5
3.0–3.9	126	15.4	1.5	13.2	13.7	14.1	14.4	15.2	16.2	17.1	17.7	17.9
4.0–4.9	147	15.5	1.7	13.3	13.6	13.8	14.3	15.4	16.3	17.1	17.7	18.6
5.0–5.9	163	15.4	2.0	13.2	13.5	13.8	14.2	15.2	16.3	16.9	17.6	18.8
6.0–6.9	72	15.4	1.8	13.6	13.9	14.0	14.2	14.8	15.9	16.5	17.0	18.5
7.0–7.9	81	15.7	1.7	13.7	14.2	14.3	14.7	15.5	16.4	17.0	17.2	18.7
8.0–8.9	54	16.1	2.1	13.7	13.9	14.5	14.8	15.5	16.9	17.8	19.8	21.1
9.0–9.9	71	16.7	2.7	13.9	14.5	14.7	14.9	15.7	17.7	18.9	20.3	23.0
10.0–10.9	62	18.2	3.9	14.3	14.4	15.0	15.7	16.9	20.2	22.2	24.0	25.2
11.0–11.9	67	19.3	4.6	14.8	15.3	15.6	16.2	18.3	21.2	22.2	24.3	28.0
12.0–12.9	72	20.1	4.9	14.6	15.1	15.4	16.1	19.2	21.8	26.6	27.0	29.9
13.0–13.9	82	20.9	4.0	16.2	16.5	17.2	18.3	19.9	23.0	24.2	26.0	28.6
14.0–14.9	79	21.3	4.7	15.8	16.4	17.1	17.8	20.2	23.4	25.4	28.1	29.9
15.0–15.9	73	21.9	4.8	16.7	17.6	18.1	18.9	20.7	22.8	25.3	29.1	35.0
16.0–16.9	54	23.5	5.0	18.5	19.0	19.5	20.1	22.4	25.3	26.8	30.1	35.7
17.0–17.9	68	22.8	5.4	16.9	17.6	18.7	19.5	21.2	23.9	25.9	30.1	34.0
18.0–24.9	474	23.9	5.6	17.5	18.5	19.1	20.3	22.7	25.7	29.0	31.4	35.0
25.0–29.9	279	25.6	6.0	18.4	19.2	19.9	21.3	24.3	28.5	31.8	34.2	38.4
30.0–34.9	237	27.3	7.1	18.2	19.5	20.6	22.0	26.0	30.7	33.8	35.4	40.9
35.0–39.9	239	28.4	6.8	18.8	19.9	21.3	23.8	27.0	32.0	34.9	38.2	41.6
40.0–44.9	232	28.4	6.4	19.8	21.2	22.2	24.0	27.5	31.9	34.3	36.5	40.0
45.0–49.9	126	28.9	8.2	20.3	21.6	22.1	23.8	27.1	31.6	34.2	36.3	44.3
50.0–54.9	136	29.5	6.6	18.9	21.3	22.8	25.3	29.2	32.8	35.2	37.6	43.0
55.0–59.9	124	30.4	8.2	19.1	21.6	23.3	25.4	29.4	33.6	37.0	40.3	48.6
60.0–64.9	153	28.9	6.1	19.9	22.5	23.4	25.0	28.1	32.2	35.0	36.7	41.0
65.0–69.9	281	28.4	5.8	19.4	21.4	22.7	24.5	27.9	32.6	34.8	35.7	37.5
70.0–74.9	198	27.6	5.9	19.2	20.8	22.2	23.7	27.1	30.3	32.8	34.2	39.8

Means, standard deviations, and percentiles of sitting height (cm) by age (yrs) for Black males and females of 2 to 74 years

Age (yrs)	N	Mean	SD	Percentiles								
				5	10	15	25	50	75	85	90	95
Males												
2.0–2.9	96	52.7	2.5	48.4	50.0	50.0	51.0	52.1	54.0	55.0	56.0	58.0
3.0–3.9	151	55.5	3.3	50.0	52.0	52.1	53.5	55.6	57.5	58.2	60.0	61.7
4.0–4.9	151	58.5	2.8	54.0	55.0	55.8	56.8	58.5	60.1	61.6	62.0	63.1
5.0–5.9	121	61.5	2.9	57.3	58.0	59.0	59.4	61.0	63.0	64.2	65.6	66.0
6.0–6.9	60	63.9	2.9	58.4	60.0	60.6	61.6	64.0	65.2	67.1	67.8	69.0
7.0–7.9	67	65.8	2.9	60.7	62.1	63.0	64.0	66.0	67.8	68.2	69.0	71.0
8.0–8.9	49	68.3	2.8	64.3	65.0	65.4	66.0	68.2	69.9	71.2	72.0	73.0
9.0–9.9	74	69.8	3.0	64.8	66.0	67.0	68.0	69.0	71.9	73.1	74.0	74.6
10.0–10.9	60	72.1	3.5	66.7	67.0	68.0	69.0	72.0	75.0	76.0	76.7	77.0
11.0–11.9	71	74.2	3.8	68.0	69.0	71.0	71.9	74.5	76.9	78.2	79.0	80.4
12.0–12.9	71	75.9	4.8	69.7	70.0	71.0	72.1	75.4	79.1	81.0	82.0	85.3
13.0–13.9	74	79.8	4.9	72.0	73.6	75.0	76.1	79.7	83.1	84.8	85.6	88.5
14.0–14.9	68	82.8	4.6	75.5	76.3	77.4	79.9	81.9	86.3	88.2	89.0	90.4
15.0–15.9	65	85.4	3.6	79.7	81.0	81.5	82.7	85.3	87.4	89.6	90.0	91.1
16.0–16.9	66	87.5	3.3	83.0	83.6	84.4	85.2	87.0	90.2	90.9	91.5	92.3
17.0–17.9	63	88.3	3.9	80.9	83.4	84.4	86.0	88.6	91.5	92.4	92.9	94.4
18.0–24.9	254	89.0	3.6	83.0	84.4	85.6	86.7	89.0	91.2	92.4	93.0	94.7
25.0–29.9	161	89.9	3.5	84.6	85.7	86.0	87.5	89.8	92.5	93.5	94.3	95.6
30.0–34.9	120	90.1	3.4	84.4	86.0	86.7	87.9	90.1	92.4	93.5	94.3	95.5
35.0–39.9	88	89.7	3.6	84.0	85.5	86.4	87.1	89.6	92.5	94.1	94.8	95.5
40.0–44.9	90	89.0	3.8	81.8	83.6	85.4	86.6	89.6	91.4	92.8	93.4	94.0
45.0–49.9	113	89.3	3.6	83.7	84.6	85.5	86.6	89.4	91.7	93.1	94.3	94.7
50.0–54.9	104	88.5	3.4	83.5	84.2	85.0	86.2	88.6	90.8	92.1	92.7	94.2
55.0–59.9	104	88.5	3.6	82.9	83.5	84.5	85.5	88.4	90.8	92.3	92.7	94.0
60.0–64.9	124	88.8	3.3	84.2	85.0	85.5	86.4	88.3	90.7	92.7	93.5	95.0
65.0–69.9	254	86.6	3.2	81.3	82.8	83.4	84.5	86.4	88.7	89.9	91.1	92.0
70.0–74.9	186	86.2	3.9	79.5	81.0	82.2	83.4	86.4	89.0	90.3	91.0	92.2
Females												
2.0–2.9	81	51.7	2.8	47.0	48.0	49.0	49.8	52.0	54.0	54.9	55.0	55.9
3.0–3.9	126	54.6	2.4	51.0	51.6	52.2	53.0	54.9	56.0	57.0	57.0	58.0
4.0–4.9	146	58.0	2.8	53.0	54.7	55.0	56.0	58.0	60.0	61.0	61.8	63.0
5.0–5.9	162	60.8	3.1	55.4	56.0	58.0	59.0	61.0	63.0	63.9	64.3	66.0
6.0–6.9	72	63.2	2.7	58.0	59.9	60.6	61.5	63.0	65.0	66.0	66.2	67.8
7.0–7.9	81	65.4	3.2	60.7	61.4	62.1	63.3	65.3	67.3	68.7	69.0	70.0
8.0–8.9	54	67.8	3.3	62.2	64.0	64.7	65.5	67.4	70.5	71.0	71.3	73.7
9.0–9.9	71	69.8	3.4	64.5	65.3	66.3	68.0	70.0	72.0	73.0	74.0	75.6
10.0–10.9	62	73.2	4.2	65.4	68.0	70.0	70.6	73.0	75.0	77.4	80.0	81.2
11.0–11.9	67	75.7	4.3	69.0	70.0	71.4	72.3	75.0	79.4	80.2	81.2	82.8
12.0–12.9	72	78.0	4.2	71.5	72.6	73.0	74.2	78.6	80.7	82.1	83.4	85.5
13.0–13.9	82	80.8	3.3	75.7	76.2	77.0	78.2	80.5	83.6	84.5	85.2	85.5
14.0–14.9	79	81.7	3.1	76.1	77.8	78.6	79.4	81.8	84.0	85.1	85.8	87.2
15.0–15.9	73	83.4	3.1	77.8	79.1	80.6	81.8	83.5	85.5	86.6	87.5	88.4
16.0–16.9	54	84.0	3.3	77.4	79.5	80.2	81.8	84.0	86.7	87.2	88.0	88.9
17.0–17.9	68	83.2	3.2	78.4	79.2	80.4	81.0	83.0	85.1	86.3	87.3	88.4
18.0–24.9	474	83.7	3.4	78.3	79.6	80.2	81.5	83.5	85.9	87.1	87.9	89.4
25.0–29.9	279	84.3	3.0	79.5	80.3	81.0	82.2	84.2	86.5	87.7	88.2	88.9
30.0–34.9	237	84.4	3.3	78.6	80.3	80.8	82.1	84.5	86.2	87.7	88.6	89.6
35.0–39.9	238	84.9	3.4	79.1	80.6	81.4	82.6	85.0	87.4	88.4	89.4	90.3
40.0–44.9	232	84.7	3.3	79.7	80.3	81.0	82.2	84.7	87.0	88.0	88.7	90.0
45.0–49.9	125	84.0	3.3	78.4	79.1	80.5	82.2	84.2	86.2	87.2	88.0	89.0
50.0–54.9	136	84.1	3.4	79.0	79.8	80.8	82.3	84.1	86.2	87.6	88.7	90.4
55.0–59.9	124	82.9	3.5	77.5	78.4	79.2	80.2	82.9	85.2	86.4	87.3	88.8
60.0–64.9	152	82.7	3.0	76.9	78.8	79.5	80.3	83.0	84.9	85.9	86.4	87.4
65.0–69.9	281	81.4	3.3	76.4	77.2	77.9	79.0	81.6	83.6	84.9	85.5	86.7
70.0–74.9	198	80.6	3.1	75.5	76.9	77.6	78.8	80.7	82.6	83.4	84.3	85.7

Means, standard deviations, and percentiles of sitting height index (sitting height / stature x 100) (cm) by age (yrs) for Black males and females of 2 to 74 years

Age (yrs)	N	Mean	SD	Percentiles								
				5	10	15	25	50	75	85	90	95
Males												
2.0–2.9	95	58.1	1.9	54.9	55.8	56.1	56.9	57.9	59.4	60.0	60.3	60.8
3.0–3.9	151	56.1	2.2	53.2	54.2	54.5	55.1	56.1	57.0	57.6	58.0	58.8
4.0–4.9	151	54.7	1.7	51.6	52.5	53.2	53.6	54.7	55.7	56.2	56.5	57.1
5.0–5.9	121	53.9	1.6	51.6	52.3	52.4	52.8	53.7	54.8	55.5	55.8	56.5
6.0–6.9	60	53.4	1.8	51.3	51.6	52.1	52.4	53.0	53.9	54.5	55.0	55.3
7.0–7.9	67	52.6	1.2	50.9	51.2	51.6	51.9	52.6	53.3	53.9	54.3	54.8
8.0–8.9	49	51.9	1.3	49.5	50.2	50.7	51.0	51.8	52.8	53.4	53.6	54.3
9.0–9.9	74	51.4	1.5	48.7	49.6	49.8	50.4	51.5	52.4	52.6	52.9	53.9
10.0–10.9	60	51.0	1.7	48.5	49.0	49.2	49.6	50.9	52.2	52.8	53.5	53.7
11.0–11.9	71	50.4	1.3	48.3	48.8	49.2	49.7	50.5	51.1	51.5	51.8	52.7
12.0–12.9	71	50.2	1.5	48.0	48.5	49.0	49.3	50.0	51.0	51.7	51.9	52.5
13.0–13.9	74	50.2	1.3	48.0	48.5	48.9	49.5	50.2	50.9	51.2	51.6	52.0
14.0–14.9	68	49.9	1.6	46.9	47.7	48.6	49.1	49.9	50.8	51.4	51.7	52.7
15.0–15.9	65	50.0	1.4	47.9	48.1	48.6	49.0	49.9	51.1	51.7	51.9	52.4
16.0–16.9	66	50.4	1.3	48.8	49.0	49.3	49.4	50.0	51.3	51.6	51.9	53.1
17.0–17.9	63	50.3	1.4	47.9	49.1	49.3	49.6	50.3	51.1	51.6	51.9	52.2
18.0–24.9	254	50.6	1.4	48.5	48.8	49.2	49.7	50.6	51.5	52.2	52.4	53.1
25.0–29.9	160	51.1	1.4	48.9	49.3	49.7	50.1	51.2	52.0	52.5	52.8	53.5
30.0–34.9	120	51.2	1.3	49.1	49.5	49.8	50.2	51.2	52.2	52.6	52.9	53.1
35.0–39.9	88	51.2	1.4	48.5	49.6	49.7	50.3	51.2	52.2	52.5	52.7	53.1
40.0–44.9	89	51.0	1.5	48.5	49.0	49.2	50.4	51.0	52.1	52.4	52.7	53.2
45.0–49.9	113	51.0	1.5	48.6	49.1	49.6	50.1	50.8	51.8	52.6	53.0	53.6
50.0–54.9	104	51.0	1.4	48.6	49.6	49.7	50.2	50.9	51.9	52.3	52.3	53.1
55.0–59.9	104	51.0	1.3	49.3	49.6	49.8	50.1	51.1	51.8	52.2	52.7	52.9
60.0–64.9	124	51.1	1.3	48.9	49.3	49.6	50.1	51.1	52.0	52.3	52.6	53.0
65.0–69.9	254	50.7	1.5	48.2	48.8	49.3	49.8	50.7	51.7	52.2	52.6	53.0
70.0–74.9	186	50.5	1.7	47.7	48.7	49.1	49.5	50.4	51.5	51.9	52.4	53.1
Females												
2.0–2.9	81	57.2	2.0	54.4	54.7	55.3	56.0	57.4	58.2	59.2	59.7	60.0
3.0–3.9	126	55.5	1.6	53.0	53.4	54.0	54.4	55.6	56.5	56.9	57.4	57.7
4.0–4.9	146	54.4	1.4	52.1	52.7	53.1	53.6	54.3	55.4	55.8	56.2	56.6
5.0–5.9	162	53.6	1.5	51.4	51.8	52.2	52.6	53.4	54.5	55.0	55.5	56.0
6.0–6.9	72	52.5	1.4	49.7	50.5	51.0	51.5	52.7	53.5	53.9	54.0	54.7
7.0–7.9	81	52.1	1.4	50.2	50.3	50.6	51.1	52.0	52.9	53.4	53.9	54.6
8.0–8.9	54	51.9	2.1	49.8	50.2	50.7	50.9	51.7	52.5	52.9	53.5	53.9
9.0–9.9	71	51.0	1.4	48.5	49.3	49.4	49.8	51.0	52.1	52.5	52.8	53.1
10.0–10.9	62	50.8	1.1	49.1	49.4	49.8	50.2	50.7	51.5	51.7	51.9	52.3
11.0–11.9	67	50.7	1.4	48.4	48.6	49.3	49.7	50.6	51.7	52.1	52.8	52.9
12.0–12.9	72	50.5	1.5	48.1	48.7	49.1	49.4	50.3	51.4	52.3	52.4	53.1
13.0–13.9	82	50.7	1.2	48.6	49.3	49.5	49.9	50.7	51.7	52.1	52.4	52.7
14.0–14.9	79	51.0	1.5	48.6	48.9	49.1	50.2	51.1	51.8	52.3	52.9	53.7
15.0–15.9	73	51.2	1.6	48.9	49.3	49.5	50.2	51.3	52.2	52.7	52.9	53.5
16.0–16.9	54	51.6	1.6	49.1	50.2	50.3	50.5	51.6	52.4	52.9	53.4	54.1
17.0–17.9	68	51.4	1.5	49.5	49.6	49.9	50.2	51.4	52.4	53.0	53.1	54.1
18.0–24.9	474	51.5	1.4	49.1	49.6	50.1	50.6	51.6	52.4	52.9	53.2	53.7
25.0–29.9	279	51.8	1.4	49.4	50.0	50.3	50.9	51.8	52.7	53.2	53.6	54.0
30.0–34.9	237	51.9	1.5	49.6	50.1	50.4	50.9	51.8	52.9	53.4	53.9	54.3
35.0–39.9	238	52.1	1.5	49.6	50.2	50.6	51.2	52.2	53.1	53.4	53.7	54.1
40.0–44.9	232	51.8	1.5	49.4	50.0	50.4	50.8	51.9	52.8	53.4	53.6	54.1
45.0–49.9	125	52.0	1.4	49.7	50.3	50.6	51.0	52.0	53.1	53.6	53.8	54.3
50.0–54.9	136	51.9	1.5	49.5	50.2	50.5	51.0	51.8	52.8	53.4	53.8	54.5
55.0–59.9	124	51.6	1.7	49.4	49.6	49.7	50.2	51.6	52.7	53.4	54.1	54.4
60.0–64.9	152	51.7	1.5	49.1	49.5	49.9	50.6	51.8	52.6	53.2	53.5	54.1
65.0–69.9	281	51.2	1.7	48.8	49.4	49.6	50.1	51.2	52.4	52.8	53.2	53.7
70.0–74.9	198	50.9	1.6	48.4	48.8	49.4	50.0	51.0	51.9	52.5	52.6	53.5

Means, standard deviations, and percentiles of bitrochanteric breadth
(cm) by age (yrs) for Black males and females of 2 to 74 years

Age (yrs)	N	Mean	SD	Percentiles								
				5	10	15	25	50	75	85	90	95
Males												
1.0–1.9	156	15.0	3.1	12.3	13.3	13.5	14.0	14.8	15.6	16.0	16.5	17.4
2.0–2.9	142	15.6	1.2	13.7	14.3	14.5	14.9	15.5	16.5	16.8	17.3	17.8
3.0–3.9	151	16.4	1.5	14.2	14.7	15.1	15.7	16.6	17.4	17.8	18.2	18.7
4.0–4.9	151	17.6	1.4	15.5	15.8	16.0	16.7	17.7	18.6	19.1	19.3	19.7
5.0–5.9	122	18.7	1.2	16.8	17.3	17.5	18.0	18.6	19.5	20.0	20.1	20.9
6.0–6.9	60	19.4	1.5	16.2	17.6	17.9	18.6	19.6	20.1	20.5	21.0	21.6
7.0–7.9	67	20.2	1.4	17.9	18.5	18.6	19.2	20.1	21.1	21.7	21.9	22.6
8.0–8.9	48	21.3	1.5	18.8	19.5	20.1	20.5	21.0	22.1	22.6	23.2	24.1
9.0–9.9	74	22.0	1.8	18.4	19.9	20.2	20.9	21.9	23.1	23.6	23.9	24.5
10.0–10.9	60	23.2	1.9	20.3	20.8	21.1	21.5	23.2	24.5	25.2	25.2	25.5
11.0–11.9	71	24.0	2.2	20.9	21.3	21.4	22.5	24.0	25.4	25.8	26.0	27.6
12.0–12.9	71	25.3	2.9	21.7	22.3	22.5	23.5	25.0	26.4	27.4	28.1	30.6
13.0–13.9	74	26.4	2.2	22.9	23.5	23.8	24.8	26.5	27.8	28.4	28.8	29.9
14.0–14.9	68	28.0	2.4	23.6	24.6	25.6	26.7	27.8	29.0	30.5	31.5	32.1
15.0–15.9	65	29.1	1.9	26.4	27.0	27.2	27.7	28.9	30.2	31.2	32.4	32.8
16.0–16.9	66	29.7	1.7	27.0	27.6	28.2	28.7	29.5	30.3	30.9	31.6	33.5
17.0–17.9	63	30.0	1.9	27.6	27.9	28.0	28.7	29.8	31.2	32.5	32.8	33.1
18.0–24.9	255	30.5	2.2	27.8	28.3	28.7	29.2	30.5	31.6	32.3	33.0	34.1
25.0–29.9	162	31.1	2.4	27.9	28.6	29.0	29.5	30.9	32.2	33.2	33.7	34.2
30.0–34.9	121	31.6	2.4	28.0	29.2	29.6	30.2	31.5	32.8	33.6	34.1	35.4
35.0–39.9	88	31.7	2.0	28.3	29.0	29.7	30.4	31.7	32.9	33.8	34.5	35.7
40.0–44.9	90	31.6	2.3	28.2	28.9	29.4	30.2	31.6	33.2	33.8	34.0	35.4
45.0–49.9	113	32.1	2.0	28.8	29.4	29.8	30.7	32.1	33.5	34.1	34.5	35.0
50.0–54.9	105	31.7	2.2	27.8	28.7	29.2	30.4	31.6	33.5	34.4	34.6	35.0
55.0–59.9	105	32.0	2.4	29.0	29.6	30.1	30.6	31.6	33.1	34.4	34.6	35.6
60.0–64.9	125	32.0	2.0	28.8	29.7	30.0	30.6	32.0	33.1	34.0	34.4	35.3
65.0–69.9	254	31.9	4.1	28.4	29.2	29.6	30.4	31.8	32.9	33.9	34.2	34.9
70.0–74.9	186	32.1	2.2	29.3	29.8	30.0	30.5	31.9	33.3	34.0	34.6	35.4
Females												
1.0–1.9	133	14.5	1.2	12.6	13.0	13.2	13.8	14.5	15.3	15.9	16.2	16.5
2.0–2.9	119	15.6	1.2	13.5	14.1	14.4	14.7	15.6	16.5	16.8	17.2	17.5
3.0–3.9	126	16.7	1.3	14.5	15.1	15.3	15.8	16.8	17.6	18.0	18.3	18.8
4.0–4.9	147	17.8	1.4	15.5	16.0	16.4	17.0	17.8	18.5	19.0	19.4	19.7
5.0–5.9	163	18.7	1.5	16.5	16.9	17.2	17.7	18.6	19.7	20.3	20.5	21.3
6.0–6.9	71	19.4	1.4	17.1	17.8	18.0	18.4	19.4	20.4	21.0	21.1	21.4
7.0–7.9	81	20.4	1.4	18.5	18.6	19.2	19.5	20.4	21.0	21.9	22.2	22.8
8.0–8.9	54	21.4	1.5	19.5	19.8	20.0	20.6	21.3	22.2	22.7	23.0	24.0
9.0–9.9	71	22.4	1.9	19.6	20.1	20.2	21.0	22.2	23.8	24.5	25.0	25.6
10.0–10.9	62	24.3	2.4	21.3	21.7	22.4	22.6	23.8	25.9	27.0	27.5	28.8
11.0–11.9	67	25.8	2.7	22.0	22.5	23.1	23.4	25.8	27.4	29.0	29.9	30.1
12.0–12.9	72	27.2	2.9	22.3	23.2	23.6	24.6	27.6	28.8	30.2	30.4	32.3
13.0–13.9	82	28.3	2.1	24.7	25.5	26.3	27.1	28.4	29.7	30.4	31.2	31.5
14.0–14.9	79	28.8	2.2	25.8	26.6	26.8	27.3	28.5	29.9	30.6	31.9	33.8
15.0–15.9	73	29.3	2.3	25.9	26.9	27.1	27.8	28.9	30.6	31.5	31.8	34.1
16.0–16.9	54	30.5	3.0	26.7	27.5	28.1	28.9	30.0	31.2	32.8	34.1	36.6
17.0–17.9	68	30.1	2.5	27.1	27.4	27.7	28.2	29.6	31.4	32.8	34.2	34.5
18.0–24.9	474	30.8	2.6	27.5	28.0	28.4	29.0	30.4	32.0	33.2	33.8	35.8
25.0–29.9	279	31.4	2.3	28.1	28.6	29.1	29.8	31.0	32.8	33.7	34.4	35.6
30.0–34.9	237	31.8	3.0	27.3	28.4	29.2	29.9	31.5	33.4	34.6	35.4	36.8
35.0–39.9	239	32.2	2.7	28.1	29.0	29.9	30.5	32.1	34.0	34.9	35.9	36.8
40.0–44.9	232	32.2	2.5	28.5	29.1	29.6	30.5	32.2	33.7	34.7	35.6	36.4
45.0–49.9	126	31.9	2.7	28.5	29.0	29.5	30.0	31.5	33.5	34.2	35.2	36.6
50.0–54.9	136	32.6	2.8	28.6	29.5	30.0	30.8	32.1	34.2	35.2	36.5	38.6
55.0–59.9	124	32.3	2.8	28.4	29.0	29.7	30.4	32.1	33.7	35.0	35.9	37.6
60.0–64.9	153	31.9	2.3	28.5	29.1	29.8	30.5	31.9	33.3	34.0	34.5	35.7
65.0–69.9	282	32.0	2.4	28.5	29.1	29.6	30.4	32.0	33.4	34.2	34.9	35.6
70.0–74.9	198	31.9	2.4	28.2	28.8	29.8	30.6	31.6	33.2	34.4	35.3	36.1

Means, standard deviations, and percentiles of elbow breadth (mm) by age (yrs) for Black males and females of 1 to 74 years

Age (yrs)	N	Mean	SD	Percentiles								
				5	10	15	25	50	75	85	90	95
Males												
1.0–1.9	157	40.5	3.0	35.0	37.0	38.0	39.0	41.0	42.0	44.0	44.0	45.0
2.0–2.9	142	42.7	2.7	38.0	39.0	40.0	41.0	43.0	44.0	45.0	46.0	48.0
3.0–3.9	151	44.5	3.0	40.0	41.0	42.0	42.0	44.0	46.0	47.0	48.0	50.0
4.0–4.9	151	46.7	3.1	42.0	43.0	43.0	45.0	47.0	49.0	50.0	51.0	52.0
5.0–5.9	122	49.3	3.6	44.0	45.0	46.0	47.0	50.0	51.0	52.0	53.0	55.0
6.0–6.9	60	51.0	2.8	46.0	47.0	47.0	49.0	51.0	52.0	53.0	53.0	55.0
7.0–7.9	67	52.1	3.6	45.0	48.0	49.0	50.0	53.0	55.0	56.0	56.0	58.0
8.0–8.9	49	54.3	4.1	48.0	49.0	51.0	51.0	54.0	57.0	58.0	59.0	61.0
9.0–9.9	74	55.3	3.6	49.0	50.0	52.0	53.0	55.0	58.0	59.0	60.0	61.0
10.0–10.9	60	58.4	4.8	52.0	52.0	53.0	54.0	57.0	62.0	63.0	65.0	66.0
11.0–11.9	71	60.4	4.5	53.0	55.0	56.0	57.0	60.0	63.0	65.0	66.0	67.0
12.0–12.9	71	62.8	6.4	53.0	55.0	56.0	59.0	61.0	68.0	70.0	72.0	75.0
13.0–13.9	74	65.7	5.3	58.0	58.0	60.0	62.0	65.0	69.0	71.0	72.0	75.0
14.0–14.9	68	67.5	5.0	60.0	61.0	63.0	64.0	67.0	70.0	73.0	75.0	77.0
15.0–15.9	65	70.1	3.8	64.0	65.0	66.0	68.0	70.0	72.0	74.0	75.0	77.0
16.0–16.9	66	70.7	4.2	65.0	65.0	67.0	68.0	71.0	73.0	75.0	76.0	78.0
17.0–17.9	63	70.9	3.8	65.0	66.0	67.0	68.0	71.0	74.0	75.0	76.0	76.0
18.0–24.9	254	71.1	4.6	64.0	65.0	67.0	69.0	71.0	74.0	76.0	77.0	78.0
25.0–29.9	162	71.7	4.6	65.0	67.0	67.0	69.0	71.0	74.0	76.0	78.0	80.0
30.0–34.9	121	72.1	4.0	66.0	68.0	69.0	69.0	72.0	75.0	76.0	76.0	78.0
35.0–39.9	88	72.8	4.7	65.0	67.0	67.0	69.0	73.0	76.0	77.0	78.0	80.0
40.0–44.9	90	73.3	4.7	66.0	67.0	69.0	70.0	73.0	76.0	78.0	80.0	82.0
45.0–49.9	113	73.7	4.7	66.0	68.0	69.0	71.0	74.0	76.0	79.0	80.0	81.0
50.0–54.9	105	73.7	4.8	66.0	69.0	70.0	71.0	73.0	77.0	79.0	80.0	83.0
55.0–59.9	105	74.2	5.3	67.0	68.0	69.0	71.0	74.0	77.0	79.0	80.0	82.0
60.0–64.9	127	74.5	4.3	68.0	70.0	70.0	72.0	74.0	77.0	79.0	81.0	82.0
65.0–69.9	254	73.3	4.4	66.0	68.0	69.0	70.0	73.0	76.0	78.0	79.0	81.0
70.0–74.9	186	73.6	4.1	68.0	69.0	70.0	71.0	73.0	76.0	77.0	79.0	80.0
Females												
1.0–1.9	134	38.9	2.6	34.0	35.0	36.0	37.0	39.0	41.0	41.0	42.0	43.0
2.0–2.9	119	40.9	3.2	36.0	37.0	38.0	39.0	41.0	43.0	44.0	45.0	46.0
3.0–3.9	127	42.6	2.8	38.0	39.0	40.0	41.0	42.0	44.0	45.0	46.0	48.0
4.0–4.9	147	44.7	3.2	40.0	41.0	42.0	43.0	45.0	47.0	48.0	49.0	50.0
5.0–5.9	163	47.0	3.4	42.0	42.0	44.0	45.0	47.0	49.0	50.0	51.0	52.0
6.0–6.9	72	48.2	3.3	43.0	44.0	45.0	46.0	48.0	50.0	52.0	53.0	54.0
7.0–7.9	81	50.9	3.3	46.0	47.0	48.0	49.0	51.0	53.0	54.0	55.0	57.0
8.0–8.9	54	51.7	2.7	47.0	48.0	49.0	50.0	52.0	53.0	54.0	55.0	57.0
9.0–9.9	71	54.1	4.0	48.0	50.0	51.0	51.0	54.0	56.0	57.0	59.0	62.0
10.0–10.9	62	56.5	4.2	50.0	51.0	52.0	55.0	56.0	59.0	60.0	62.0	63.0
11.0–11.9	67	58.3	3.6	54.0	54.0	55.0	56.0	58.0	61.0	62.0	64.0	65.0
12.0–12.9	72	59.9	4.1	51.0	55.0	56.0	57.0	60.0	62.0	64.0	66.0	67.0
13.0–13.9	82	60.4	4.1	54.0	56.0	56.0	58.0	60.0	63.0	64.0	65.0	66.0
14.0–14.9	79	60.8	3.6	54.0	56.0	57.0	58.0	61.0	64.0	64.0	65.0	66.0
15.0–15.9	73	61.2	3.7	56.0	57.0	58.0	59.0	61.0	63.0	66.0	66.0	67.0
16.0–16.9	54	61.9	4.0	55.0	57.0	59.0	60.0	61.0	65.0	66.0	67.0	70.0
17.0–17.9	68	61.7	4.1	56.0	57.0	58.0	59.0	61.0	64.0	66.0	68.0	68.0
18.0–24.9	474	61.7	4.1	56.0	57.0	58.0	59.0	62.0	64.0	66.0	67.0	68.0
25.0–29.9	279	62.8	4.3	56.0	58.0	59.0	60.0	62.0	65.0	67.0	69.0	70.0
30.0–34.9	237	62.9	4.9	55.0	57.0	58.0	60.0	63.0	66.0	67.0	70.0	72.0
35.0–39.9	239	64.5	5.1	57.0	58.0	60.0	61.0	64.0	67.0	69.0	72.0	74.0
40.0–44.9	232	64.9	4.7	59.0	60.0	60.0	61.0	64.0	68.0	70.0	70.0	73.0
45.0–49.9	126	64.9	4.8	59.0	60.0	60.0	62.0	64.0	67.0	69.0	71.0	74.0
50.0–54.9	135	66.5	5.8	57.0	59.0	60.0	63.0	66.0	70.0	73.0	75.0	77.0
55.0–59.9	124	66.5	5.0	60.0	60.0	61.0	63.0	66.0	70.0	72.0	73.0	74.0
60.0–64.9	153	65.8	4.4	60.0	60.0	61.0	63.0	66.0	69.0	71.0	72.0	73.0
65.0–69.9	282	66.4	4.8	59.0	60.0	61.0	63.0	66.0	69.0	71.0	73.0	75.0
70.0–74.9	197	65.6	4.3	59.0	60.0	61.0	62.0	65.0	68.0	70.0	71.0	73.0

Means, standard deviations, and percentiles of upper arm circumference
(cm) by age (yrs) for Black males and females of 1 to 74 years

Age (yrs)	N	Mean	SD	Percentiles								
				5	10	15	25	50	75	85	90	95
Males												
1.0–1.9	157	16.0	1.3	14.0	14.3	14.8	15.3	16.0	16.9	17.2	17.6	18.6
2.0–2.9	142	16.3	1.2	14.4	14.7	14.9	15.4	16.3	17.1	17.5	17.8	18.2
3.0–3.9	151	16.6	1.4	14.6	15.1	15.2	15.7	16.5	17.4	18.0	18.2	18.9
4.0–4.9	150	16.8	1.4	14.3	15.2	15.5	16.0	16.9	17.8	18.5	18.6	18.9
5.0–5.9	122	17.6	1.6	15.8	16.0	16.2	16.6	17.3	18.2	19.0	19.5	20.2
6.0–6.9	60	18.3	2.2	16.0	16.2	16.5	17.0	17.7	18.6	19.6	20.7	23.0
7.0–7.9	67	18.7	2.4	15.6	16.6	17.0	17.3	18.4	19.7	20.3	21.0	22.6
8.0–8.9	49	19.2	1.9	17.1	17.1	17.3	17.6	19.0	20.3	20.9	21.8	23.1
9.0–9.9	74	20.0	2.3	17.0	17.5	18.4	18.7	19.6	21.0	21.9	22.2	25.0
10.0–10.9	60	21.3	3.0	18.0	18.5	19.1	19.7	20.4	21.8	23.3	25.0	27.3
11.0–11.9	71	22.2	3.2	18.2	19.2	19.4	20.5	21.3	22.8	26.0	27.2	28.7
12.0–12.9	71	23.3	4.1	19.2	20.1	20.4	20.8	22.3	24.0	27.1	27.9	29.0
13.0–13.9	74	24.2	3.4	19.8	20.3	20.9	21.7	23.4	25.9	28.1	28.8	29.9
14.0–14.9	68	25.5	2.9	21.5	22.2	22.5	23.4	25.4	26.9	28.2	28.7	31.5
15.0–15.9	65	27.6	3.2	23.0	24.0	24.7	25.4	27.3	29.0	30.9	31.1	33.2
16.0–16.9	66	28.8	2.6	25.2	25.7	25.9	27.2	28.6	30.1	31.5	32.5	34.0
17.0–17.9	63	28.5	3.2	24.3	25.3	25.6	26.4	28.0	29.8	32.0	32.6	36.2
18.0–24.9	254	30.8	3.8	25.9	27.0	27.4	28.2	30.2	32.6	33.8	34.8	38.0
25.0–29.9	162	32.3	4.3	26.8	28.0	28.5	29.5	31.7	34.5	36.2	37.2	39.8
30.0–34.9	121	33.4	4.1	28.0	29.4	29.9	31.0	32.6	35.3	36.8	38.0	39.3
35.0–39.9	88	33.8	3.9	27.2	27.7	29.6	31.1	33.9	36.5	37.6	38.2	39.3
40.0–44.9	90	33.2	3.9	26.3	28.0	29.0	30.3	33.2	36.1	37.1	37.7	40.0
45.0–49.9	113	33.0	4.1	26.8	27.8	28.8	30.1	32.7	35.6	37.2	38.5	40.1
50.0–54.9	105	33.1	4.5	26.5	27.9	28.3	29.9	32.7	35.7	38.6	39.4	40.1
55.0–59.9	105	32.9	4.1	26.9	27.9	28.7	30.0	32.3	35.3	37.4	38.1	39.1
60.0–64.9	127	32.4	3.8	26.0	27.8	28.8	30.0	32.8	34.1	36.1	37.9	39.0
65.0–69.9	254	31.3	4.0	25.7	26.6	27.4	28.5	31.0	34.0	35.5	36.5	38.6
70.0–74.9	186	30.4	3.7	25.1	25.9	26.5	27.5	30.3	32.5	34.3	35.2	37.0
Females												
1.0–1.9	134	15.5	1.3	13.5	14.0	14.3	14.7	15.6	16.3	16.7	17.0	17.6
2.0–2.9	119	16.1	1.4	13.8	14.3	14.7	15.2	16.0	17.0	17.5	17.8	18.4
3.0–3.9	126	16.3	1.4	14.3	14.7	14.9	15.4	16.2	17.1	17.5	18.4	19.0
4.0–4.9	147	16.9	1.7	14.1	14.8	15.2	15.8	16.8	17.8	18.6	19.1	19.8
5.0–5.9	163	17.6	2.0	14.8	15.5	16.0	16.3	17.2	18.5	19.4	20.2	21.6
6.0–6.9	72	18.2	2.4	15.7	16.0	16.3	16.8	17.5	18.8	19.9	20.2	22.0
7.0–7.9	80	18.8	2.0	16.4	16.7	16.8	17.3	18.6	19.9	20.3	21.0	22.0
8.0–8.9	54	19.3	2.2	16.0	17.0	17.4	17.9	19.0	20.0	21.6	22.5	23.6
9.0–9.9	71	20.2	2.5	16.9	17.8	17.9	18.6	19.6	21.3	23.1	23.7	25.1
10.0–10.9	62	22.1	3.5	18.3	18.7	19.0	19.5	21.2	23.8	26.0	26.8	28.9
11.0–11.9	67	23.3	4.0	18.8	19.6	20.1	20.7	22.1	25.1	26.6	29.6	30.0
12.0–12.9	72	24.2	4.5	17.9	19.1	19.3	20.7	23.9	26.3	29.0	30.1	33.0
13.0–13.9	82	25.1	3.5	20.5	21.3	21.8	22.8	24.5	26.7	27.8	30.1	31.3
14.0–14.9	79	25.6	4.4	20.8	21.2	21.8	22.3	24.7	27.2	29.5	31.6	33.4
15.0–15.9	73	26.0	4.1	21.7	22.3	22.6	23.2	25.0	27.8	29.1	31.2	37.1
16.0–16.9	54	27.6	4.3	22.8	23.3	23.9	24.7	26.4	29.3	31.4	33.8	38.3
17.0–17.9	68	26.9	4.3	21.8	22.5	23.6	24.2	26.0	28.2	30.1	34.6	35.6
18.0–24.9	474	28.0	4.6	22.4	23.2	24.0	24.9	27.0	30.2	32.2	34.5	37.3
25.0–29.9	279	29.9	5.0	23.4	24.3	25.1	26.0	29.3	32.3	34.6	37.2	40.1
30.0–34.9	237	31.2	5.3	23.9	25.0	25.9	27.2	30.9	34.5	36.5	37.8	41.4
35.0–39.9	239	32.5	5.7	24.0	25.1	26.5	28.4	32.0	36.0	37.7	39.5	43.7
40.0–44.9	232	32.7	5.7	24.6	25.6	27.4	29.1	32.1	35.9	37.8	39.7	41.1
45.0–49.9	126	33.0	6.2	24.8	26.4	27.2	29.2	31.6	35.8	38.4	41.0	44.2
50.0–54.9	135	33.7	5.2	24.8	27.2	28.4	30.7	33.7	36.7	39.3	40.2	43.6
55.0–59.9	124	34.2	7.0	24.0	27.3	28.4	29.5	33.5	36.8	39.5	42.9	48.2
60.0–64.9	153	33.0	5.0	25.1	26.3	28.1	29.3	32.7	36.0	38.0	39.1	41.8
65.0–69.9	282	32.0	4.7	24.0	26.1	27.6	29.0	31.8	35.1	36.8	37.7	39.4
70.0–74.9	197	31.0	4.4	23.3	25.5	26.3	27.7	31.5	34.0	35.0	36.2	39.0

Means, standard deviations, and percentiles of total upper arm area
(cm^2) by age (yrs) for Black males and females of 1 to 74 years

Age (yrs)	N	Mean	SD	\multicolumn{9}{c}{Percentiles}
				5	10	15	25	50	75	85	90	95
\multicolumn{13}{c}{Males}
1.0–1.9	157	20.6	3.5	15.6	16.3	17.4	18.6	20.4	22.7	23.5	24.6	27.5
2.0–2.9	142	21.3	3.3	16.5	17.2	17.7	18.9	21.1	23.3	24.4	25.2	26.4
3.0–3.9	151	22.2	3.9	17.0	18.1	18.4	19.6	21.7	24.1	25.8	26.4	28.4
4.0–4.9	150	22.7	3.8	16.3	18.4	19.1	20.4	22.7	25.2	27.2	27.5	28.4
5.0–5.9	122	24.8	4.8	19.9	20.4	20.9	21.9	23.8	26.4	28.7	30.3	32.5
6.0–6.9	60	27.0	7.3	20.4	20.9	21.7	23.0	24.9	27.5	30.6	34.1	42.1
7.0–7.9	67	28.4	7.9	19.4	21.9	23.0	23.8	26.9	30.9	32.8	35.1	40.6
8.0–8.9	49	29.7	5.9	23.3	23.3	23.8	24.6	28.7	32.8	34.8	37.8	42.5
9.0–9.9	74	32.3	7.9	23.0	24.4	26.9	27.8	30.6	35.1	38.2	39.2	49.7
10.0–10.9	60	36.9	11.5	25.8	27.2	29.0	30.9	33.1	37.8	43.2	49.7	59.3
11.0–11.9	71	40.0	12.5	26.4	29.3	29.9	33.4	36.1	41.4	53.8	58.9	65.5
12.0–12.9	71	44.4	18.0	29.3	32.2	33.1	34.4	39.6	45.8	58.4	61.9	66.9
13.0–13.9	74	47.4	13.7	31.2	32.8	34.8	37.5	43.6	53.4	62.8	66.0	71.1
14.0–14.9	68	52.5	12.4	36.8	39.2	40.3	43.6	51.3	57.6	63.3	65.5	79.0
15.0–15.9	65	61.6	14.7	42.1	45.8	48.5	51.3	59.3	66.9	76.0	77.0	87.7
16.0–16.9	66	66.4	12.1	50.5	52.6	53.4	58.9	65.1	72.1	79.0	84.1	92.0
17.0–17.9	63	65.5	15.2	47.0	50.9	52.2	55.5	62.4	70.7	81.5	84.6	104.3
18.0–24.9	254	76.6	20.2	53.4	58.0	59.7	63.3	72.6	84.6	90.9	96.4	114.9
25.0–29.9	162	84.4	24.4	57.2	62.4	64.6	69.3	80.0	94.7	104.3	110.1	126.1
30.0–34.9	121	90.1	24.1	62.4	68.8	71.1	76.5	84.6	99.2	107.8	114.9	122.9
35.0–39.9	88	92.2	20.8	58.9	61.1	69.7	77.0	91.5	106.0	112.5	116.1	122.9
40.0–44.9	90	88.8	20.8	55.0	62.4	66.9	73.1	87.7	103.7	109.5	113.1	127.3
45.0–49.9	113	88.1	21.7	57.2	61.5	66.0	72.1	85.1	100.9	110.1	118.0	128.0
50.0–54.9	105	88.8	24.5	55.9	61.9	63.7	71.1	85.1	101.4	118.6	123.5	128.0
55.0–59.9	105	87.3	21.6	57.6	61.9	65.5	71.6	83.0	99.2	111.3	115.5	121.7
60.0–64.9	127	84.5	19.7	53.8	61.5	66.0	71.6	85.6	92.5	103.7	114.3	121.0
65.0–69.9	254	79.4	20.5	52.6	56.3	59.7	64.6	76.5	92.0	100.3	106.0	118.6
70.0–74.9	186	74.8	18.2	50.1	53.4	55.9	60.2	73.1	84.1	93.6	98.6	108.9
\multicolumn{13}{c}{Females}
1.0–1.9	134	19.4	3.2	14.5	15.6	16.3	17.2	19.4	21.1	22.2	23.0	24.6
2.0–2.9	119	20.7	3.5	15.2	16.3	17.2	18.4	20.4	23.0	24.4	25.2	26.9
3.0–3.9	126	21.4	3.9	16.3	17.2	17.7	18.9	20.9	23.3	24.4	26.9	28.7
4.0–4.9	147	23.1	4.9	15.8	17.4	18.4	19.9	22.5	25.2	27.5	29.0	31.2
5.0–5.9	163	24.9	6.0	17.4	19.1	20.4	21.1	23.5	27.2	29.9	32.5	37.1
6.0–6.9	72	26.8	8.2	19.6	20.4	21.1	22.5	24.4	28.1	31.5	32.5	38.5
7.0–7.9	80	28.5	6.3	21.4	22.2	22.5	23.8	27.5	31.5	32.8	35.1	38.5
8.0–8.9	54	30.1	7.0	20.4	23.0	24.1	25.5	28.7	31.8	37.1	40.3	44.3
9.0–9.9	71	33.1	8.8	22.7	25.2	25.5	27.5	30.6	36.1	42.5	44.7	50.1
10.0–10.9	62	40.0	13.6	26.6	27.8	28.7	30.3	35.8	45.1	53.8	57.2	66.5
11.0–11.9	67	44.4	16.7	28.1	30.6	32.2	34.1	38.9	50.1	56.3	69.7	71.6
12.0–12.9	72	48.0	18.4	25.5	29.0	29.6	34.1	45.5	55.0	66.9	72.1	86.7
13.0–13.9	82	51.1	14.9	33.4	36.1	37.8	41.4	47.8	56.7	61.5	72.1	78.0
14.0–14.9	79	53.5	20.2	34.4	35.8	37.8	39.6	48.5	58.9	69.3	79.5	88.8
15.0–15.9	73	55.1	18.8	37.5	39.6	40.6	42.8	49.7	61.5	67.4	77.5	109.5
16.0–16.9	54	62.2	20.9	41.4	43.2	45.5	48.5	55.5	68.3	78.5	90.9	116.7
17.0–17.9	68	59.2	20.8	37.8	40.3	44.3	46.6	53.8	63.3	72.1	95.3	100.9
18.0–24.9	474	64.2	22.7	39.9	42.8	45.8	49.3	58.0	72.6	82.5	94.7	110.7
25.0–29.9	279	72.9	25.6	43.6	47.0	50.1	53.8	68.3	83.0	95.3	110.1	128.0
30.0–34.9	237	79.7	28.2	45.5	49.7	53.4	58.9	76.0	94.7	106.0	113.7	136.4
35.0–39.9	239	86.6	30.8	45.8	50.1	55.9	64.2	81.5	103.1	113.1	124.2	152.0
40.0–44.9	232	87.6	33.5	48.2	52.2	59.7	67.4	82.0	102.6	113.7	125.4	134.4
45.0–49.9	126	89.8	36.8	48.9	55.5	58.9	67.9	79.5	102.0	117.3	133.8	155.5
50.0–54.9	135	92.7	28.4	48.9	58.9	64.2	75.0	90.4	107.2	122.9	128.6	151.3
55.0–59.9	124	97.0	43.5	45.8	59.3	64.2	69.3	89.3	107.8	124.2	146.5	184.9
60.0–64.9	153	88.3	27.0	50.1	55.0	62.8	68.3	85.1	103.1	114.9	121.7	139.0
65.0–69.9	282	83.3	24.7	45.8	54.2	60.6	66.9	80.5	98.0	107.8	113.1	123.5
70.0–74.9	197	78.3	22.1	43.2	51.7	55.0	61.1	79.0	92.0	97.5	104.3	121.0

Means, standard deviations, and percentiles of upper arm muscle area
(cm^2) by age (yrs) for Black males and females of 1 to 74 years

Age (yrs)	N	Mean	SD	Percentiles								
				5	10	15	25	50	75	85	90	95
Males												
1.0–1.9	157	13.2	2.5	9.0	10.3	10.8	11.5	13.2	14.7	15.6	16.6	17.4
2.0–2.9	142	14.1	2.5	10.4	11.1	11.8	12.6	13.9	15.7	16.3	17.0	19.1
3.0–3.9	151	15.3	2.8	11.9	12.2	12.7	13.5	14.9	16.8	17.9	18.9	20.4
4.0–4.9	149	16.4	2.8	11.7	13.0	13.7	14.7	16.3	18.0	19.0	20.0	21.3
5.0–5.9	122	18.5	2.9	14.8	15.2	15.8	16.4	18.4	20.3	21.5	22.3	23.5
6.0–6.9	60	20.5	4.8	15.3	16.2	16.4	17.8	19.3	22.8	24.4	25.0	26.3
7.0–7.9	67	21.9	5.4	16.4	16.7	17.5	18.9	21.1	23.7	25.3	27.2	28.8
8.0–8.9	49	22.5	3.3	18.1	18.4	19.2	19.8	22.1	25.1	26.1	26.9	28.5
9.0–9.9	74	24.9	5.5	18.5	19.3	20.3	22.5	23.9	27.4	28.8	29.9	32.2
10.0–10.9	60	27.0	5.2	19.7	21.3	22.0	23.6	26.1	29.7	31.2	32.4	35.1
11.0–11.9	71	29.4	6.9	21.0	23.0	24.0	25.1	27.7	32.2	34.8	36.9	40.2
12.0–12.9	71	32.8	8.5	22.7	25.1	25.7	27.3	30.4	36.7	39.9	41.2	49.7
13.0–13.9	74	38.0	11.4	24.8	26.5	27.5	30.4	35.2	44.0	47.4	50.9	58.5
14.0–14.9	68	43.2	9.7	28.6	31.7	32.7	34.9	42.8	47.5	51.2	53.9	59.4
15.0–15.9	64	48.9	9.7	33.3	36.6	39.7	42.2	49.4	54.9	57.2	59.1	65.6
16.0–16.9	66	55.2	9.3	42.0	44.4	46.1	49.5	54.7	57.9	63.7	66.9	70.5
17.0–17.9	62	54.0	10.0	38.9	42.3	44.9	46.9	52.8	59.3	63.7	66.1	71.7
18.0–24.9	253	52.0	11.8	35.5	38.3	40.1	44.2	51.0	59.4	63.1	65.3	73.0
25.0–29.9	160	56.9	12.6	36.9	40.9	44.3	48.8	55.6	63.2	68.7	74.5	81.1
30.0–34.9	120	60.3	14.0	42.9	45.8	47.7	50.1	57.3	67.1	73.6	76.7	80.0
35.0–39.9	83	61.6	13.6	39.3	41.8	46.0	52.8	61.2	70.8	77.3	80.5	85.4
40.0–44.9	89	59.6	13.8	36.9	41.2	44.2	50.3	59.0	68.4	74.5	79.4	83.7
45.0–49.9	112	58.8	13.7	39.0	42.7	46.5	49.4	56.8	66.9	72.8	75.0	82.5
50.0–54.9	105	60.6	17.1	39.1	41.3	44.7	47.7	60.1	69.3	72.7	81.3	88.8
55.0–59.9	104	58.7	13.4	36.6	42.0	44.6	50.8	57.6	66.8	73.6	76.5	80.6
60.0–64.9	126	55.5	12.3	34.4	39.6	45.1	48.3	55.0	62.7	66.3	70.7	77.0
65.0–69.9	254	53.1	14.3	33.4	36.9	40.4	43.2	51.0	62.2	67.5	71.4	80.1
70.0–74.9	186	50.2	13.2	30.7	34.3	37.7	41.2	48.9	58.9	63.2	67.1	72.3
Females												
1.0–1.9	134	12.2	2.3	8.1	9.8	10.3	10.8	12.3	13.7	14.5	15.2	16.7
2.0–2.9	119	13.6	2.5	9.9	10.4	10.8	12.0	13.3	14.8	16.2	17.1	18.3
3.0–3.9	126	14.4	2.3	11.2	11.5	11.8	12.8	14.2	15.9	16.5	17.2	18.8
4.0–4.9	147	15.7	2.8	11.4	12.4	12.8	13.8	15.6	17.6	18.3	18.9	19.9
5.0–5.9	163	17.0	3.5	12.0	13.5	14.1	14.8	16.6	18.3	19.3	22.4	23.5
6.0–6.9	72	19.0	5.2	14.0	14.8	15.2	15.9	18.2	20.2	22.3	22.9	27.5
7.0–7.9	80	19.7	3.5	14.4	16.0	16.4	17.3	19.1	21.4	22.9	24.1	25.5
8.0–8.9	54	20.7	3.8	15.7	16.6	17.9	19.2	20.6	23.0	23.7	25.4	27.2
9.0–9.9	71	22.5	3.8	16.9	18.7	19.2	20.1	21.4	25.5	26.9	27.9	28.3
10.0–10.9	61	26.0	6.2	18.9	19.8	20.6	21.9	24.7	29.5	31.3	32.2	34.0
11.0–11.9	67	29.0	6.3	22.2	22.9	23.2	24.9	27.5	31.7	33.2	35.7	42.1
12.0–12.9	71	30.6	8.6	18.0	20.9	22.0	23.6	30.8	35.8	39.6	40.1	40.8
13.0–13.9	82	32.0	5.7	24.5	25.1	26.0	27.8	31.2	36.2	37.6	39.3	42.8
14.0–14.9	79	34.6	9.0	23.3	25.2	27.6	29.2	33.0	37.1	40.6	44.2	57.2
15.0–15.9	73	35.3	7.2	25.3	27.5	27.8	30.2	33.5	40.0	43.5	46.9	49.1
16.0–16.9	54	37.9	9.7	26.5	28.1	29.2	31.7	35.5	41.0	44.9	48.6	61.6
17.0–17.9	66	37.2	8.2	26.1	28.4	29.7	32.3	35.5	40.0	46.3	49.2	52.6
18.0–24.9	473	32.3	9.8	21.0	23.0	24.2	25.8	30.2	35.9	40.3	43.6	49.4
25.0–29.9	275	34.6	10.5	21.8	23.5	25.6	27.4	33.0	40.3	44.6	47.6	53.2
30.0–34.9	236	37.3	11.2	22.8	24.6	27.3	29.9	35.0	42.9	47.1	51.5	58.3
35.0–39.9	235	40.2	13.8	23.4	27.1	28.4	31.2	37.7	44.9	51.6	56.7	68.0
40.0–44.9	231	41.5	18.6	23.9	26.5	28.2	30.9	38.5	48.4	53.3	56.5	70.8
45.0–49.9	125	41.6	15.3	27.3	28.9	30.4	32.6	37.2	43.4	52.0	60.1	65.8
50.0–54.9	134	41.9	12.9	23.9	27.9	29.0	32.6	40.2	48.7	51.6	56.2	68.9
55.0–59.9	119	43.4	18.9	24.6	26.5	29.7	33.1	41.2	47.3	53.9	62.1	65.7
60.0–64.9	152	40.6	12.1	23.1	26.0	29.3	32.3	38.7	47.0	50.1	56.8	63.7
65.0–69.9	282	40.0	11.9	22.6	25.6	28.7	32.5	39.6	46.6	50.5	53.6	58.1
70.0–74.9	196	37.6	11.3	21.9	24.4	26.6	29.2	36.3	44.7	48.4	51.3	55.5

Note: Values for males and females aged 18 years and older have been adjusted for bone area by subtracting 10.0 cm² and 6.5 cm² respectively from the calculated mid upper arm muscle area.

Means, standard deviations, and percentiles of upper arm muscle area
(cm^2) by height (cm) for Black boys and girls of 2 to 17 years

Height (cm)	N	Mean	SD	Percentiles								
				5	10	15	25	50	75	85	90	95
Boys: 2 to 11 years												
87–092	32	13.5	2.2	10.4	10.8	11.1	12.2	13.1	14.5	16.0	16.0	17.5
93–098	78	14.1	2.6	10.5	11.5	11.9	12.3	13.7	15.3	16.0	17.0	19.2
99–104	118	14.5	2.4	10.7	11.9	12.0	13.1	14.6	15.8	16.4	16.9	19.3
105–110	94	15.8	2.3	12.6	13.1	13.6	14.2	15.3	17.3	18.3	19.2	19.9
111–116	112	16.7	2.6	12.8	13.9	14.5	15.2	16.6	18.0	19.1	19.9	20.7
117–122	106	18.6	2.9	14.5	15.4	16.1	16.6	18.1	20.2	21.1	21.7	23.9
123–128	83	19.5	2.6	15.9	16.1	16.6	17.3	19.3	21.2	22.5	22.9	24.4
129–134	76	22.6	5.9	15.5	18.2	18.9	19.4	21.6	24.7	25.3	27.5	30.1
135–140	70	23.3	3.0	18.2	19.2	20.2	21.1	23.3	25.1	25.7	26.2	28.6
141–146	57	24.8	4.4	19.3	19.7	20.7	22.0	24.8	26.9	28.0	29.7	31.0
147–152	55	27.2	3.6	20.0	22.2	23.5	25.1	27.4	29.9	30.7	31.8	32.4
153–158	36	31.4	9.1	22.0	22.9	24.5	25.1	28.4	34.8	36.9	39.0	57.8
159–164	21	31.5	5.6	24.2	24.5	25.3	26.7	31.6	35.1	37.8	39.7	40.2
Boys: 12 to 17 years												
153–158	32	30.7	5.7	22.7	25.1	25.1	27.5	29.3	32.5	39.1	39.4	42.4
159–164	46	37.3	10.1	27.3	28.2	29.3	31.3	34.8	41.2	45.2	50.8	54.7
165–170	62	44.0	11.9	29.1	30.5	32.5	35.7	42.2	49.7	56.4	57.7	63.4
171–176	93	47.7	10.0	32.7	35.1	38.1	40.2	46.5	53.0	56.2	59.1	66.9
177–182	74	51.8	9.0	38.0	40.7	42.3	44.7	51.0	57.2	62.1	63.7	70.1
183–188	44	54.5	10.7	36.9	42.2	45.8	47.5	54.6	59.0	64.3	65.6	72.7
Girls: 2 to 10 years												
87–092	31	12.3	2.2	9.6	9.7	9.9	10.7	12.3	13.5	15.4	15.5	16.3
93–098	61	13.7	2.3	10.2	10.9	11.4	12.0	13.6	14.4	15.8	17.0	17.8
99–104	99	14.2	2.1	11.1	11.6	12.2	12.6	14.0	15.6	16.3	17.2	18.1
105–110	110	14.4	2.4	10.5	11.3	11.6	12.8	14.3	15.9	16.8	17.8	18.7
111–116	109	15.9	2.4	12.3	12.7	13.6	14.3	15.7	17.3	17.9	18.6	19.1
117–122	117	17.1	2.8	13.5	14.2	14.8	15.5	16.7	18.5	19.3	20.3	22.6
123–128	96	18.3	3.2	14.1	15.0	15.5	16.2	17.9	19.6	20.4	21.9	22.9
129–134	88	20.6	4.5	15.8	16.8	17.1	17.6	19.8	22.1	23.5	24.2	27.2
135–140	63	21.1	3.7	16.6	18.1	18.7	19.2	20.5	23.4	24.4	25.5	27.3
141–146	50	23.6	3.4	17.9	19.2	19.8	20.8	23.2	25.8	27.7	28.0	29.7
147–152	39	24.6	4.4	18.7	20.6	20.8	21.4	23.9	27.2	30.0	32.1	32.7
Girls: 11 to 17 years												
147–152	27	24.3	4.0	16.8	20.9	21.5	22.0	23.3	26.4	27.5	29.3	31.4
153–158	67	30.2	6.7	22.1	23.0	24.4	25.4	28.1	33.9	37.6	39.9	42.0
159–164	129	33.4	8.6	23.3	24.6	26.3	27.9	31.8	36.4	39.1	41.2	51.5
165–170	154	35.5	7.9	25.6	27.5	28.4	30.8	33.7	38.8	40.6	44.5	50.8
171–176	80	35.6	6.7	27.0	27.6	28.1	30.4	35.0	40.5	42.8	45.3	46.5

Appendix A: Table 14.

Means, standard deviations, and percentiles of upper arm fat area (cm^2)
by age (yrs) for Black males and females of 1 to 74 years

Age (yrs)	N	Mean	SD	Percentiles								
				5	10	15	25	50	75	85	90	95
Males												
1.0–1.9	157	7.4	2.3	3.9	4.7	5.3	5.8	7.2	8.5	9.5	10.2	11.6
2.0–2.9	142	7.1	2.4	3.7	4.1	4.8	5.3	7.0	8.3	9.9	10.6	11.5
3.0–3.9	151	6.9	2.2	4.2	4.6	4.9	5.1	6.7	8.2	9.0	9.4	10.3
4.0–4.9	149	6.4	2.1	3.6	3.8	4.5	5.0	6.1	7.5	8.3	8.9	10.4
5.0–5.9	122	6.3	3.0	3.6	3.8	4.0	4.5	5.6	7.0	8.2	9.3	11.5
6.0–6.9	60	6.5	4.6	3.3	3.5	3.9	4.2	5.4	6.9	7.8	8.4	12.8
7.0–7.9	67	6.5	4.1	3.3	3.6	4.1	4.3	5.3	7.1	8.8	10.2	12.5
8.0–8.9	49	7.1	4.1	3.2	3.4	4.1	4.9	6.2	7.8	9.1	11.5	15.6
9.0–9.9	74	7.4	4.0	3.4	3.8	4.2	5.3	6.1	8.7	10.6	11.5	17.8
10.0–10.9	60	9.9	7.5	4.5	4.8	5.1	5.6	7.4	10.3	14.4	16.7	24.2
11.0–11.9	71	10.6	8.1	4.0	4.9	5.1	5.6	8.0	10.6	16.1	22.7	28.5
12.0–12.9	71	11.7	11.1	4.0	4.4	4.7	5.9	8.1	12.1	19.9	22.9	30.3
13.0–13.9	74	9.4	5.6	3.4	4.3	4.8	5.9	7.7	10.7	13.0	15.6	25.5
14.0–14.9	68	9.4	5.6	4.3	4.6	5.3	6.2	7.8	10.1	12.4	16.3	21.1
15.0–15.9	64	12.4	10.2	5.6	5.8	6.4	7.0	9.2	12.7	14.4	25.4	31.4
16.0–16.9	66	11.2	7.8	5.5	5.7	6.1	6.9	8.8	12.1	15.4	17.3	25.4
17.0–17.9	62	10.8	7.9	4.7	5.4	5.7	6.2	8.5	12.5	14.8	18.1	31.8
18.0–24.9	253	14.6	12.8	4.5	5.4	5.8	7.4	10.3	17.8	22.5	28.7	37.2
25.0–29.9	160	16.3	13.9	5.0	5.7	6.2	7.3	11.9	18.6	26.2	35.2	40.8
30.0–34.9	120	19.1	13.9	5.1	5.9	7.1	9.0	16.1	24.6	30.0	33.9	42.1
35.0–39.9	83	18.9	13.4	5.7	6.7	7.8	10.1	15.6	24.6	27.4	29.0	39.3
40.0–44.9	89	18.7	12.6	5.8	6.9	8.3	9.3	16.8	24.5	26.9	30.3	42.2
45.0–49.9	112	19.0	13.2	4.9	6.6	7.8	9.5	15.1	23.8	32.0	34.1	47.5
50.0–54.9	105	18.2	11.8	4.7	5.9	6.7	8.9	16.4	24.4	27.8	35.7	43.6
55.0–59.9	104	18.0	12.5	4.3	5.7	6.6	8.9	13.7	24.1	29.5	36.0	45.6
60.0–64.9	126	18.5	12.1	5.0	6.9	7.9	9.1	15.7	23.4	30.1	35.6	40.7
65.0–69.9	254	16.3	11.5	5.2	6.2	7.1	8.2	13.7	19.5	24.9	30.7	40.9
70.0–74.9	186	14.6	8.8	5.1	6.1	6.7	7.7	12.4	19.0	23.1	25.8	29.1
Females												
1.0–1.9	134	7.1	2.2	3.9	4.3	5.0	5.5	7.1	8.6	9.1	9.5	11.0
2.0–2.9	119	7.1	2.2	3.9	4.5	4.8	5.5	7.1	8.2	9.5	10.1	11.0
3.0–3.9	126	7.0	2.8	3.9	4.3	4.7	5.4	6.5	8.1	9.3	9.5	12.0
4.0–4.9	147	7.4	3.0	3.5	4.2	4.9	5.3	6.7	8.7	10.0	11.6	12.9
5.0–5.9	163	7.9	3.9	3.7	4.2	4.7	5.4	6.8	9.5	11.1	12.6	17.0
6.0–6.9	72	7.8	4.3	3.6	4.4	4.9	5.3	6.8	8.5	9.4	11.2	17.8
7.0–7.9	80	8.8	4.6	4.0	5.0	5.1	6.0	7.6	10.0	11.6	13.8	15.6
8.0–8.9	54	9.4	4.8	4.2	5.2	5.7	6.1	7.9	11.2	13.3	16.6	19.4
9.0–9.9	71	10.6	6.6	4.1	5.1	5.4	6.0	9.1	13.2	15.8	18.8	24.1
10.0–10.9	61	13.6	9.0	5.4	6.2	6.7	7.2	9.7	19.7	22.9	25.5	28.1
11.0–11.9	67	15.4	11.5	4.5	6.5	7.3	7.8	11.7	19.3	25.9	29.3	36.7
12.0–12.9	71	16.9	11.1	5.3	6.1	6.9	8.4	13.5	21.3	31.0	33.0	40.2
13.0–13.9	82	19.0	11.7	6.5	7.7	8.5	11.2	16.5	24.0	27.2	33.1	42.6
14.0–14.9	79	19.0	12.7	6.7	8.1	8.9	11.3	14.8	21.3	30.3	34.8	48.0
15.0–15.9	73	19.8	14.0	6.4	8.7	9.9	11.5	15.8	22.6	30.1	33.9	57.0
16.0–16.9	54	24.2	12.9	9.5	12.6	13.0	14.1	21.6	29.8	34.0	45.3	54.5
17.0–17.9	66	19.7	10.7	7.1	9.5	10.3	12.9	16.3	23.9	30.4	35.7	42.3
18.0–24.9	473	25.2	15.0	8.3	10.3	11.9	14.3	21.1	31.8	40.2	46.2	55.0
25.0–29.9	275	31.2	17.9	9.8	12.2	14.5	17.7	27.3	39.8	45.5	53.4	66.4
30.0–34.9	236	35.3	19.3	9.4	11.6	16.0	20.3	32.6	46.3	53.1	62.9	71.4
35.0–39.9	235	39.1	20.1	11.5	14.7	17.6	23.6	36.1	51.4	60.2	64.9	75.4
40.0–44.9	231	39.5	19.2	12.2	17.1	19.1	26.7	37.8	51.6	58.3	63.0	73.6
45.0–49.9	125	40.6	23.4	12.0	13.8	17.8	25.1	37.5	52.1	63.7	66.6	76.6
50.0–54.9	134	44.0	19.7	13.9	18.2	21.0	30.3	42.8	55.4	63.0	70.8	77.7
55.0–59.9	119	44.0	25.5	9.1	16.2	19.8	27.9	39.1	57.3	64.4	71.6	94.5
60.0–64.9	152	40.7	18.3	14.5	17.0	22.4	27.2	38.9	50.9	61.6	67.3	76.1
65.0–69.9	282	36.8	16.9	12.1	16.2	20.1	25.4	34.6	46.3	54.3	60.7	68.9
70.0–74.9	196	33.9	15.3	12.3	14.6	17.7	22.5	33.6	43.6	48.6	51.7	60.1

157

Means, standard deviations, and percentiles of arm fat index (arm fat area / total arm area x 100) by age (yrs) for Black males and females of 1 to 74 years

Age (yrs)	N	Mean	SD	Percentiles 5	10	15	25	50	75	85	90	95
Males												
1.0–1.9	157	35.6	8.2	23.1	25.5	27.1	29.6	36.0	41.0	42.9	44.6	46.7
2.0–2.9	142	33.1	8.7	20.4	22.0	24.2	26.7	33.5	38.5	41.1	44.8	48.0
3.0–3.9	151	30.8	7.1	21.5	22.4	23.7	25.5	30.5	35.8	38.3	39.6	43.2
4.0–4.9	149	27.8	6.6	18.7	19.8	21.9	23.6	26.7	32.0	35.6	37.5	39.0
5.0–5.9	122	24.6	7.0	15.8	17.1	17.8	19.6	23.2	28.9	31.7	33.5	37.3
6.0–6.9	60	23.1	8.3	13.1	13.5	15.5	17.6	21.4	26.5	31.0	31.4	34.6
7.0–7.9	67	21.9	7.1	14.0	14.2	15.7	17.1	20.3	25.2	28.4	30.7	33.9
8.0–8.9	49	23.0	8.0	13.8	14.7	16.9	18.7	21.9	24.7	29.2	30.7	36.6
9.0–9.9	74	22.0	7.5	12.3	13.1	15.4	17.1	19.7	25.3	28.0	32.1	38.8
10.0–10.9	60	24.7	9.1	15.2	15.6	16.3	17.7	21.6	29.6	34.1	37.4	40.7
11.0–11.9	71	24.6	10.2	12.0	14.0	14.3	16.3	23.4	29.9	36.3	39.4	49.4
12.0–12.9	71	23.5	10.2	11.1	11.9	13.1	16.3	20.7	28.1	36.0	37.7	45.2
13.0–13.9	74	19.4	8.3	8.6	10.9	11.7	12.6	17.6	23.3	27.8	32.6	35.9
14.0–14.9	68	17.4	7.1	9.4	10.2	10.8	11.9	16.4	20.2	23.0	26.1	33.9
15.0–15.9	64	19.0	10.5	10.3	10.9	11.5	12.9	15.1	20.3	26.2	33.2	42.8
16.0–16.9	66	16.3	7.9	8.4	9.4	10.2	11.9	14.3	19.1	21.8	23.2	30.2
17.0–17.9	62	15.8	7.8	8.9	9.1	10.2	10.8	13.9	18.1	21.8	22.8	31.5
18.0–24.9	253	17.6	9.5	6.8	8.9	9.5	11.1	14.9	21.8	26.7	31.0	36.6
25.0–29.9	160	18.0	10.1	7.3	8.2	8.7	10.3	15.4	21.8	27.7	32.1	36.2
30.0–34.9	120	20.0	10.1	6.8	8.2	9.2	11.9	19.1	27.8	30.3	33.9	35.7
35.0–39.9	83	19.7	9.6	8.3	9.4	10.5	12.5	18.3	24.3	28.1	30.9	37.0
40.0–44.9	89	20.0	9.4	9.1	10.4	11.4	12.6	19.2	23.9	28.3	34.9	38.5
45.0–49.9	112	20.1	10.0	7.9	9.2	10.7	12.6	18.5	26.1	30.4	33.7	42.0
50.0–54.9	105	19.3	8.8	7.4	8.2	10.2	12.7	18.4	24.2	28.1	32.2	36.4
55.0–59.9	104	19.3	10.0	7.1	8.5	9.7	11.5	17.7	23.9	30.5	35.5	38.3
60.0–64.9	126	20.7	9.8	8.0	9.6	11.1	13.5	18.6	26.2	32.4	35.2	37.4
65.0–69.9	254	19.4	9.6	8.5	9.3	10.1	13.0	17.1	23.4	28.6	31.7	40.0
70.0–74.9	186	18.6	7.9	8.5	10.1	11.1	12.7	17.6	22.9	25.7	28.3	33.8
Females												
1.0–1.9	134	36.5	8.3	22.7	24.6	27.6	31.5	37.4	40.9	44.6	46.4	50.9
2.0–2.9	119	34.2	7.3	23.1	24.9	25.7	28.4	34.1	38.4	41.9	43.7	47.8
3.0–3.9	126	32.2	7.8	21.8	23.6	24.9	26.7	31.9	36.9	39.6	42.3	45.9
4.0–4.9	147	31.2	7.5	20.6	23.3	24.0	26.0	30.3	35.9	38.6	40.3	44.8
5.0–5.9	163	30.7	8.8	18.6	20.3	22.0	24.3	28.9	35.4	39.8	41.5	48.6
6.0–6.9	72	28.2	8.3	16.2	19.3	20.4	23.3	26.4	33.2	37.5	38.6	45.5
7.0–7.9	80	29.9	9.0	17.7	18.7	21.2	24.1	27.2	34.3	38.5	40.5	48.2
8.0–8.9	54	30.1	9.7	18.5	19.5	21.4	24.1	27.5	35.4	39.3	43.9	51.6
9.0–9.9	71	30.1	10.4	17.5	20.1	20.8	22.2	28.1	36.2	42.0	43.8	50.1
10.0–10.9	61	31.8	11.4	17.0	21.7	22.0	23.4	27.5	40.7	44.2	48.3	49.7
11.0–11.9	67	31.4	10.9	16.7	19.0	20.8	23.1	29.7	40.5	43.6	47.0	50.6
12.0–12.9	71	33.0	10.7	16.9	20.1	22.2	24.3	31.5	41.6	45.8	47.6	51.4
13.0–13.9	82	35.0	11.3	16.8	19.8	22.9	26.6	35.0	42.2	44.8	49.0	56.2
14.0–14.9	79	33.0	9.8	18.3	20.2	23.4	25.5	32.3	39.6	42.3	47.8	53.8
15.0–15.9	73	33.3	11.3	16.2	19.7	20.7	24.6	33.1	41.1	46.7	47.8	55.9
16.0–16.9	54	37.3	9.3	20.6	25.5	26.0	29.5	39.0	44.7	47.3	48.5	51.1
17.0–17.9	66	33.0	9.5	17.5	21.5	22.5	26.6	31.5	40.7	44.4	45.5	48.4
18.0–24.9	473	37.0	11.1	19.2	22.5	25.1	28.6	36.3	45.4	49.5	52.5	55.6
25.0–29.9	275	40.6	11.5	22.7	24.9	27.1	31.5	41.5	48.5	52.5	54.0	60.1
30.0–34.9	236	42.1	12.3	19.8	24.0	28.4	33.4	44.3	50.5	54.3	56.1	60.1
35.0–39.9	235	43.4	11.0	23.6	28.1	31.0	37.0	44.5	50.3	54.4	57.1	61.0
40.0–44.9	231	43.5	11.1	22.4	28.3	32.7	36.5	45.1	51.8	54.5	56.0	58.7
45.0–49.9	125	43.3	11.8	21.7	26.2	31.1	35.0	45.1	51.9	54.2	56.7	59.4
50.0–54.9	134	45.7	11.4	24.6	28.7	33.1	39.3	47.3	53.6	57.4	59.0	63.4
55.0–59.9	119	44.4	11.7	22.6	27.3	29.9	35.5	46.7	53.0	57.4	59.3	60.4
60.0–64.9	152	44.6	10.6	24.5	30.5	34.0	37.9	45.8	51.1	55.7	57.3	62.1
65.0–69.9	282	42.5	10.8	22.8	28.1	31.5	34.7	43.5	49.8	52.7	54.8	60.0
70.0–74.9	196	41.8	11.0	23.0	27.0	30.8	34.2	41.9	49.6	54.1	56.5	60.0

Means, standard deviations, and percentiles of triceps skinfold thickness
(mm) by age (yrs) for Black males and females of 1 to 74 years

Age (yrs)	N	Mean	SD	Percentiles								
				5	10	15	25	50	75	85	90	95
Males												
1.0–1.9	157	10.2	3.0	6.0	7.0	7.0	8.0	10.0	12.0	12.5	13.5	15.0
2.0–2.9	142	9.6	3.1	5.0	6.0	6.5	7.0	10.0	11.0	13.0	14.0	15.0
3.0–3.9	151	9.0	2.6	6.0	6.0	6.5	7.0	9.0	10.5	12.0	12.0	13.5
4.0–4.9	150	8.2	2.4	5.0	5.5	6.0	7.0	7.5	9.5	11.0	11.0	12.0
5.0–5.9	122	7.5	3.0	4.5	5.0	5.0	5.5	7.0	8.5	10.0	11.0	13.0
6.0–6.9	60	7.4	4.1	4.0	4.0	5.0	5.0	6.5	8.0	9.5	10.0	13.0
7.0–7.9	67	7.1	3.6	4.0	4.0	5.0	5.0	6.0	8.0	9.0	11.0	13.0
8.0–8.9	49	7.8	3.9	4.0	4.0	5.0	6.0	7.0	8.0	10.0	11.5	15.0
9.0–9.9	74	7.6	3.5	3.5	4.0	5.0	6.0	6.5	9.0	10.5	12.0	17.0
10.0–10.9	60	9.5	5.5	5.0	5.0	5.5	6.0	7.5	11.0	13.0	16.5	20.0
11.0–11.9	71	9.8	6.0	4.0	5.0	5.0	6.0	8.0	11.0	15.0	18.0	25.0
12.0–12.9	71	10.0	6.9	4.0	4.0	4.5	6.0	8.0	11.0	17.0	18.0	24.0
13.0–13.9	74	8.0	4.2	3.0	4.0	5.0	5.0	6.5	9.0	11.5	14.0	19.0
14.0–14.9	68	7.6	3.9	3.5	4.0	4.5	5.0	7.0	8.5	10.0	12.5	17.0
15.0–15.9	64	9.3	6.9	4.5	5.0	5.0	6.0	6.7	9.0	12.0	18.0	28.0
16.0–16.9	66	8.0	5.1	4.0	4.0	4.5	5.5	6.5	9.0	11.0	12.0	17.0
17.0–17.9	62	7.8	5.1	4.0	4.0	4.5	5.0	6.5	8.5	10.0	12.0	20.0
18.0–24.9	253	9.6	7.0	3.0	4.0	4.5	5.0	7.0	12.0	15.0	18.5	23.5
25.0–29.9	160	10.3	7.7	3.5	4.0	4.3	5.0	8.0	12.0	17.0	21.0	24.0
30.0–34.9	120	11.8	7.4	3.5	4.0	5.0	6.0	11.0	15.5	18.5	20.0	23.5
35.0–39.9	83	11.7	7.7	4.0	4.5	5.0	7.0	10.0	15.0	17.0	19.0	24.0
40.0–44.9	89	11.7	7.1	4.0	5.0	6.0	6.0	10.0	14.2	17.0	20.5	25.5
45.0–49.9	112	11.8	7.5	3.0	4.5	5.5	6.0	10.0	15.0	18.0	21.0	30.0
50.0–54.9	105	11.2	6.4	3.5	4.0	5.0	6.0	10.0	15.0	16.0	19.0	25.5
55.0–59.9	104	11.2	7.2	3.0	4.0	5.0	5.5	10.0	14.0	19.0	22.0	28.0
60.0–64.9	126	11.8	7.0	4.0	5.0	5.5	7.0	10.0	16.0	20.0	22.0	24.5
65.0–69.9	254	10.7	6.8	4.0	4.5	5.0	6.0	9.0	13.0	15.0	19.0	25.0
70.0–74.9	186	9.8	5.3	4.0	4.5	5.0	6.0	9.0	12.0	15.0	16.0	19.0
Females												
1.0–1.9	134	10.2	2.9	6.0	6.0	7.0	8.0	10.0	12.0	13.0	14.0	15.0
2.0–2.9	119	9.8	2.7	6.0	6.5	7.0	8.0	10.0	11.0	12.0	13.0	16.0
3.0–3.9	127	9.4	3.2	5.5	6.0	7.0	7.0	9.0	11.0	12.0	13.0	15.0
4.0–4.9	147	9.4	3.2	5.0	6.0	6.5	7.0	9.0	11.0	12.0	13.5	16.0
5.0–5.9	163	9.6	4.0	5.0	5.5	6.5	7.0	8.5	11.5	13.0	15.0	18.0
6.0–6.9	72	9.1	3.9	4.5	5.5	6.0	7.0	8.0	10.0	12.0	12.0	18.5
7.0–7.9	81	10.0	4.4	5.0	6.0	6.5	7.5	9.0	12.0	13.0	15.0	18.0
8.0–8.9	54	10.4	4.5	5.0	6.0	7.0	7.0	9.0	12.0	15.0	17.5	19.0
9.0–9.9	71	11.1	5.7	5.5	6.0	6.5	7.0	10.0	13.0	17.0	20.0	21.0
10.0–10.9	61	13.0	7.0	5.5	6.5	7.5	8.0	10.0	17.5	19.5	22.0	24.5
11.0–11.9	67	13.6	7.7	5.0	6.5	7.5	8.0	11.5	17.5	22.0	23.0	30.0
12.0–12.9	71	14.7	7.6	6.0	7.0	7.0	9.0	12.5	19.0	25.0	26.0	31.0
13.0–13.9	82	16.3	8.1	6.0	8.0	8.5	10.5	15.5	20.5	24.0	25.0	34.0
14.0–14.9	79	15.5	7.7	6.5	8.0	9.0	10.5	13.5	19.0	24.0	27.0	32.0
15.0–15.9	73	16.1	8.8	6.0	8.0	9.0	10.0	14.0	20.0	23.0	27.5	40.0
16.0–16.9	54	18.9	7.5	8.0	11.0	11.5	12.0	18.5	24.0	26.0	31.0	33.0
17.0–17.9	66	15.9	6.9	7.0	9.0	9.0	12.0	14.0	20.0	24.0	27.0	28.0
18.0–24.9	473	19.3	8.9	8.0	9.0	10.5	12.5	17.0	25.0	30.0	32.0	36.0
25.0–29.9	275	22.8	10.2	8.5	10.5	12.0	15.0	22.0	29.0	32.2	35.0	40.5
30.0–34.9	236	25.0	11.0	8.0	10.0	13.0	16.0	24.0	32.0	35.5	40.0	45.0
35.0–39.9	235	26.6	10.7	10.0	12.0	15.0	18.0	26.0	33.5	37.0	40.8	46.0
40.0–44.9	231	26.8	10.0	11.0	14.0	15.5	20.0	27.0	35.0	37.0	40.5	42.0
45.0–49.9	125	27.1	11.7	10.0	12.0	14.0	19.0	26.0	34.0	40.0	42.0	50.0
50.0–54.9	135	29.5	10.9	10.0	13.5	16.5	22.0	30.5	37.5	41.0	42.5	46.0
55.0–59.9	119	28.7	12.0	8.5	13.0	15.0	20.0	28.0	37.5	41.0	43.0	50.0
60.0–64.9	152	27.7	10.1	12.0	15.0	17.0	21.0	27.0	34.5	39.5	40.5	46.0
65.0–69.9	282	25.6	9.6	10.0	13.0	15.5	18.5	25.5	31.0	35.0	38.0	44.0
70.0–74.9	196	24.3	9.3	10.0	13.0	15.0	17.0	24.0	30.0	33.0	37.0	40.5

Means, standard deviations, and percentiles of subscapular skinfold thickness
(mm) by age (yrs) for Black males and females of 1 to 74 years

Age (yrs)	N	Mean	SD	Percentiles								
				5	10	15	25	50	75	85	90	95
Males												
1.0–1.9	157	6.6	2.0	4.0	4.0	4.5	5.0	6.0	8.0	8.5	9.0	10.5
2.0–2.9	142	6.1	2.1	4.0	4.0	4.5	5.0	6.0	7.0	8.0	9.0	10.0
3.0–3.9	151	5.4	1.7	3.5	4.0	4.0	4.5	5.0	6.0	6.5	7.0	8.5
4.0–4.9	151	5.0	1.4	3.0	3.5	4.0	4.0	5.0	5.5	6.0	6.5	7.5
5.0–5.9	122	5.0	2.2	3.0	3.0	3.5	4.0	4.5	5.0	6.0	7.0	8.0
6.0–6.9	60	5.1	3.5	3.0	3.0	3.0	4.0	4.0	5.0	5.5	6.5	11.0
7.0–7.9	67	5.2	3.0	3.0	3.5	3.5	4.0	4.5	5.0	6.0	7.0	10.0
8.0–8.9	49	5.7	3.0	3.5	3.5	4.0	4.0	5.0	6.0	7.5	9.0	11.0
9.0–9.9	74	5.6	3.6	3.0	3.5	3.7	4.0	5.0	6.0	7.0	8.0	11.0
10.0–10.9	60	7.3	5.7	4.0	4.0	4.0	4.5	5.0	7.0	8.0	12.0	19.0
11.0–11.9	71	7.6	5.9	4.0	4.0	4.5	5.0	5.5	7.0	10.5	14.5	21.0
12.0–12.9	71	8.3	7.3	4.0	4.0	4.0	4.5	5.5	7.0	16.0	18.0	22.0
13.0–13.9	74	6.9	3.8	3.0	4.5	5.0	5.0	6.0	8.0	8.5	9.5	17.0
14.0–14.9	68	7.4	4.6	4.0	4.5	5.0	5.0	6.0	8.0	8.0	11.0	16.0
15.0–15.9	65	10.4	8.4	5.0	5.0	6.0	6.5	8.0	10.0	14.5	17.0	24.0
16.0–16.9	66	9.6	4.7	5.5	6.5	7.0	7.0	8.0	10.0	13.0	14.5	17.5
17.0–17.9	63	9.5	4.9	5.0	6.0	6.0	6.5	8.0	10.5	12.0	14.0	16.0
18.0–24.9	253	12.7	7.9	6.0	6.5	7.0	8.0	10.0	15.0	18.5	22.5	29.0
25.0–29.9	159	14.5	9.4	6.5	7.0	7.5	8.0	11.0	17.0	24.0	28.0	38.0
30.0–34.9	120	17.4	9.9	6.0	8.0	9.0	10.0	15.0	22.0	25.0	30.0	36.0
35.0–39.9	88	19.0	10.1	7.0	8.0	10.0	11.0	17.0	24.0	26.5	33.0	35.5
40.0–44.9	87	17.2	9.4	6.5	7.5	8.5	10.0	15.0	22.0	25.0	30.0	35.0
45.0–49.9	111	17.9	10.7	5.0	6.5	7.0	9.0	16.0	25.0	29.0	31.5	35.0
50.0–54.9	103	17.4	10.1	6.0	7.0	7.5	9.0	15.0	25.0	28.0	30.0	36.0
55.0–59.9	103	17.7	10.0	5.0	6.5	7.0	9.5	15.0	24.0	27.0	30.5	35.0
60.0–64.9	126	18.0	9.6	6.0	7.5	8.0	10.5	16.0	24.0	27.0	30.5	39.5
65.0–69.9	253	16.3	9.6	5.0	6.0	7.0	9.0	14.0	21.0	25.5	30.0	37.5
70.0–74.9	185	15.8	9.2	6.0	6.0	7.0	8.0	13.5	21.0	26.0	30.5	35.0
Females												
1.0–1.9	134	6.6	1.9	4.0	5.0	5.0	5.0	6.5	8.0	8.5	9.0	10.0
2.0–2.9	119	6.4	2.9	4.0	4.0	4.5	5.0	6.0	7.0	8.5	9.5	12.0
3.0–3.9	127	5.7	2.2	3.0	4.0	4.0	4.5	5.0	6.5	7.0	7.5	9.0
4.0–4.9	147	6.0	2.7	3.5	4.0	4.0	4.5	5.0	7.0	8.0	9.0	11.0
5.0–5.9	163	6.0	3.1	3.5	4.0	4.0	4.0	5.0	6.5	8.0	10.0	12.0
6.0–6.9	72	6.1	4.1	3.0	4.0	4.0	4.0	5.0	6.5	7.0	7.5	12.0
7.0–7.9	81	6.4	2.9	3.5	4.0	4.0	5.0	5.5	7.0	8.0	10.0	12.0
8.0–8.9	54	7.1	4.7	4.0	4.0	4.0	4.5	5.0	7.0	11.5	14.0	16.0
9.0–9.9	71	7.9	5.5	4.0	4.0	4.5	5.0	6.0	8.0	10.0	13.5	24.0
10.0–10.9	61	9.5	6.8	4.0	4.5	5.0	5.5	6.5	11.0	16.0	17.0	23.6
11.0–11.9	67	10.8	8.4	5.0	5.0	5.0	6.0	8.0	12.0	15.0	20.0	30.5
12.0–12.9	71	13.4	10.1	5.0	5.5	5.5	6.5	9.0	16.0	26.5	30.0	36.0
13.0–13.9	82	13.5	7.6	5.5	6.5	7.0	8.0	12.0	16.5	20.0	25.0	28.4
14.0–14.9	79	13.1	8.1	6.0	6.0	6.0	7.5	10.0	17.0	19.5	27.0	33.5
15.0–15.9	72	13.8	9.1	6.0	7.0	7.5	8.0	10.0	16.5	20.0	26.5	35.0
16.0–16.9	54	17.1	10.0	7.0	8.0	9.0	10.5	14.0	20.0	27.0	33.0	40.5
17.0–17.9	66	14.9	7.9	6.5	7.0	8.0	9.0	12.0	20.0	24.0	27.0	30.0
18.0–24.9	472	17.9	10.2	6.5	7.5	8.0	10.0	15.0	24.0	29.0	32.0	38.0
25.0–29.9	272	21.6	11.3	7.0	8.5	10.0	12.0	20.5	28.0	34.5	37.0	41.5
30.0–34.9	235	25.2	13.1	7.0	9.0	11.0	14.5	25.0	34.5	40.0	43.0	49.0
35.0–39.9	233	26.1	11.9	7.0	9.5	12.0	16.5	27.5	34.0	38.0	40.6	45.0
40.0–44.9	227	27.2	12.3	8.0	11.0	13.0	18.0	27.5	35.0	40.0	44.0	48.0
45.0–49.9	122	27.8	12.9	9.5	11.0	12.5	17.0	28.0	37.0	41.0	44.0	50.0
50.0–54.9	131	30.7	12.5	10.0	13.5	16.0	22.0	30.5	38.0	43.1	47.8	52.5
55.0–59.9	118	28.8	13.1	7.0	9.0	13.0	21.0	28.0	37.0	44.0	47.5	54.5
60.0–64.9	149	28.0	12.0	8.5	12.0	14.0	20.0	28.0	35.5	39.0	44.0	50.0
65.0–69.9	277	25.1	11.5	7.5	9.5	11.0	16.0	25.0	32.0	37.0	40.4	45.5
70.0–74.9	197	22.9	10.5	7.5	9.9	11.0	14.0	22.0	31.0	35.0	37.0	40.0

Appendix A: Table 18.

Means, standard deviations, and percentiles of sum of triceps and subscapular skinfold thicknesses (mm) by age (yrs) for Black males and females of 1 to 74 years

Age (yrs)	N	Mean	SD	Percentiles								
				5	10	15	25	50	75	85	90	95
Males												
1.0–1.9	157	16.8	4.5	10.0	12.0	12.0	14.0	16.5	19.0	21.0	22.0	24.0
2.0–2.9	142	15.7	4.6	9.0	10.5	11.0	12.5	15.5	18.0	20.5	21.0	24.5
3.0–3.9	151	14.4	3.7	9.5	10.5	11.0	11.5	14.0	17.0	18.0	19.0	21.5
4.0–4.9	150	13.2	3.4	8.5	9.5	10.0	11.0	12.5	15.0	16.5	17.5	19.5
5.0–5.9	122	12.5	4.7	7.5	8.5	9.0	10.0	11.5	14.0	15.0	16.5	21.0
6.0–6.9	60	12.6	7.3	7.0	7.0	8.0	9.0	11.0	13.0	15.0	16.0	24.0
7.0–7.9	67	12.3	6.4	8.0	8.0	8.5	9.0	10.5	13.0	14.5	17.0	24.0
8.0–8.9	49	13.5	6.8	7.5	8.0	9.0	10.0	12.0	14.0	16.5	20.0	26.0
9.0–9.9	74	13.3	6.6	7.0	8.0	9.0	10.0	11.0	15.0	18.0	19.0	27.5
10.0–10.9	60	16.8	10.8	9.0	10.0	10.0	11.0	13.0	17.0	22.0	27.0	40.0
11.0–11.9	71	17.4	11.6	8.0	9.5	10.0	11.0	14.0	17.0	23.5	38.0	46.0
12.0–12.9	71	18.3	14.0	7.5	8.5	9.5	11.0	13.0	18.0	34.0	38.0	43.0
13.0–13.9	74	15.0	7.5	7.0	9.0	9.5	10.5	13.0	17.0	18.5	22.5	34.5
14.0–14.9	68	15.0	8.0	8.5	9.0	9.5	11.0	13.0	15.0	19.0	23.0	27.0
15.0–15.9	64	19.7	14.9	10.0	10.0	11.0	12.0	14.5	19.0	23.0	35.0	45.0
16.0–16.9	66	17.6	9.3	10.0	11.0	12.0	13.0	15.5	18.0	23.0	27.5	28.5
17.0–17.9	62	17.0	9.0	9.5	10.5	11.0	11.5	14.0	19.5	22.5	24.5	31.0
18.0–24.9	252	22.3	14.3	10.0	11.0	11.5	13.0	17.0	27.0	33.0	39.0	51.0
25.0–29.9	159	24.7	16.3	10.5	11.0	12.0	14.0	19.0	29.5	40.0	49.0	61.0
30.0–34.9	120	29.2	16.6	10.0	12.5	14.0	17.5	26.0	37.0	43.0	49.0	59.5
35.0–39.9	83	30.1	16.8	11.0	13.0	14.5	19.0	26.5	38.0	43.0	47.0	57.0
40.0–44.9	86	28.3	14.8	12.0	13.0	14.0	16.5	27.0	35.0	41.0	47.0	50.5
45.0–49.9	110	29.3	16.9	10.0	11.0	12.0	16.0	26.0	39.5	44.5	48.0	59.0
50.0–54.9	103	28.5	15.6	10.0	11.5	13.0	15.0	26.0	41.0	43.5	49.0	56.0
55.0–59.9	103	28.8	16.0	9.0	10.0	12.0	15.5	25.5	38.0	45.5	52.0	57.0
60.0–64.9	126	29.9	15.7	10.0	13.0	15.0	18.0	25.5	37.0	46.0	53.0	61.0
65.0–69.9	253	26.9	15.4	10.0	11.0	13.0	15.0	23.5	33.5	41.5	48.0	57.0
70.0–74.9	185	25.5	13.1	10.0	11.5	12.5	15.0	23.0	32.5	41.0	46.0	49.5
Females												
1.0–1.9	134	16.8	4.3	10.0	12.0	12.5	13.5	17.0	19.0	21.0	22.0	24.5
2.0–2.9	119	16.2	4.6	10.5	11.0	12.0	13.0	15.5	18.5	20.5	24.0	25.0
3.0–3.9	127	15.0	4.9	9.0	10.5	11.0	12.0	14.0	17.0	18.5	20.5	22.0
4.0–4.9	147	15.4	5.5	9.0	10.0	11.0	12.0	14.0	18.0	20.0	22.5	26.0
5.0–5.9	163	15.6	6.7	9.0	10.0	11.0	11.0	13.5	18.0	20.0	25.0	29.0
6.0–6.9	72	15.2	7.5	8.0	10.0	10.0	11.0	14.0	17.0	18.5	19.0	33.5
7.0–7.9	81	16.4	6.9	9.0	11.0	11.5	12.5	14.5	18.0	22.0	23.0	29.0
8.0–8.9	54	17.5	8.9	9.5	10.5	11.5	12.0	14.0	18.5	28.5	31.0	33.0
9.0–9.9	71	19.0	10.7	10.0	10.5	11.0	12.0	15.5	23.0	25.5	32.0	42.0
10.0–10.9	61	22.5	13.3	10.5	12.0	12.5	13.5	18.0	28.0	36.0	39.0	54.0
11.0–11.9	67	24.5	15.7	9.5	12.5	13.0	14.5	19.0	28.5	37.5	43.0	55.0
12.0–12.9	71	28.1	17.3	11.5	13.0	13.0	16.0	21.5	34.0	50.0	55.0	67.0
13.0–13.9	82	29.8	15.2	13.0	14.0	15.5	19.0	25.5	35.5	45.0	50.0	60.5
14.0–14.9	79	28.7	15.5	12.5	14.0	16.0	19.0	24.0	35.0	42.5	53.5	65.5
15.0–15.9	72	29.5	16.8	13.0	15.0	16.5	18.0	24.0	33.0	42.5	52.0	66.2
16.0–16.9	54	36.0	16.8	18.0	20.0	21.5	23.0	32.5	41.0	52.5	62.0	72.5
17.0–17.9	66	30.8	14.2	14.0	17.0	18.0	21.0	25.0	36.5	48.0	49.0	58.0
18.0–24.9	472	37.2	18.3	15.5	18.0	19.0	22.5	32.5	47.5	57.7	63.0	74.0
25.0–29.9	271	44.0	20.1	17.5	20.0	22.0	28.0	42.0	57.0	64.0	68.0	77.5
30.0–34.9	235	50.1	23.2	15.0	22.0	24.5	30.5	50.0	66.0	75.0	84.0	91.0
35.0–39.9	232	52.5	21.3	18.0	22.0	28.0	36.5	53.2	67.0	75.0	79.0	86.0
40.0–44.9	227	53.9	21.3	19.0	26.0	30.5	39.0	54.0	68.0	76.0	82.0	89.0
45.0–49.9	122	54.3	22.7	18.5	24.0	29.0	36.5	55.0	70.5	79.0	81.5	91.0
50.0–54.9	131	59.9	22.1	21.0	30.0	37.0	45.5	60.2	76.5	83.0	86.5	93.8
55.0–59.9	117	57.1	23.7	17.0	23.0	34.0	41.0	57.0	71.5	83.0	87.0	98.5
60.0–64.9	148	55.2	20.6	21.5	27.5	35.0	40.0	55.5	67.5	76.0	81.5	92.0
65.0–69.9	277	50.5	19.7	18.0	24.5	31.5	36.5	49.5	62.0	71.5	77.5	85.5
70.0–74.9	196	47.1	18.2	19.0	24.0	28.0	33.0	46.5	61.0	65.0	69.5	78.5

Appendix B
Anthropometric Tables for Whites

Based on a cross-sectional sample of 35,436 subjects aged 1 to 74 years derived from the first and second National Health and Nutrition Examination Surveys (NHANES I and II) of the United States conducted during 1971–74 and 1976–80.

Means, standard deviations, and percentiles of stature (cm) by age (yrs) for White males and females of 1 to 74 years

Age (yrs)	N	Mean	SD	Percentiles								
				5	10	15	25	50	75	85	90	95
Males												
1.0–1.9	277	82.5	5.0	75.7	76.8	77.9	79.4	82.2	85.6	87.2	88.0	89.2
2.0–2.9	504	91.7	4.2	85.8	86.8	87.5	88.9	91.7	94.4	95.8	97.0	98.3
3.0–3.9	540	99.1	4.5	92.0	94.0	94.8	96.3	98.8	102.0	103.8	104.8	106.3
4.0–4.9	547	105.7	4.8	98.3	99.6	100.6	102.6	105.7	108.9	110.5	112.0	113.7
5.0–5.9	533	112.3	5.1	103.4	105.6	106.8	109.0	112.4	115.6	117.8	119.1	120.7
6.0–6.9	231	119.1	5.4	109.4	111.9	113.0	115.5	119.3	122.8	124.9	125.6	127.7
7.0–7.9	240	125.2	5.6	115.6	118.3	119.6	121.9	125.4	128.6	130.6	131.6	133.4
8.0–8.9	240	129.5	6.2	119.9	122.0	123.7	125.4	129.9	133.7	135.2	136.7	138.2
9.0–9.9	242	135.9	5.8	126.7	129.1	130.0	131.5	136.0	140.1	142.0	142.8	145.4
10.0–10.9	269	140.9	6.7	130.3	132.4	134.0	136.3	140.7	145.8	147.5	149.6	151.9
11.0–11.9	248	146.1	7.3	134.7	136.6	138.1	141.2	145.7	151.0	153.7	154.7	157.7
12.0–12.9	273	152.4	7.8	139.9	142.4	144.2	146.9	151.8	157.8	160.3	162.0	166.0
13.0–13.9	268	159.3	8.6	145.3	147.6	149.5	152.8	159.5	165.6	169.2	170.8	173.1
14.0–14.9	287	167.4	8.0	153.9	157.0	159.7	162.8	167.4	172.9	175.9	178.1	179.7
15.0–15.9	288	170.9	7.5	158.1	161.1	162.4	165.6	171.4	176.2	178.0	180.0	183.4
16.0–16.9	278	174.7	7.0	162.8	164.8	167.3	170.3	174.4	179.1	182.0	183.8	186.7
17.0–17.9	266	175.8	6.7	165.3	167.4	168.8	171.0	175.6	181.0	183.0	184.3	187.3
18.0–24.9	1465	176.9	7.0	166.2	168.3	169.9	172.2	176.8	181.3	183.9	185.9	188.9
25.0–29.9	1073	177.0	6.9	166.0	168.5	170.0	172.3	176.7	181.8	184.3	185.8	188.4
30.0–34.9	799	176.5	6.8	165.4	167.5	169.6	172.0	176.4	181.0	183.5	185.0	187.4
35.0–39.9	734	176.4	7.1	164.6	167.1	169.0	172.2	176.4	181.3	183.7	185.2	187.6
40.0–44.9	723	176.2	6.6	165.3	167.8	169.3	171.7	176.4	180.5	183.0	184.5	187.3
45.0–49.9	748	175.2	7.0	163.8	166.8	168.2	170.7	174.9	180.0	182.6	184.4	186.5
50.0–54.9	767	174.8	6.5	164.4	166.5	167.8	170.2	174.7	179.0	181.9	183.6	185.6
55.0–59.9	693	174.0	6.7	163.5	165.3	166.9	169.5	173.7	178.7	181.2	182.5	184.6
60.0–64.9	1122	173.0	6.6	161.9	164.9	166.3	168.7	173.0	177.4	179.7	181.1	183.5
65.0–69.9	1488	171.8	6.8	160.5	163.4	164.9	167.0	171.8	176.5	178.8	180.5	183.1
70.0–74.9	1057	170.6	6.8	159.5	162.2	163.6	165.8	170.6	175.1	177.6	179.5	181.6
Females												
1.0–1.9	264	80.5	4.9	73.0	74.7	75.6	76.9	80.2	83.6	85.8	86.8	88.4
2.0–2.9	479	90.2	4.4	83.4	84.9	85.7	86.9	90.2	93.0	94.5	95.7	97.4
3.0–3.9	509	97.5	4.5	90.1	91.6	92.7	94.6	97.4	100.5	102.3	103.4	104.5
4.0–4.9	519	104.5	4.8	96.2	98.3	99.4	101.3	104.5	107.7	109.3	110.7	112.2
5.0–5.9	504	111.5	5.2	103.1	105.2	106.7	108.3	111.5	114.7	116.4	118.5	120.3
6.0–6.9	218	117.8	5.7	109.5	111.2	111.9	113.3	118.2	121.7	123.4	124.5	127.1
7.0–7.9	245	123.7	5.9	115.3	116.9	117.8	120.0	124.0	127.7	129.4	130.7	133.6
8.0–8.9	221	129.6	5.8	120.1	122.2	123.7	125.5	129.6	133.0	135.4	137.3	139.0
9.0–9.9	248	135.3	7.3	124.5	127.1	128.3	130.4	135.4	140.1	141.8	143.6	147.2
10.0–10.9	266	140.9	7.1	129.7	132.0	133.6	135.9	141.0	145.2	147.7	150.2	152.5
11.0–11.9	230	148.0	8.2	134.6	138.2	139.6	142.2	148.1	153.2	156.2	157.7	162.7
12.0–12.9	247	154.6	7.2	142.6	145.6	147.3	149.7	154.8	159.2	162.5	164.4	165.5
13.0–13.9	276	158.6	6.6	148.0	150.4	152.4	155.1	158.8	163.0	164.9	165.8	168.3
14.0–14.9	287	161.2	6.2	151.0	153.0	154.7	157.0	161.2	165.3	167.3	169.0	171.9
15.0–15.9	234	163.3	6.3	153.4	155.6	157.2	158.9	162.7	167.3	169.9	172.4	175.3
16.0–16.9	284	162.2	6.4	151.9	154.0	155.9	157.7	162.1	166.1	169.0	171.3	172.8
17.0–17.9	223	162.9	6.2	152.5	155.6	156.9	159.6	162.8	166.8	169.0	170.6	173.9
18.0–24.9	2061	163.3	6.4	152.6	155.2	156.8	159.0	163.4	167.4	169.7	171.2	173.7
25.0–29.9	1618	163.0	6.3	152.9	155.3	156.7	158.7	162.9	167.2	169.5	171.2	173.9
30.0–34.9	1374	162.7	6.2	153.1	155.2	156.5	158.5	162.5	167.0	169.3	171.2	173.2
35.0–39.9	1198	162.9	6.4	152.4	155.2	156.4	158.4	162.8	167.1	169.5	171.0	173.5
40.0–44.9	1142	162.6	6.3	152.3	154.7	156.4	158.3	162.7	166.7	168.6	170.3	173.2
45.0–49.9	832	162.2	6.1	152.2	154.2	155.5	158.2	162.2	166.4	168.5	169.9	172.4
50.0–54.9	863	161.1	5.9	151.6	153.9	155.4	156.9	161.1	164.9	167.2	168.7	170.6
55.0–59.9	756	160.2	6.0	150.2	152.8	154.4	156.7	160.2	164.3	166.1	167.5	169.9
60.0–64.9	1225	159.6	6.3	149.2	151.4	153.1	155.7	160.0	163.7	166.0	167.3	169.4
65.0–69.9	1651	158.6	6.0	148.4	150.7	152.4	154.7	158.9	162.6	164.8	166.2	168.2
70.0–74.9	1262	157.5	6.1	147.2	150.0	151.6	153.6	157.3	161.5	163.7	165.5	167.4

Appendix B: Table 2.

Means, standard deviations, and percentiles of weight (kg) by age (yrs) for White males and females of 1 to 74 years

Age (yrs)	N	Mean	SD	Percentiles								
				5	10	15	25	50	75	85	90	95
Males												
1.0–1.9	508	11.8	1.7	9.5	10.0	10.3	10.7	11.6	12.6	13.1	13.6	14.2
2.0–2.9	513	13.6	1.7	11.0	11.6	12.0	12.6	13.6	14.6	15.2	15.5	16.6
3.0–3.9	541	15.7	2.0	12.9	13.6	13.9	14.4	15.5	16.8	17.5	18.0	18.9
4.0–4.9	547	17.7	2.4	14.3	15.1	15.4	16.1	17.5	18.9	19.8	20.5	21.4
5.0–5.9	534	19.8	2.9	15.9	16.6	17.1	17.7	19.5	21.4	22.3	23.5	24.6
6.0–6.9	231	22.5	3.7	17.2	18.8	19.3	20.1	21.9	24.0	26.0	27.7	30.0
7.0–7.9	240	25.3	4.2	19.0	21.1	21.3	22.4	24.8	27.2	28.7	29.9	33.3
8.0–8.9	240	27.6	5.3	21.0	22.7	23.3	24.3	26.6	29.7	31.8	33.3	37.0
9.0–9.9	242	31.7	6.5	23.8	25.3	26.2	27.3	30.5	33.6	38.4	40.7	43.5
10.0–10.9	269	35.5	7.7	26.8	27.9	28.5	30.4	33.9	38.4	42.1	45.6	52.3
11.0–11.9	248	40.0	10.2	28.2	29.8	31.5	33.3	37.6	43.9	49.4	52.4	59.9
12.0–12.9	273	44.5	10.1	31.3	33.0	34.5	37.5	42.6	49.6	54.1	59.0	65.7
13.0–13.9	266	50.7	12.0	35.3	37.6	38.9	42.9	48.9	57.4	61.7	66.3	71.1
14.0–14.9	287	57.6	12.3	41.6	44.4	46.5	49.7	56.1	63.3	67.4	71.0	77.1
15.0–15.9	288	60.7	11.3	44.0	48.3	50.6	53.8	60.0	65.9	70.2	73.9	80.3
16.0–16.9	278	67.0	12.3	51.1	53.9	55.4	58.8	65.0	73.4	78.0	81.1	89.0
17.0–17.9	267	68.0	11.9	51.4	55.3	57.0	60.0	66.1	73.1	78.2	83.3	91.4
18.0–24.9	1467	74.3	13.0	56.8	60.3	61.9	65.3	71.9	81.0	86.9	92.1	99.9
25.0–29.9	1073	78.3	14.0	59.4	62.5	65.0	68.9	76.7	85.2	90.6	95.1	102.6
30.0–34.9	800	80.1	13.5	60.4	64.3	66.9	70.4	79.1	87.4	93.5	96.7	102.7
35.0–39.9	735	80.6	13.0	59.2	64.6	68.0	72.7	80.1	87.8	92.4	96.3	102.1
40.0–44.9	723	81.4	13.5	61.7	65.7	68.5	72.6	79.9	89.4	94.2	99.6	104.8
45.0–49.9	748	80.9	13.6	60.2	64.2	67.1	72.0	79.8	88.7	93.8	96.7	103.0
50.0–54.9	767	79.6	13.6	59.1	64.4	66.4	70.6	78.3	87.2	92.8	98.8	102.7
55.0–59.9	694	79.5	13.3	59.1	64.0	66.7	70.8	78.7	86.9	92.8	96.4	102.6
60.0–64.9	1124	77.4	12.9	58.2	62.0	64.9	69.1	76.8	84.9	89.5	92.3	99.3
65.0–69.9	1489	75.6	12.7	55.6	59.5	62.5	67.5	75.3	83.5	87.9	91.2	96.7
70.0–74.9	1057	74.1	12.4	54.0	58.5	62.0	66.2	73.5	81.4	86.3	90.3	95.4
Females												
1.0–1.9	470	10.9	1.4	8.8	9.2	9.5	9.9	10.8	11.8	12.4	12.8	13.4
2.0–2.9	483	13.0	1.6	10.8	11.2	11.6	12.0	12.8	13.9	14.6	15.0	15.9
3.0–3.9	509	15.0	2.0	11.8	12.6	13.0	13.6	14.9	16.2	17.1	17.6	18.5
4.0–4.9	523	16.9	2.2	13.7	14.3	14.6	15.3	16.7	18.3	19.0	19.7	20.9
5.0–5.9	505	19.4	3.0	15.4	16.3	16.8	17.3	18.9	20.6	21.9	22.9	24.9
6.0–6.9	218	21.7	3.6	17.0	17.5	18.4	19.3	21.3	23.5	24.5	26.9	29.5
7.0–7.9	245	24.6	4.6	19.2	19.7	20.6	21.8	23.5	26.2	28.2	29.9	32.8
8.0–8.9	221	28.2	6.5	20.8	21.8	22.6	24.0	27.0	30.5	33.1	36.3	39.9
9.0–9.9	248	32.2	7.8	23.7	24.8	25.6	26.9	31.0	34.7	38.9	42.8	47.6
10.0–10.9	266	35.1	7.7	25.6	27.0	27.9	29.4	33.6	38.9	43.7	45.7	49.7
11.0–11.9	230	41.6	10.4	29.5	30.5	31.6	34.3	39.5	46.3	52.2	56.6	60.0
12.0–12.9	247	46.8	9.9	33.0	34.9	37.1	39.5	45.8	52.3	57.3	60.4	66.0
13.0–13.9	276	51.1	12.0	36.1	38.6	40.3	43.2	49.0	55.3	60.9	66.7	75.2
14.0–14.9	287	54.8	10.5	40.5	43.7	45.0	47.5	53.0	60.0	64.1	69.1	75.2
15.0–15.9	234	56.0	10.8	43.4	45.1	46.5	48.4	54.3	60.2	64.3	67.6	76.5
16.0–16.9	284	57.5	11.0	43.2	45.8	47.5	50.7	55.3	62.5	68.5	72.2	76.8
17.0–17.9	223	59.5	12.8	43.8	46.4	49.6	52.0	57.6	62.7	69.2	74.3	81.8
18.0–24.9	2061	60.4	12.2	45.9	48.6	50.1	52.6	57.9	65.0	70.3	74.6	82.4
25.0–29.9	1618	62.1	13.8	46.4	48.8	50.5	53.1	58.7	67.4	74.5	80.4	88.2
30.0–34.9	1374	64.5	15.2	47.6	50.1	52.0	54.5	60.7	70.1	78.0	84.5	95.6
35.0–39.9	1198	65.5	14.6	48.4	51.6	53.6	56.1	61.9	71.3	78.5	84.6	94.5
40.0–44.9	1142	66.4	15.1	49.3	51.6	53.5	56.4	62.4	72.1	80.5	86.0	95.8
45.0–49.9	832	67.3	15.2	47.7	51.4	53.5	56.9	64.3	74.7	81.8	86.5	97.0
50.0–54.9	863	67.1	13.7	48.6	51.9	54.3	57.4	64.8	73.8	80.6	85.5	93.7
55.0–59.9	757	67.7	14.6	48.5	51.5	54.3	57.5	64.9	75.1	82.8	87.7	94.8
60.0–64.9	1226	67.4	13.8	48.3	51.4	53.9	57.9	65.2	75.0	80.6	84.6	92.6
65.0–69.9	1652	66.9	13.9	48.0	51.4	53.4	57.1	65.0	74.2	79.6	84.4	92.5
70.0–74.9	1263	65.6	13.1	46.6	50.2	52.5	56.9	64.1	73.9	79.0	82.5	87.4

Means, standard deviations, and percentiles of weight (kg) by height (cm) for White males of 2 to 74 years

Height (cm)	N	Mean	SD	Percentiles								
				5	10	15	25	50	75	85	90	95
Boys: 2 to 11 years												
84–086	43	12.0	1.0	10.7	10.9	11.0	11.3	12.0	12.7	12.8	13.1	13.5
87–089	127	12.8	1.1	11.2	11.4	11.7	12.0	12.8	13.4	13.8	14.2	14.6
90–092	158	13.5	1.0	11.9	12.4	12.6	12.8	13.6	14.2	14.6	14.9	15.0
93–095	222	14.4	1.2	12.7	13.0	13.4	13.7	14.3	15.0	15.4	15.6	16.2
96–098	233	15.0	1.2	13.1	13.6	13.8	14.3	15.0	15.5	16.1	16.4	16.9
99–101	243	16.0	1.3	14.1	14.4	14.7	15.1	15.9	16.8	17.3	17.8	18.4
102–104	235	16.9	1.3	15.1	15.5	15.6	15.9	16.8	17.7	18.0	18.5	19.3
105–107	237	17.7	1.7	15.4	15.9	16.2	16.7	17.5	18.4	18.9	19.4	20.1
108–110	226	18.7	1.9	16.6	16.9	17.1	17.5	18.4	19.5	20.0	20.6	21.3
111–113	210	20.1	2.3	17.2	17.8	18.0	18.8	19.6	21.1	21.8	22.3	23.4
114–116	171	20.9	2.1	18.3	18.9	19.2	19.6	20.5	21.5	22.3	22.7	23.6
117–119	152	22.1	2.4	19.3	19.8	20.3	20.9	21.7	23.0	23.9	24.6	26.2
120–122	133	23.4	2.3	20.2	21.0	21.4	22.1	23.1	24.5	25.5	26.3	27.3
123–125	132	24.8	2.6	21.4	21.9	22.4	23.1	24.3	26.0	27.0	28.0	29.1
126–128	139	26.6	4.0	22.2	23.0	23.7	24.3	26.1	27.9	29.5	30.6	33.8
129–131	132	27.9	3.2	23.6	24.6	24.9	25.7	27.4	29.3	30.6	31.8	33.2
132–134	147	29.5	3.5	25.2	25.7	26.1	26.9	28.8	31.3	33.1	34.4	35.4
135–137	141	31.6	4.7	26.4	27.3	27.7	28.6	30.6	33.2	36.5	38.0	41.5
138–140	123	33.5	4.6	28.0	29.0	29.4	30.4	32.3	35.6	38.6	40.3	42.0
141–143	120	36.5	5.1	30.5	31.5	32.0	33.2	35.4	38.6	40.5	43.3	45.4
144–146	91	39.4	7.2	31.6	32.3	33.0	35.1	38.1	42.1	45.0	47.3	55.2
147–149	62	40.6	6.7	33.6	34.5	35.3	35.6	38.6	43.3	47.3	50.6	53.4
Boys: 12 to 17 years												
144–146	48	38.4	5.7	31.3	32.4	33.6	34.6	37.1	40.5	42.1	46.1	53.0
147–149	63	41.4	7.6	33.6	34.0	34.7	36.3	38.9	44.7	48.1	50.5	59.8
150–152	82	44.0	6.9	36.3	37.2	38.0	38.9	41.7	46.8	53.5	55.4	57.0
153–155	83	46.3	8.1	36.5	38.0	38.9	40.6	44.4	50.6	53.1	55.2	59.3
156–158	84	48.9	9.4	40.4	41.2	41.6	42.5	46.4	50.0	57.9	63.2	67.3
159–161	112	51.9	9.9	40.8	43.4	44.0	45.9	49.0	54.2	61.7	66.9	71.3
162–164	141	54.4	9.0	45.0	46.0	46.9	48.9	53.0	58.1	61.3	64.3	68.9
165–167	141	57.5	9.7	47.2	48.1	49.7	51.4	55.4	61.1	65.3	68.6	73.3
168–170	188	61.2	9.8	49.2	51.5	52.8	55.0	59.9	65.3	69.6	72.5	77.1
171–173	190	62.9	9.2	51.4	53.1	54.8	56.9	61.2	66.1	71.7	75.1	79.8
174–176	165	66.4	9.9	52.8	55.8	57.4	60.0	65.0	71.0	74.5	78.0	85.7
177–179	135	69.3	12.8	56.6	58.8	59.9	61.6	66.2	72.3	76.3	83.1	94.3
180–182	88	71.8	9.4	60.5	61.0	62.1	63.7	70.1	79.5	81.6	84.8	87.9
183–185	50	73.5	9.2	62.4	63.4	65.4	68.3	72.1	77.8	79.4	85.3	94.8
186–188	31	80.9	17.2	60.9	63.6	64.6	68.5	78.1	91.7	95.8	104.4	119.8
Males: 18 to 74 years												
153–155	45	62.8	9.8	48.6	50.7	53.6	57.1	61.7	66.6	73.1	76.9	80.6
156–158	103	66.9	11.1	49.0	54.0	55.2	58.1	66.9	74.3	78.0	79.7	86.0
159–161	226	67.5	10.0	50.7	55.8	57.4	60.6	67.0	73.4	79.3	80.6	84.6
162–164	523	68.4	10.4	52.5	55.6	57.4	60.9	68.3	74.7	79.6	81.6	86.5
165–167	958	71.1	11.2	53.0	57.1	60.2	63.8	71.0	77.7	82.3	84.9	90.0
168–170	1332	73.9	11.9	56.0	59.4	62.1	66.4	73.3	80.4	84.7	88.1	93.9
171–173	1757	76.4	12.0	58.6	61.9	64.0	68.1	75.5	83.3	88.1	91.7	97.4
174–176	1769	78.4	12.2	60.3	64.3	66.6	70.2	77.4	84.9	89.7	93.5	99.3
177–179	1523	80.4	12.3	62.3	65.5	68.0	71.8	79.5	87.3	92.2	96.0	101.8
180–182	1094	82.4	13.1	63.4	67.7	69.8	73.1	81.2	89.9	94.3	98.7	104.5
183–185	729	85.4	13.6	65.5	69.7	72.1	75.6	83.7	93.2	99.0	102.6	110.4
186–188	358	87.8	12.5	69.3	72.6	75.1	79.9	86.6	94.8	100.1	103.4	107.7
189–191	143	91.6	15.3	71.3	75.3	77.8	80.5	89.9	99.4	104.3	110.3	123.7
192–194	62	96.3	16.0	71.8	78.6	80.2	86.6	94.6	105.2	109.1	111.8	123.8

Means, standard deviations, and percentiles of weight (kg) by height (cm) for White females of 2 to 74 years

Height (cm)	N	Mean	SD	Percentiles								
				5	10	15	25	50	75	85	90	95
Girls: 2 to 10 years												
81–083	28	11.1	.8	10.1	10.2	10.3	10.5	10.9	11.6	12.1	12.6	12.6
84–086	91	12.0	.9	10.7	10.9	11.0	11.4	12.0	12.5	12.8	13.0	13.4
87–089	122	12.5	1.0	11.1	11.4	11.6	11.8	12.4	12.9	13.5	13.7	14.4
90–092	190	13.2	1.2	11.6	11.8	11.9	12.3	13.0	13.7	14.3	14.6	15.3
93–095	205	14.0	1.2	12.3	12.6	12.8	13.1	13.8	14.6	15.3	15.6	16.1
96–098	220	15.0	1.3	13.3	13.6	13.7	14.2	14.9	15.6	16.3	16.7	17.2
99–101	211	15.8	1.5	13.9	14.2	14.4	14.7	15.5	16.6	17.2	17.6	18.4
102–104	218	16.7	2.0	14.4	15.0	15.1	15.5	16.4	17.3	17.9	18.3	19.4
105–107	215	17.7	1.6	15.6	16.0	16.2	16.7	17.5	18.5	19.3	19.6	20.2
108–110	213	18.2	1.6	15.8	16.6	16.8	17.2	18.1	19.0	19.7	20.1	21.0
111–113	195	19.4	1.8	16.3	17.2	17.5	18.4	19.4	20.4	21.2	21.8	22.8
114–116	150	20.8	2.6	17.3	18.3	18.6	19.0	20.2	21.8	23.0	24.1	25.9
117–119	133	21.8	2.1	19.0	19.5	19.6	20.2	21.4	22.7	23.7	24.6	26.0
120–122	135	23.2	2.6	19.7	20.4	20.9	21.5	22.8	24.4	25.3	26.3	28.5
123–125	118	24.4	2.4	21.0	21.8	22.2	22.8	24.0	25.9	26.5	27.3	29.3
126–128	123	26.5	3.0	22.6	23.0	23.6	24.0	25.8	28.0	29.6	30.3	31.5
129–131	127	28.3	3.9	23.7	24.4	24.9	25.6	27.6	29.7	31.1	33.6	37.0
132–134	115	30.7	4.6	24.6	25.8	26.2	27.2	30.3	32.7	35.0	38.0	39.9
135–137	105	31.9	5.2	26.4	27.3	27.6	28.2	30.8	33.3	35.7	38.8	43.3
138–140	102	35.1	7.9	27.3	28.8	29.3	30.8	32.5	36.5	42.6	44.7	47.6
141–143	76	36.2	6.4	28.8	29.9	31.0	32.3	34.9	37.9	41.2	45.6	49.9
144–146	45	39.4	6.6	32.7	32.9	33.0	35.0	37.6	42.4	46.3	49.7	51.8
147–149	33	39.9	7.2	29.6	32.0	33.9	35.5	38.9	44.2	46.7	48.0	56.5
Girls: 11 to 17 years												
141–143	43	37.0	7.1	29.8	30.0	31.2	33.2	35.3	38.2	42.2	44.0	51.0
144–146	47	39.0	6.8	30.5	31.1	31.6	33.4	38.7	41.5	44.1	46.5	52.4
147–149	98	43.1	8.4	32.7	34.3	35.6	37.6	40.7	46.1	51.0	56.4	62.4
150–152	136	45.0	8.2	34.8	36.3	37.3	38.9	43.4	49.4	52.5	54.8	59.0
153–155	176	48.3	8.2	38.0	39.7	40.6	42.9	46.1	52.8	56.5	59.9	64.1
156–158	272	52.2	9.7	40.3	42.4	43.5	45.3	50.0	58.1	62.5	65.9	71.1
159–161	285	54.8	10.4	42.5	44.3	46.1	48.3	52.4	58.7	62.6	67.1	75.6
162–164	274	55.9	9.2	44.6	46.4	47.5	49.9	54.2	60.1	64.1	66.9	71.9
165–167	183	59.8	12.5	46.1	48.8	50.0	52.7	57.5	62.7	69.5	74.7	84.1
168–170	102	60.8	10.0	48.9	49.2	51.3	53.5	59.0	64.8	72.6	74.6	78.7
171–173	63	67.2	15.2	53.2	54.3	54.9	57.7	61.7	70.8	79.5	89.7	104.2
Females: 18 to 74 years												
141–143	60	55.6	10.4	38.1	40.9	42.4	48.3	55.9	63.2	64.9	67.7	70.6
144–146	139	57.3	14.2	38.7	42.0	44.1	48.5	54.7	64.2	70.9	74.4	77.7
147–149	329	59.1	12.8	42.3	44.9	47.6	50.1	56.6	66.0	71.8	75.8	83.2
150–152	776	60.7	13.1	43.1	46.4	48.1	51.4	58.6	67.8	73.7	78.0	86.4
153–155	1421	62.3	13.3	45.1	47.5	49.7	52.8	60.2	69.5	76.3	80.4	86.8
156–158	2222	62.8	13.6	46.6	49.0	50.7	53.3	60.0	69.7	76.1	80.1	88.3
159–161	2568	64.7	13.9	47.8	50.3	52.0	54.9	61.7	71.8	78.7	83.5	91.4
162–164	2387	65.9	13.8	49.4	51.4	53.3	56.3	62.7	72.6	79.5	83.6	92.4
165–167	1971	67.4	14.5	50.2	52.7	54.5	57.5	63.5	73.6	81.4	86.8	96.4
168–170	1102	68.1	13.9	52.6	54.5	56.3	59.0	64.9	73.6	79.7	86.2	94.5
171–173	578	70.6	15.1	54.0	55.7	57.4	60.1	66.9	77.3	84.0	91.6	103.9
174–176	281	71.4	15.7	56.1	57.9	59.4	61.7	67.6	75.6	80.8	88.4	105.6
177–179	78	72.4	14.3	57.6	59.9	60.7	63.5	68.4	77.1	83.3	88.8	109.4

Means, standard deviations, and percentiles of Body mass index (w/s^2) by age (yrs) for White males and females of 1 to 74 years

Age (yrs)	N	Mean	SD	Percentiles								
				5	10	15	25	50	75	85	90	95
Males												
1.0–1.9	277	17.3	2.6	15.3	15.6	15.9	16.4	17.1	17.9	18.6	18.9	19.6
2.0–2.9	504	16.2	1.3	14.3	14.5	15.0	15.4	16.2	17.0	17.4	17.7	18.2
3.0–3.9	540	16.0	1.3	14.2	14.5	14.8	15.2	15.8	16.6	17.1	17.5	18.2
4.0–4.9	547	15.8	1.4	14.0	14.4	14.6	14.9	15.6	16.4	16.8	17.2	17.8
5.0–5.9	533	15.6	1.5	13.8	14.1	14.3	14.7	15.5	16.3	16.8	17.2	18.1
6.0–6.9	231	15.8	1.8	13.7	14.0	14.3	14.6	15.3	16.4	17.1	17.9	19.1
7.0–7.9	240	16.1	1.8	13.6	14.1	14.5	15.0	15.7	16.8	17.7	18.2	19.2
8.0–8.9	240	16.4	2.2	13.9	14.3	14.6	15.0	16.0	17.1	18.1	19.1	20.1
9.0–9.9	242	17.0	2.5	14.3	14.6	14.9	15.4	16.4	18.0	19.4	20.2	21.8
10.0–10.9	269	17.7	2.8	14.6	15.0	15.4	15.8	17.1	18.8	20.0	21.2	23.3
11.0–11.9	248	18.6	3.8	14.6	15.1	15.6	16.2	17.5	20.2	21.7	22.7	26.0
12.0–12.9	273	19.0	3.4	15.1	15.8	16.1	16.7	18.1	20.4	22.1	23.7	25.9
13.0–13.9	266	19.8	3.7	15.7	16.5	16.8	17.5	19.0	21.2	23.4	24.6	26.7
14.0–14.9	287	20.4	3.5	16.6	17.1	17.6	18.1	19.6	21.8	23.6	24.4	27.0
15.0–15.9	288	20.7	3.1	16.6	17.4	18.0	19.0	20.4	21.9	23.0	24.0	26.6
16.0–16.9	278	21.9	3.4	17.8	18.4	18.8	19.6	21.3	23.0	25.0	26.0	27.6
17.0–17.9	266	21.9	3.4	17.9	18.6	19.0	19.7	21.2	23.5	24.9	26.0	27.6
18.0–24.9	1465	23.7	3.7	18.8	19.6	20.2	21.1	23.2	25.6	27.2	28.6	30.9
25.0–29.9	1073	25.0	4.1	19.5	20.6	21.3	22.1	24.4	27.0	28.5	29.9	32.4
30.0–34.9	799	25.7	3.9	20.0	21.2	22.0	23.1	25.2	27.9	29.3	30.5	32.8
35.0–39.9	734	25.9	3.8	20.3	21.2	22.1	23.5	25.6	27.9	29.4	30.5	32.6
40.0–44.9	723	26.2	3.9	20.6	21.8	22.3	23.5	26.0	28.5	29.8	30.8	32.5
45.0–49.9	748	26.3	4.1	20.1	21.5	22.5	23.7	26.0	28.6	30.0	31.0	33.3
50.0–54.9	767	26.0	4.1	20.0	21.2	22.2	23.4	25.9	28.2	29.9	31.2	33.1
55.0–59.9	693	26.2	4.1	19.9	21.3	22.2	23.7	26.2	28.5	30.1	31.5	33.2
60.0–64.9	1122	25.8	3.8	20.1	21.3	22.1	23.4	25.7	28.0	29.4	30.4	32.2
65.0–69.9	1488	25.6	3.9	19.1	20.6	21.6	23.0	25.7	27.9	29.6	30.7	32.1
70.0–74.9	1057	25.4	3.9	19.3	20.6	21.7	23.0	25.2	27.8	29.3	30.5	32.2
Females												
1.0–1.9	264	16.8	1.6	14.3	14.9	15.2	15.8	16.7	17.6	18.2	18.8	19.3
2.0–2.9	479	16.0	1.4	14.1	14.5	14.7	15.1	15.9	16.8	17.3	17.8	18.5
3.0–3.9	509	15.7	1.3	13.8	14.2	14.5	14.8	15.6	16.4	17.1	17.5	18.0
4.0–4.9	519	15.5	1.3	13.7	13.9	14.2	14.6	15.3	16.2	16.7	17.0	17.7
5.0–5.9	504	15.5	1.6	13.4	13.8	14.1	14.6	15.3	16.3	16.9	17.5	18.6
6.0–6.9	218	15.5	1.7	13.3	13.7	13.9	14.3	15.3	16.4	17.2	17.6	18.7
7.0–7.9	245	16.0	2.0	13.9	14.0	14.2	14.8	15.4	16.8	17.6	18.5	19.7
8.0–8.9	221	16.6	2.9	13.9	14.2	14.4	14.9	15.9	17.6	18.8	19.7	22.0
9.0–9.9	248	17.5	3.2	14.0	14.6	15.0	15.5	16.7	18.2	19.9	21.8	23.9
10.0–10.9	266	17.6	2.9	14.0	14.6	15.0	15.6	16.8	18.8	20.5	21.9	23.7
11.0–11.9	230	18.8	3.5	14.8	15.2	15.7	16.5	18.1	20.2	21.7	23.4	25.8
12.0–12.9	247	19.4	3.3	15.2	15.8	16.4	17.1	18.7	21.0	22.7	23.9	26.1
13.0–13.9	276	20.2	4.1	15.3	16.1	16.7	17.5	19.2	21.6	23.7	24.8	28.7
14.0–14.9	287	21.0	3.7	16.7	17.3	17.8	18.5	20.4	22.7	24.3	26.2	28.5
15.0–15.9	234	20.9	3.4	17.0	17.5	18.0	18.8	20.1	22.1	23.4	25.4	26.9
16.0–16.9	284	21.8	3.8	17.6	18.2	18.6	19.2	20.9	23.4	25.6	26.4	29.1
17.0–17.9	223	22.4	4.4	17.1	17.9	18.7	19.6	21.4	24.0	25.8	27.4	30.7
18.0–24.9	2061	22.6	4.4	17.8	18.5	19.0	19.9	21.7	24.2	26.0	27.7	31.3
25.0–29.9	1618	23.4	5.0	18.0	18.7	19.1	19.9	22.1	25.3	27.6	30.2	33.6
30.0–34.9	1374	24.4	5.5	18.5	19.3	19.9	20.7	22.8	26.4	29.5	31.6	35.9
35.0–39.9	1198	24.7	5.4	18.7	19.4	20.1	21.2	23.2	26.8	29.8	32.0	35.3
40.0–44.9	1142	25.1	5.7	18.8	19.7	20.3	21.3	23.6	27.5	30.6	32.9	36.2
45.0–49.9	832	25.6	5.7	18.9	20.0	20.7	21.8	24.1	28.2	30.8	32.9	36.6
50.0–54.9	863	25.8	5.1	19.2	20.3	20.9	22.2	24.8	28.4	31.1	33.1	36.0
55.0–59.9	756	26.3	5.5	19.2	20.5	21.2	22.5	25.2	29.3	32.1	33.7	37.2
60.0–64.9	1225	26.5	5.4	19.2	20.6	21.3	22.7	25.6	29.6	31.8	33.4	36.2
65.0–69.9	1651	26.6	5.4	19.5	20.7	21.6	22.8	25.8	29.1	31.4	33.4	36.3
70.0–74.9	1262	26.4	5.2	19.3	20.5	21.5	22.9	25.9	29.4	31.6	33.0	35.5

ns, standard deviations, and percentiles of sitting height (cm) by age (yrs) for White males and females of 2 to 74 years

Age (yrs)	N	Mean	SD	Percentiles								
				5	10	15	25	50	75	85	90	95
Males												
2.0–2.9	406	54.4	1.8	51.0	51.5	52.0	53.0	54.4	56.0	57.0	57.0	58.0
3.0–3.9	538	57.3	1.5	54.0	54.0	55.0	55.7	57.1	59.0	60.0	60.0	61.0
4.0–4.9	547	60.1	2.0	56.0	56.5	57.0	58.0	60.0	62.0	63.0	63.5	64.6
5.0–5.9	533	62.5	1.6	58.0	59.0	59.6	60.6	62.9	64.1	65.1	66.0	67.3
6.0–6.9	231	65.3	1.2	59.9	62.0	62.4	63.4	65.0	67.3	68.4	69.0	69.6
7.0–7.9	240	67.6	1.7	62.3	64.0	64.4	66.0	67.8	69.8	70.6	71.0	72.0
8.0–8.9	240	69.6	1.9	64.1	65.9	66.4	67.7	69.6	72.0	72.9	73.1	74.9
9.0–9.9	242	72.2	1.3	67.0	68.0	69.0	70.0	72.0	74.0	75.0	76.0	77.1
10.0–10.9	267	74.1	1.6	68.9	70.0	70.7	72.0	74.0	76.3	77.6	78.5	79.8
11.0–11.9	248	76.1	1.3	70.0	71.1	72.0	73.5	76.0	78.1	79.8	81.0	82.4
12.0–12.9	273	78.7	1.2	73.0	74.0	74.5	76.0	78.4	81.2	82.5	84.3	86.2
13.0–13.9	267	82.3	1.3	74.6	75.1	77.0	78.4	82.4	85.9	88.0	89.0	90.8
14.0–14.9	286	86.2	1.5	77.6	80.3	81.5	83.3	86.5	89.4	90.9	91.8	93.0
15.0–15.9	287	88.7	1.4	80.5	82.9	84.6	86.1	88.9	91.5	93.4	94.1	95.3
16.0–16.9	275	91.1	1.4	84.9	86.2	87.4	88.6	91.4	93.7	94.7	95.3	97.1
17.0–17.9	266	91.6	1.3	85.7	87.0	88.0	89.4	91.7	93.9	95.3	96.4	97.6
18.0–24.9	1459	92.9	1.4	87.3	88.6	89.4	90.6	92.9	95.3	96.6	97.5	98.8
25.0–29.9	1072	93.3	1.3	87.6	88.9	89.8	91.1	93.3	95.5	97.0	97.9	99.1
30.0–34.9	796	93.1	1.4	87.6	88.6	89.6	90.8	93.1	95.5	96.8	97.7	99.2
35.0–39.9	732	92.8	1.3	87.0	88.2	89.0	90.5	92.8	95.3	96.6	97.3	98.4
40.0–44.9	720	92.8	1.3	87.1	88.6	89.5	90.6	92.8	94.9	96.3	97.2	98.3
45.0–49.9	748	92.3	1.3	86.4	88.1	88.8	90.1	92.4	94.5	95.8	96.6	98.0
50.0–54.9	766	91.9	1.3	86.0	87.4	88.4	89.8	91.9	94.0	95.4	96.3	97.4
55.0–59.9	692	91.4	1.3	85.6	87.1	87.9	89.1	91.4	93.7	94.8	95.6	96.8
60.0–64.9	1120	90.6	1.4	85.0	86.3	87.1	88.3	90.7	93.1	94.2	94.9	96.1
65.0–69.9	1485	89.8	1.3	84.0	85.3	86.2	87.5	89.9	92.2	93.5	94.4	95.5
70.0–74.9	1051	89.0	1.4	83.1	84.2	85.4	86.6	89.0	91.3	92.7	93.6	94.5
Females												
2.0–2.9	369	53.0	1.6	49.4	50.0	50.6	51.0	53.0	54.6	55.3	56.0	57.0
3.0–3.9	509	55.9	1.5	51.3	53.0	53.0	54.0	56.0	57.7	58.8	59.0	60.0
4.0–4.9	519	58.9	1.4	54.2	55.1	56.0	57.0	59.0	61.0	61.5	62.0	63.0
5.0–5.9	503	61.8	1.8	57.0	58.0	59.0	60.0	62.0	63.4	64.6	65.0	66.1
6.0–6.9	218	64.3	1.9	60.0	60.7	61.0	62.0	64.3	66.4	67.3	68.0	69.1
7.0–7.9	245	66.8	1.4	62.0	63.0	63.8	65.0	66.8	69.0	70.0	70.7	72.0
8.0–8.9	221	69.3	1.3	64.0	65.4	66.0	67.0	69.3	71.0	72.0	73.4	74.1
9.0–9.9	248	71.6	2.1	66.0	67.0	68.0	69.0	71.0	73.9	75.6	76.1	77.3
10.0–10.9	266	73.8	1.2	68.4	69.3	70.2	71.5	73.6	76.0	77.3	78.9	80.9
11.0–11.9	229	77.2	1.2	71.0	72.0	73.0	74.3	77.0	80.1	81.3	82.6	84.3
12.0–12.9	247	80.8	1.4	74.0	75.0	76.4	78.0	81.0	83.7	84.9	85.7	86.7
13.0–13.9	276	83.0	1.4	77.4	78.4	79.4	80.6	83.0	85.5	86.6	87.4	88.2
14.0–14.9	286	84.9	1.3	79.0	80.4	81.2	82.4	85.0	87.4	88.4	89.0	89.7
15.0–15.9	233	86.1	1.3	81.0	82.2	83.0	84.0	86.1	87.9	89.3	91.0	91.8
16.0–16.9	283	86.0	1.3	79.6	81.4	82.4	83.9	86.1	88.2	89.2	90.1	91.5
17.0–17.9	223	86.7	1.2	81.3	82.7	83.7	84.9	86.7	88.6	90.0	90.8	92.5
18.0–24.9	2059	86.9	1.3	81.9	83.0	83.6	84.8	87.0	88.9	90.2	90.9	92.1
25.0–29.9	1617	86.9	1.4	81.3	82.8	83.7	85.0	86.8	89.0	90.3	91.0	92.3
30.0–34.9	1368	87.1	1.3	81.8	82.9	83.7	85.0	86.9	89.3	90.4	91.3	92.4
35.0–39.9	1193	87.0	1.3	81.6	82.9	83.6	85.0	87.0	89.1	90.4	91.1	92.4
40.0–44.9	1141	86.7	1.4	81.6	82.7	83.5	84.5	86.6	88.8	89.9	90.7	91.9
45.0–49.9	831	86.6	1.3	81.3	82.6	83.5	84.5	86.7	88.7	89.8	90.5	91.7
50.0–54.9	862	85.8	1.4	81.0	82.0	82.6	83.7	85.8	87.8	89.0	89.8	90.8
55.0–59.9	756	85.1	1.4	79.5	81.2	81.9	83.1	85.3	87.3	88.5	89.3	90.1
60.0–64.9	1221	84.5	1.5	78.9	80.3	81.2	82.3	84.6	86.7	87.9	88.7	89.9
65.0–69.9	1644	83.5	1.4	77.8	79.3	80.1	81.4	83.6	85.8	86.9	87.6	88.8
70.0–74.9	1257	82.5	1.5	76.7	78.1	79.0	80.3	82.7	84.7	86.0	86.7	87.7

Means, standard deviations, and percentiles of sitting height index (sitting height / stature x 100)(cm) by age (yrs) for White males and females of 2 to 74 years

Age (yrs)	N	Mean	SD	Percentiles								
				5	10	15	25	50	75	85	90	95
Males												
2.0–2.9	406	59.1	1.8	56.2	56.9	57.4	58.1	59.2	60.2	60.8	61.3	61.9
3.0–3.9	538	57.8	1.5	55.6	56.0	56.4	56.9	57.9	58.8	59.3	59.7	60.4
4.0–4.9	547	56.9	2.0	54.4	54.9	55.5	56.1	56.9	57.7	58.1	58.4	58.9
5.0–5.9	533	55.7	1.6	53.5	54.1	54.3	54.9	55.7	56.6	57.1	57.5	58.1
6.0–6.9	231	54.8	1.2	52.8	53.3	53.6	54.0	54.9	55.6	56.1	56.3	56.7
7.0–7.9	240	54.0	1.7	52.1	52.4	52.8	53.3	54.1	54.9	55.4	55.7	56.2
8.0–8.9	240	53.8	1.9	51.5	51.9	52.2	52.8	53.8	54.5	55.1	55.4	55.7
9.0–9.9	242	53.1	1.3	51.0	51.3	51.7	52.4	53.2	54.0	54.3	54.5	55.0
10.0–10.9	267	52.6	1.6	50.6	51.0	51.4	51.8	52.6	53.4	53.8	54.1	54.4
11.0–11.9	248	52.1	1.3	50.0	50.5	50.8	51.2	52.1	52.8	53.3	53.8	54.2
12.0–12.9	273	51.7	1.2	49.8	50.2	50.5	50.9	51.6	52.5	52.9	53.2	53.6
13.0–13.9	267	51.6	1.3	49.7	49.9	50.3	50.7	51.6	52.4	52.9	53.2	53.8
14.0–14.9	286	51.5	1.5	49.5	49.9	50.2	50.7	51.5	52.3	52.9	53.3	53.6
15.0–15.9	287	51.9	1.4	49.7	50.1	50.4	50.9	51.8	52.7	53.3	53.8	54.2
16.0–16.9	275	52.2	1.4	50.1	50.6	51.0	51.3	52.2	53.1	53.5	53.7	54.2
17.0–17.9	266	52.1	1.3	50.0	50.5	50.9	51.3	52.0	52.9	53.4	53.7	54.3
18.0–24.9	1459	52.6	1.4	50.5	51.0	51.3	51.8	52.6	53.4	53.9	54.2	54.8
25.0–29.9	1072	52.7	1.3	50.7	51.2	51.4	51.9	52.7	53.6	54.0	54.4	54.8
30.0–34.9	796	52.8	1.4	50.9	51.3	51.6	51.9	52.8	53.6	54.1	54.4	54.9
35.0–39.9	732	52.6	1.3	50.5	51.0	51.3	51.8	52.7	53.5	54.0	54.2	54.6
40.0–44.9	720	52.7	1.3	50.6	51.1	51.4	51.9	52.7	53.5	53.9	54.2	54.6
45.0–49.9	748	52.7	1.3	50.7	51.1	51.5	51.9	52.7	53.5	53.9	54.2	54.7
50.0–54.9	766	52.6	1.3	50.3	50.9	51.3	51.7	52.6	53.5	53.9	54.2	54.7
55.0–59.9	692	52.5	1.3	50.4	50.8	51.2	51.7	52.6	53.4	53.9	54.2	54.7
60.0–64.9	1120	52.4	1.4	50.2	50.8	51.2	51.6	52.5	53.2	53.7	54.0	54.5
65.0–69.9	1485	52.3	1.3	50.1	50.6	50.9	51.4	52.3	53.2	53.6	53.9	54.4
70.0–74.9	1051	52.2	1.4	50.0	50.5	50.8	51.3	52.3	53.1	53.5	53.9	54.3
Females												
2.0–2.9	369	58.8	1.6	56.3	56.7	57.1	57.8	58.8	59.9	60.3	60.8	61.3
3.0–3.9	509	57.4	1.5	54.9	55.6	55.9	56.5	57.4	58.3	58.8	59.1	59.6
4.0–4.9	519	56.3	1.4	54.1	54.7	55.0	55.5	56.4	57.2	57.6	57.9	58.6
5.0–5.9	503	55.4	1.8	53.1	53.6	54.0	54.6	55.4	56.2	56.7	57.0	57.7
6.0–6.9	218	54.6	1.9	52.6	53.1	53.3	53.8	54.6	55.5	55.8	56.0	56.7
7.0–7.9	245	54.0	1.4	52.2	52.6	52.8	53.2	53.9	54.8	55.3	55.6	55.9
8.0–8.9	221	53.5	1.3	51.5	51.9	52.1	52.7	53.4	54.2	54.7	55.1	55.7
9.0–9.9	248	52.9	2.1	50.6	51.2	51.5	51.9	52.8	53.8	54.3	54.6	55.0
10.0–10.9	266	52.4	1.2	50.6	50.9	51.2	51.6	52.3	53.1	53.6	53.9	54.3
11.0–11.9	229	52.2	1.2	50.2	50.7	51.1	51.4	52.1	53.0	53.5	53.8	54.2
12.0–12.9	247	52.2	1.4	50.1	50.4	50.9	51.3	52.1	53.1	53.7	54.3	54.6
13.0–13.9	276	52.3	1.4	50.0	50.6	51.0	51.4	52.2	53.1	53.7	54.2	54.6
14.0–14.9	286	52.7	1.3	50.6	50.9	51.3	51.7	52.6	53.6	54.1	54.4	54.8
15.0–15.9	233	52.8	1.3	50.8	51.2	51.5	51.8	52.7	53.6	54.1	54.5	55.1
16.0–16.9	283	53.0	1.3	50.8	51.4	51.7	52.2	53.1	53.9	54.3	54.5	55.0
17.0–17.9	223	53.2	1.2	51.4	51.8	52.0	52.4	53.2	54.0	54.5	54.8	55.3
18.0–24.9	2059	53.3	1.3	51.2	51.7	52.0	52.4	53.2	54.1	54.6	54.9	55.4
25.0–29.9	1617	53.3	1.4	51.3	51.8	52.1	52.5	53.3	54.1	54.6	55.0	55.6
30.0–34.9	1368	53.5	1.3	51.6	52.0	52.3	52.7	53.5	54.3	54.8	55.1	55.6
35.0–39.9	1193	53.4	1.3	51.3	51.8	52.1	52.5	53.4	54.3	54.8	55.1	55.7
40.0–44.9	1141	53.3	1.4	51.2	51.6	51.9	52.4	53.3	54.2	54.6	55.0	55.6
45.0–49.9	831	53.4	1.3	51.3	51.7	52.0	52.5	53.4	54.2	54.7	55.0	55.5
50.0–54.9	862	53.2	1.4	51.1	51.6	51.9	52.4	53.2	54.1	54.6	54.9	55.3
55.0–59.9	756	53.2	1.4	51.0	51.5	51.8	52.2	53.1	54.1	54.5	54.8	55.4
60.0–64.9	1221	52.9	1.5	50.7	51.3	51.6	52.1	52.9	53.8	54.3	54.6	55.1
65.0–69.9	1644	52.7	1.4	50.4	51.0	51.3	51.8	52.7	53.6	54.0	54.4	54.9
70.0–74.9	1257	52.4	1.5	49.9	50.5	50.9	51.5	52.4	53.3	53.8	54.2	54.6

Means, standard deviations, and percentiles of bitrochanteric breadth
(cm) by age (yrs) for White males and females of 1 to 74 years

Age (yrs)	N	Mean	SD	Percentiles									
				5	10	15	25	50	75	85	90	95
Males													
1.0–1.9	507	14.8	2.0	12.7	13.3	13.6	14.0	14.7	15.5	16.0	16.2	16.5
2.0–2.9	506	15.8	1.2	13.9	14.3	14.7	15.2	15.8	16.5	17.0	17.3	17.6
3.0–3.9	534	16.9	1.2	14.9	15.4	15.8	16.1	16.8	17.6	18.0	18.2	18.7
4.0–4.9	544	17.7	1.2	16.0	16.4	16.6	17.0	17.7	18.5	18.9	19.2	19.6
5.0–5.9	533	18.6	1.3	16.6	17.1	17.3	17.7	18.6	19.4	19.9	20.2	20.8
6.0–6.9	230	19.6	1.3	17.4	18.1	18.5	18.9	19.5	20.4	20.9	21.3	22.1
7.0–7.9	240	20.6	1.4	18.3	18.8	19.1	19.6	20.5	21.5	21.8	22.2	22.7
8.0–8.9	240	21.4	1.6	19.0	19.5	19.7	20.3	21.3	22.3	23.0	23.5	24.2
9.0–9.9	242	22.5	1.7	20.3	20.6	20.8	21.4	22.3	23.5	24.3	24.6	25.2
10.0–10.9	269	23.7	1.9	21.1	21.6	22.0	22.4	23.5	24.7	25.5	26.2	26.8
11.0–11.9	248	24.9	2.4	21.6	22.4	22.8	23.2	24.5	26.1	27.0	27.8	29.1
12.0–12.9	272	26.0	2.2	22.7	23.5	24.0	24.5	25.8	27.3	28.3	28.8	30.0
13.0–13.9	268	27.5	2.4	24.0	24.4	25.2	25.7	27.5	29.0	30.2	30.6	31.5
14.0–14.9	287	29.1	2.3	25.2	26.0	26.7	27.6	29.3	30.6	31.4	31.8	32.3
15.0–15.9	288	29.9	2.1	26.3	27.1	27.7	28.5	30.1	31.3	32.0	32.4	33.1
16.0–16.9	279	30.9	2.0	27.7	28.5	29.1	29.7	30.9	32.3	32.7	33.3	34.1
17.0–17.9	267	31.0	1.9	28.1	28.6	29.4	30.0	31.1	32.1	32.8	33.4	34.1
18.0–24.9	1466	31.8	1.9	28.7	29.4	29.8	30.6	31.7	32.9	33.6	34.2	34.9
25.0–29.9	1073	32.3	1.9	29.4	30.0	30.4	31.1	32.3	33.4	34.0	34.5	35.5
30.0–34.9	798	32.4	2.1	29.5	30.2	30.5	31.1	32.3	33.5	34.3	34.7	35.6
35.0–39.9	733	32.6	1.9	29.6	30.2	30.6	31.4	32.6	33.9	34.5	35.1	35.7
40.0–44.9	723	32.9	2.0	29.8	30.5	31.0	31.6	33.0	34.0	34.7	35.1	35.9
45.0–49.9	748	32.9	1.8	30.1	30.5	31:1	31.6	32.8	34.0	34.7	35.2	35.9
50.0–54.9	767	33.0	2.0	30.0	30.7	31.2	31.8	33.0	34.0	34.6	35.1	36.0
55.0–59.9	694	33.0	3.5	30.0	30.7	31.3	31.7	32.9	34.2	34.7	35.2	36.0
60.0–64.9	1123	33.0	2.4	30.2	30.8	31.2	31.9	32.9	34.0	34.6	35.0	35.8
65.0–69.9	1487	33.1	1.9	30.1	30.8	31.2	31.9	33.1	34.3	35.0	35.6	36.1
70.0–74.9	1052	33.2	3.0	30.4	31.0	31.4	31.9	33.1	34.3	34.9	35.4	36.3
Females													
1.0–1.9	468	14.4	1.3	12.4	12.8	13.2	13.6	14.4	15.3	15.6	15.9	16.4
2.0–2.9	477	15.7	1.1	14.0	14.3	14.5	14.9	15.6	16.3	16.7	16.9	17.5
3.0–3.9	509	16.7	1.2	14.6	15.1	15.4	15.9	16.8	17.5	17.9	18.2	18.6
4.0–4.9	514	17.6	1.3	15.7	16.2	16.4	16.8	17.6	18.3	18.7	19.1	19.6
5.0–5.9	502	18.6	1.5	16.5	17.1	17.4	17.8	18.5	19.4	19.7	20.3	20.9
6.0–6.9	218	19.6	1.3	17.4	18.0	18.4	18.6	19.7	20.4	20.9	21.4	22.0
7.0–7.9	245	20.6	1.8	18.2	18.8	19.2	19.7	20.5	21.4	21.8	22.4	23.5
8.0–8.9	220	21.8	1.9	19.2	19.8	20.2	20.6	21.6	22.7	23.3	23.9	24.6
9.0–9.9	248	23.2	2.3	20.4	21.0	21.2	21.6	22.9	24.2	25.0	25.8	26.9
10.0–10.9	266	24.1	2.2	21.1	21.6	22.0	22.6	23.8	25.4	26.1	26.9	28.3
11.0–11.9	229	25.8	2.5	22.0	22.5	23.3	24.0	25.7	27.4	28.4	28.9	30.3
12.0–12.9	247	27.6	2.3	23.8	24.3	25.2	25.9	27.5	29.3	30.0	30.5	31.1
13.0–13.9	276	28.7	2.3	25.1	25.9	26.4	27.3	28.8	30.1	31.0	31.5	32.0
14.0–14.9	287	29.6	2.2	26.3	27.0	27.7	28.4	29.6	30.8	31.5	31.9	32.6
15.0–15.9	234	30.0	1.8	27.2	27.8	28.2	29.0	29.9	31.2	31.6	31.9	32.8
16.0–16.9	284	30.5	2.0	27.9	28.1	28.5	29.1	30.2	31.6	32.5	33.4	34.1
17.0–17.9	223	30.9	1.9	27.9	28.6	29.2	29.7	30.8	32.0	32.6	33.1	33.9
18.0–24.9	2061	31.2	2.1	28.3	28.9	29.2	29.9	31.1	32.4	33.2	33.6	34.8
25.0–29.9	1619	31.7	3.0	28.4	29.0	29.6	30.2	31.4	32.8	33.8	34.4	35.5
30.0–34.9	1373	32.1	3.2	28.6	29.3	29.8	30.5	31.8	33.3	34.2	34.9	36.1
35.0–39.9	1197	32.1	2.2	28.8	29.5	30.0	30.7	32.0	33.4	34.2	34.8	35.9
40.0–44.9	1142	32.3	2.3	29.0	29.7	30.2	30.8	32.1	33.6	34.5	35.1	36.2
45.0–49.9	832	32.4	2.3	29.0	29.6	30.1	31.0	32.3	33.6	34.5	35.2	36.0
50.0–54.9	863	32.5	2.2	29.0	29.9	30.4	31.1	32.3	33.9	34.6	35.3	36.4
55.0–59.9	754	32.3	2.9	28.9	29.6	30.2	31.0	32.2	33.5	34.2	34.8	35.6
60.0–64.9	1226	32.3	2.1	29.1	29.7	30.2	30.9	32.3	33.6	34.5	35.0	35.8
65.0–69.9	1647	32.4	2.5	29.1	29.8	30.3	31.0	32.4	33.7	34.5	35.2	36.0
70.0–74.9	1262	32.5	3.0	29.1	29.8	30.4	31.1	32.4	33.8	34.4	34.9	35.8

Means, standard deviations, and percentiles of elbow breadth (mm) by age (yrs) for White males and females of 1 to 74 years

Age (yrs)	N	Mean	SD	Percentiles								
				5	10	15	25	50	75	85	90	95
Males												
1.0–1.9	508	40.4	2.8	36.0	37.0	37.0	39.0	40.0	42.0	43.0	44.0	45.0
2.0–2.9	513	42.5	2.7	38.0	39.0	40.0	41.0	42.0	44.0	45.0	46.0	47.0
3.0–3.9	541	44.5	2.8	40.0	41.0	42.0	43.0	44.0	46.0	47.0	48.0	50.0
4.0–4.9	547	46.3	3.0	42.0	43.0	43.0	44.0	46.0	48.0	49.0	50.0	52.0
5.0–5.9	534	48.1	3.1	43.0	44.0	45.0	46.0	48.0	50.0	51.0	52.0	53.0
6.0–6.9	231	50.3	3.5	45.0	46.0	47.0	48.0	50.0	52.0	54.0	55.0	56.0
7.0–7.9	240	51.9	3.6	47.0	48.0	49.0	49.0	52.0	54.0	55.0	56.0	57.0
8.0–8.9	240	53.6	3.6	48.0	49.0	50.0	51.0	54.0	56.0	57.0	58.0	60.0
9.0–9.9	242	56.0	3.9	50.0	51.0	52.0	53.0	56.0	58.0	60.0	61.0	63.0
10.0–10.9	269	58.0	4.0	51.0	53.0	54.0	56.0	58.0	60.0	62.0	63.0	65.0
11.0–11.9	248	59.7	4.3	53.0	54.0	56.0	57.0	60.0	62.0	64.0	65.0	67.0
12.0–12.9	273	62.9	4.6	55.0	57.0	58.0	60.0	63.0	66.0	68.0	68.0	72.0
13.0–13.9	268	65.9	4.6	59.0	61.0	61.0	63.0	66.0	69.0	71.0	72.0	74.0
14.0–14.9	286	68.7	4.2	62.0	64.0	64.0	66.0	69.0	71.0	73.0	74.0	75.0
15.0–15.9	288	69.8	4.2	63.0	64.0	65.0	67.0	70.0	72.0	74.0	75.0	77.0
16.0–16.9	279	70.5	4.0	64.0	66.0	66.0	68.0	70.0	73.0	74.0	76.0	77.0
17.0–17.9	267	70.7	4.0	64.0	66.0	67.0	68.0	71.0	73.0	75.0	76.0	77.0
18.0–24.9	1467	71.3	4.0	65.0	66.0	67.0	69.0	71.0	74.0	75.0	76.0	78.0
25.0–29.9	1073	71.7	4.0	65.0	67.0	68.0	69.0	72.0	74.0	76.0	77.0	78.0
30.0–34.9	798	71.9	4.1	65.0	67.0	68.0	69.0	72.0	74.0	76.0	77.0	79.0
35.0–39.9	733	72.4	4.1	66.0	67.0	69.0	70.0	72.0	75.0	77.0	77.0	79.0
40.0–44.9	723	72.8	3.9	67.0	68.0	69.0	70.0	73.0	75.0	77.0	78.0	80.0
45.0–49.9	748	73.1	4.2	66.0	68.0	69.0	70.0	73.0	76.0	78.0	78.0	80.0
50.0–54.9	767	73.4	4.0	67.0	68.0	70.0	71.0	73.0	76.0	77.0	78.0	80.0
55.0–59.9	695	73.7	4.3	67.0	68.0	69.0	71.0	73.0	77.0	78.0	80.0	81.0
60.0–64.9	1123	73.5	4.3	67.0	68.0	69.0	71.0	73.0	76.0	78.0	79.0	81.0
65.0–69.9	1489	73.3	4.3	66.0	68.0	69.0	71.0	73.0	76.0	78.0	79.0	81.0
70.0–74.9	1052	73.5	4.3	67.0	68.0	69.0	71.0	73.0	76.0	78.0	79.0	81.0
Females												
1.0–1.9	470	38.7	2.8	34.0	35.0	36.0	37.0	39.0	41.0	42.0	42.0	43.0
2.0–2.9	483	40.7	2.8	36.0	37.0	38.0	39.0	41.0	42.0	44.0	44.0	45.0
3.0–3.9	509	42.5	2.9	38.0	39.0	40.0	41.0	43.0	44.0	45.0	46.0	47.0
4.0–4.9	522	44.0	2.8	40.0	41.0	41.0	42.0	44.0	46.0	47.0	48.0	49.0
5.0–5.9	505	46.2	3.0	42.0	43.0	43.0	44.0	46.0	48.0	49.0	50.0	51.0
6.0–6.9	218	47.8	3.1	43.0	44.0	45.0	46.0	48.0	50.0	51.0	52.0	53.0
7.0–7.9	245	49.8	3.4	44.0	45.0	46.0	48.0	50.0	52.0	53.0	54.0	55.0
8.0–8.9	221	51.5	3.9	46.0	47.0	48.0	49.0	51.0	54.0	55.0	56.0	58.0
9.0–9.9	248	53.9	3.9	48.0	50.0	50.0	51.0	54.0	56.0	57.0	59.0	60.0
10.0–10.9	266	55.5	3.8	50.0	51.0	51.0	53.0	55.0	58.0	60.0	61.0	62.0
11.0–11.9	229	57.8	4.1	52.0	53.0	53.0	55.0	58.0	61.0	63.0	63.0	64.0
12.0–12.9	247	59.1	3.6	54.0	55.0	55.0	57.0	59.0	61.0	62.0	64.0	65.0
13.0–13.9	276	60.0	3.7	54.0	55.0	56.0	57.0	60.0	62.0	63.0	64.0	66.0
14.0–14.9	287	60.3	3.4	55.0	56.0	57.0	58.0	60.0	62.0	64.0	65.0	66.0
15.0–15.9	234	60.7	4.0	54.0	56.0	57.0	58.0	61.0	63.0	65.0	66.0	66.0
16.0–16.9	284	60.9	3.8	55.0	56.0	57.0	58.0	61.0	63.0	65.0	66.0	67.0
17.0–17.9	223	61.1	4.0	54.0	56.0	57.0	58.0	61.0	64.0	65.0	66.0	67.0
18.0–24.9	2060	61.0	3.7	55.0	56.0	57.0	59.0	61.0	63.0	64.0	66.0	67.0
25.0–29.9	1617	61.3	3.8	55.0	57.0	57.0	59.0	61.0	63.0	65.0	66.0	68.0
30.0–34.9	1371	61.9	4.1	56.0	57.0	58.0	59.0	62.0	64.0	66.0	67.0	69.0
35.0–39.9	1197	62.4	4.2	56.0	58.0	59.0	60.0	62.0	65.0	66.0	67.0	69.0
40.0–44.9	1142	62.9	4.3	57.0	58.0	59.0	60.0	62.0	65.0	67.0	68.0	70.0
45.0–49.9	831	63.6	4.3	57.0	59.0	59.0	61.0	63.0	66.0	68.0	69.0	71.0
50.0–54.9	863	63.8	4.4	57.0	59.0	60.0	61.0	63.0	67.0	68.0	69.0	71.0
55.0–59.9	756	64.4	4.7	58.0	59.0	60.0	61.0	64.0	67.0	69.0	70.0	73.0
60.0–64.9	1227	64.5	4.4	58.0	60.0	61.0	62.0	64.0	67.0	69.0	70.0	72.0
65.0–69.9	1648	64.4	4.4	58.0	59.0	60.0	61.0	64.0	67.0	69.0	70.0	72.0
70.0–74.9	1260	64.7	4.4	58.0	60.0	60.0	62.0	64.0	67.0	69.0	71.0	72.0

Appendix B: Table 10.
Means, standard deviations, and percentiles of upper arm circumference
(cm) by age (yrs) for White males and females of 1 to 74 years

Age (yrs)	N	Mean	SD	Percentiles								
				5	10	15	25	50	75	85	90	95
Males												
1.0–1.9	508	16.1	1.2	14.3	14.7	14.9	15.2	16.0	16.9	17.4	17.8	18.2
2.0–2.9	508	16.4	1.5	14.3	14.8	15.2	15.5	16.3	17.2	17.6	18.0	18.6
3.0–3.9	539	16.9	1.5	15.1	15.3	15.6	16.0	16.8	17.6	18.1	18.4	19.0
4.0–4.9	547	17.3	1.4	15.3	15.6	15.9	16.2	17.2	18.0	18.5	19.0	19.4
5.0–5.9	534	17.7	1.8	15.4	15.9	16.1	16.6	17.5	18.6	19.1	19.6	20.5
6.0–6.9	231	18.3	2.1	15.8	16.1	16.4	16.9	18.0	19.1	19.8	20.6	22.7
7.0–7.9	240	19.1	2.0	16.2	16.8	17.1	17.7	18.8	20.1	21.0	22.1	22.9
8.0–8.9	240	19.7	2.3	16.5	17.2	17.6	18.3	19.3	20.5	21.6	22.8	24.4
9.0–9.9	242	20.9	2.8	17.5	18.0	18.4	19.1	20.3	22.1	23.5	24.9	26.0
10.0–10.9	268	22.0	3.0	18.2	18.7	19.1	19.8	21.4	23.2	24.9	26.2	27.9
11.0–11.9	248	23.0	3.5	18.6	19.3	19.8	20.5	22.3	24.6	26.1	27.8	29.8
12.0–12.9	273	23.9	3.3	19.4	20.1	20.7	21.6	23.2	25.5	27.3	28.5	30.5
13.0–13.9	268	25.0	3.3	20.0	21.3	22.0	22.8	24.7	26.7	28.2	29.5	31.0
14.0–14.9	286	26.4	3.5	21.8	22.7	23.3	23.9	26.0	28.3	29.2	30.2	32.3
15.0–15.9	288	27.2	3.2	22.3	23.2	23.8	25.1	27.1	28.9	30.1	31.2	32.5
16.0–16.9	279	28.7	3.3	24.0	24.8	25.6	26.6	28.1	30.8	32.2	33.3	34.7
17.0–17.9	267	29.1	3.3	24.5	25.1	26.1	27.0	28.7	30.8	32.3	33.3	34.5
18.0–24.9	1467	31.1	3.4	26.2	27.2	27.8	28.8	30.8	33.1	34.4	35.5	37.2
25.0–29.9	1072	32.1	3.4	27.1	28.2	28.8	29.9	31.9	34.2	35.4	36.5	38.1
30.0–34.9	797	32.7	3.2	27.8	28.8	29.4	30.5	32.5	34.9	35.8	36.6	38.2
35.0–39.9	733	32.9	3.2	27.9	28.9	29.7	30.7	32.8	34.9	36.1	36.7	37.9
40.0–44.9	723	32.9	3.1	28.2	29.0	29.8	31.0	32.8	34.8	35.9	36.6	37.9
45.0–49.9	748	32.7	3.3	27.4	28.7	29.5	30.7	32.7	34.8	36.0	36.8	38.1
50.0–54.9	767	32.3	3.2	27.2	28.4	29.2	30.2	32.3	34.3	35.6	36.5	37.8
55.0–59.9	695	32.2	3.2	26.8	28.1	29.2	30.4	32.3	34.2	35.2	36.1	37.4
60.0–64.9	1123	31.9	3.3	26.7	27.8	28.6	29.7	32.0	34.0	35.1	35.8	37.1
65.0–69.9	1488	31.1	3.3	25.3	26.8	27.8	29.1	31.2	33.2	34.4	35.1	36.5
70.0–74.9	1051	30.6	3.3	25.1	26.3	27.3	28.6	30.7	32.6	33.7	34.6	35.9
Females												
1.0–1.9	470	15.7	1.3	13.7	14.2	14.4	14.9	15.7	16.5	17.0	17.3	17.9
2.0–2.9	483	16.2	1.3	14.3	14.7	15.0	15.4	16.1	17.0	17.4	18.0	18.5
3.0–3.9	509	16.7	1.4	14.5	15.1	15.3	15.8	16.6	17.5	18.1	18.4	19.0
4.0–4.9	521	17.1	1.4	15.1	15.5	15.8	16.2	17.1	18.0	18.5	18.9	19.4
5.0–5.9	504	17.8	1.7	15.4	15.8	16.2	16.6	17.5	18.5	19.3	20.0	20.8
6.0–6.9	218	18.2	1.9	15.7	16.2	16.5	17.0	17.9	19.1	20.0	20.6	22.1
7.0–7.9	245	19.1	2.3	16.4	16.7	17.1	17.5	18.6	20.1	21.1	21.8	23.4
8.0–8.9	220	20.1	2.7	16.9	17.2	17.6	18.4	19.5	21.3	22.4	23.3	25.3
9.0–9.9	247	21.3	2.8	17.8	18.3	18.8	19.4	21.0	22.3	24.3	25.3	26.9
10.0–10.9	266	21.7	3.0	17.8	18.4	18.9	19.6	21.2	23.4	24.7	25.7	27.2
11.0–11.9	229	23.2	3.5	18.8	19.6	20.0	20.7	22.4	25.2	26.5	27.9	30.3
12.0–12.9	247	23.9	3.1	19.5	20.3	20.8	21.6	23.7	25.7	27.2	28.1	29.4
13.0–13.9	276	25.0	3.8	20.0	20.8	21.5	22.3	24.3	26.7	28.5	30.1	33.4
14.0–14.9	287	26.0	3.4	21.2	22.2	23.0	23.9	25.2	27.6	29.6	30.9	32.2
15.0–15.9	234	25.9	3.3	21.4	22.3	23.0	23.9	25.3	27.7	28.8	30.0	32.0
16.0–16.9	284	26.7	3.3	22.1	23.0	23.6	24.3	26.1	28.4	29.9	31.4	32.8
17.0–17.9	223	27.3	4.0	22.2	23.1	23.7	24.5	27.0	29.1	30.7	32.4	34.7
18.0–24.9	2060	27.4	3.8	22.5	23.3	24.0	24.9	26.8	29.1	30.8	32.1	34.7
25.0–29.9	1617	28.3	4.1	23.1	23.9	24.5	25.4	27.4	30.2	32.1	33.8	36.5
30.0–34.9	1371	29.3	4.5	23.8	24.7	25.4	26.3	28.4	31.3	33.5	35.4	37.9
35.0–39.9	1197	29.8	4.5	24.2	25.2	25.7	26.5	29.0	31.8	34.2	35.9	38.4
40.0–44.9	1141	30.1	4.5	24.2	25.4	26.1	27.0	29.3	32.4	34.9	36.4	38.1
45.0–49.9	831	30.6	4.7	24.2	25.5	26.2	27.3	29.9	33.2	35.2	37.0	39.3
50.0–54.9	862	30.8	4.3	24.8	26.0	26.7	27.9	30.3	33.1	35.3	36.8	38.5
55.0–59.9	756	31.2	4.6	24.8	26.0	26.7	28.1	30.6	33.8	36.3	37.4	39.5
60.0–64.9	1227	31.2	4.5	25.0	26.1	27.1	28.3	30.6	33.8	35.5	37.1	39.4
65.0–69.9	1648	30.7	4.4	24.3	25.7	26.6	27.8	30.3	33.1	34.9	36.2	38.3
70.0–74.9	1261	30.4	4.3	23.8	25.3	26.3	27.6	30.2	33.0	34.5	35.8	37.3

Appendix B: Table 11.
Means, standard deviations, and percentiles of total upper arm area
(cm^2) by age (yrs) for White males and females of 1 to 74 years

Age (yrs)	N	Mean	SD	Percentiles 5	10	15	25	50	75	85	90	95
Males												
1.0–1.9	508	20.7	3.2	16.3	17.2	17.7	18.4	20.4	22.7	24.1	25.2	26.4
2.0–2.9	508	21.7	4.4	16.3	17.4	18.4	19.1	21.1	23.5	24.6	25.8	27.5
3.0–3.9	539	22.9	4.3	18.1	18.6	19.4	20.4	22.5	24.6	26.1	26.9	28.7
4.0–4.9	547	23.8	3.9	18.6	19.4	20.1	20.9	23.5	25.8	27.2	28.7	29.9
5.0–5.9	534	25.3	5.7	18.9	20.1	20.6	21.9	24.4	27.5	29.0	30.6	33.4
6.0–6.9	231	27.0	6.7	19.9	20.6	21.4	22.7	25.8	29.0	31.2	33.8	41.0
7.0–7.9	240	29.4	6.4	20.9	22.5	23.3	24.9	28.1	32.2	35.1	38.9	41.7
8.0–8.9	240	31.3	8.0	21.7	23.5	24.6	26.6	29.6	33.4	37.1	41.4	47.4
9.0–9.9	242	35.4	9.9	24.4	25.8	26.9	29.0	32.8	38.9	43.9	49.3	53.8
10.0–10.9	268	39.1	11.3	26.4	27.8	29.0	31.2	36.4	42.8	49.3	54.6	61.9
11.0–11.9	248	43.1	14.1	27.5	29.6	31.2	33.4	39.6	48.2	54.2	61.5	70.7
12.0–12.9	273	46.3	13.4	29.9	32.2	34.1	37.1	42.8	51.7	59.3	64.6	74.0
13.0–13.9	268	50.6	13.8	31.8	36.1	38.5	41.4	48.5	56.7	63.3	69.3	76.5
14.0–14.9	286	56.5	16.5	37.8	41.0	43.2	45.5	53.8	63.7	67.9	72.6	83.0
15.0–15.9	288	59.8	14.8	39.6	42.8	45.1	50.1	58.4	66.5	72.1	77.5	84.1
16.0–16.9	279	66.4	15.9	45.8	48.9	52.2	56.3	62.8	75.5	82.5	88.2	95.8
17.0–17.9	267	68.4	16.5	47.8	50.1	54.2	58.0	65.5	75.5	83.0	88.2	94.7
18.0–24.9	1467	77.9	17.3	54.6	58.9	61.5	66.0	75.5	87.2	94.2	100.3	110.1
25.0–29.9	1072	83.1	17.8	58.4	63.3	66.0	71.1	81.0	93.1	99.7	106.0	115.5
30.0–34.9	797	86.1	17.1	61.5	66.0	68.8	74.0	84.1	96.9	102.0	106.6	116.1
35.0–39.9	733	86.7	16.7	61.9	66.5	70.2	75.0	85.6	96.9	103.7	107.2	114.3
40.0–44.9	723	87.0	16.5	63.3	66.9	70.7	76.5	85.6	96.4	102.6	106.6	114.3
45.0–49.9	748	86.1	17.3	59.7	65.5	69.3	75.0	85.1	96.4	103.1	107.8	115.5
50.0–54.9	767	84.0	16.7	58.9	64.2	67.9	72.6	83.0	93.6	100.9	106.0	113.7
55.0–59.9	695	83.6	16.4	57.2	62.8	67.9	73.5	83.0	93.1	98.6	103.7	111.3
60.0–64.9	1123	81.9	17.2	56.7	61.5	65.1	70.2	81.5	92.0	98.0	102.0	109.5
65.0–69.9	1488	77.7	16.5	50.9	57.2	61.5	67.4	77.5	87.7	94.2	98.0	106.0
70.0–74.9	1051	75.5	16.1	50.1	55.0	59.3	65.1	75.0	84.6	90.4	95.3	102.6
Females												
1.0–1.9	470	19.8	3.2	14.9	16.0	16.5	17.7	19.6	21.7	23.0	23.8	25.5
2.0–2.9	483	21.1	3.4	16.3	17.2	17.9	18.9	20.6	23.0	24.1	25.8	27.2
3.0–3.9	509	22.3	3.7	16.7	18.1	18.6	19.9	21.9	24.4	26.1	26.9	28.7
4.0–4.9	521	23.4	3.8	18.1	19.1	19.9	20.9	23.3	25.8	27.2	28.4	29.9
5.0–5.9	504	25.3	5.1	18.9	19.9	20.9	21.9	24.4	27.2	29.6	31.8	34.4
6.0–6.9	218	26.7	5.8	19.6	20.9	21.7	23.0	25.5	29.0	31.8	33.8	38.9
7.0–7.9	245	29.4	7.4	21.4	22.2	23.3	24.4	27.5	32.2	35.4	37.8	43.6
8.0–8.9	220	32.9	9.7	22.7	23.5	24.6	26.9	30.3	36.1	39.9	43.2	50.9
9.0–9.9	247	36.9	10.5	25.2	26.6	28.1	29.9	35.1	39.6	47.0	50.9	57.6
10.0–10.9	266	38.1	10.8	25.2	26.9	28.4	30.6	35.8	43.6	48.5	52.6	58.9
11.0–11.9	229	43.9	13.9	28.1	30.6	31.8	34.1	39.9	50.5	55.9	61.9	73.1
12.0–12.9	247	46.4	12.4	30.3	32.8	34.4	37.1	44.7	52.6	58.9	62.8	68.8
13.0–13.9	276	50.9	16.3	31.8	34.4	36.8	39.6	47.0	56.7	64.6	72.1	88.8
14.0–14.9	287	54.6	14.9	35.8	39.2	42.1	45.5	50.5	60.6	69.7	76.0	82.5
15.0–15.9	234	54.3	14.9	36.4	39.6	42.1	45.5	50.9	61.1	66.0	71.6	81.5
16.0–16.9	284	57.7	15.2	38.9	42.1	44.3	47.0	54.2	64.2	71.1	78.5	85.6
17.0–17.9	223	60.6	18.9	39.2	42.5	44.7	47.8	58.0	67.4	75.0	83.5	95.8
18.0–24.9	2060	61.0	18.3	40.3	43.2	45.8	49.3	57.2	67.4	75.5	82.0	95.8
25.0–29.9	1617	64.9	20.2	42.5	45.5	47.8	51.3	59.7	72.6	82.0	90.9	106.0
30.0–34.9	1371	70.0	23.2	45.1	48.5	51.3	55.0	64.2	78.0	89.3	99.7	114.3
35.0–39.9	1197	72.2	23.5	46.6	50.5	52.6	55.9	66.9	80.5	93.1	102.6	117.3
40.0–44.9	1141	73.8	23.5	46.6	51.3	54.2	58.0	68.3	83.5	96.9	105.4	115.5
45.0–49.9	831	76.2	24.1	46.6	51.7	54.6	59.3	71.1	87.7	98.6	108.9	122.9
50.0–54.9	862	77.1	22.2	48.9	53.8	56.7	61.9	73.1	87.2	99.2	107.8	118.0
55.0–59.9	756	79.2	24.4	48.9	53.8	56.7	62.8	74.5	90.9	104.9	111.3	124.2
60.0–64.9	1227	79.3	23.9	49.7	54.2	58.4	63.7	74.5	90.9	100.3	109.5	123.5
65.0–69.9	1648	76.6	22.6	47.0	52.6	56.3	61.5	73.1	87.2	96.9	104.3	116.7
70.0–74.9	1261	75.1	21.8	45.1	50.9	55.0	60.6	72.6	86.7	94.7	102.0	110.7

Means, standard deviations, and percentiles of upper arm muscle area
(cm^2) by age (yrs) for White males and females of 1 to 74 years

Age (yrs)	N	Mean	SD	Percentiles									
				5	10	15	25	50	75	85	90	95
Males													
1.0–1.9	508	13.1	2.3	9.7	10.4	10.8	11.6	12.9	14.5	15.4	16.3	17.1
2.0–2.9	508	14.1	3.5	10.1	10.9	11.2	12.2	13.8	15.6	16.5	16.9	18.4
3.0–3.9	539	15.2	3.2	11.1	12.0	12.6	13.5	15.1	16.4	17.4	18.1	19.2
4.0–4.9	547	16.3	2.7	12.0	12.8	13.5	14.5	16.2	18.0	18.8	19.8	20.9
5.0–5.9	534	17.6	3.9	13.0	14.0	14.5	15.3	17.4	19.2	20.5	21.4	23.1
6.0–6.9	231	19.0	3.8	14.1	15.1	15.5	16.3	18.5	21.3	22.5	23.2	24.9
7.0–7.9	240	20.8	4.2	15.1	16.0	16.8	18.5	20.5	22.4	24.2	24.9	27.3
8.0–8.9	240	22.1	4.4	16.2	17.4	18.2	19.5	21.4	23.9	25.5	26.6	29.4
9.0–9.9	242	24.4	5.1	18.1	19.3	20.3	21.6	23.5	26.7	28.7	30.4	33.1
10.0–10.9	268	26.6	6.1	19.6	20.6	21.4	22.8	25.5	29.0	32.2	34.2	36.6
11.0–11.9	248	28.6	6.7	20.9	21.7	22.7	24.5	27.7	31.5	33.4	35.9	41.4
12.0–12.9	272	31.7	7.1	22.2	23.9	24.9	26.8	30.7	35.8	39.0	40.8	44.1
13.0–13.9	268	36.5	8.2	24.4	26.8	28.1	30.4	36.0	41.2	44.6	47.8	51.5
14.0–14.9	286	42.2	9.0	28.5	30.9	33.1	36.3	41.2	47.4	51.3	54.0	56.8
15.0–15.9	286	46.3	9.4	31.8	34.6	35.8	40.1	45.9	52.6	56.1	57.3	61.5
16.0–16.9	279	51.9	10.1	36.2	40.7	41.8	44.9	51.0	57.8	63.6	66.2	69.9
17.0–17.9	266	54.9	10.6	40.2	42.7	44.3	48.3	53.5	60.6	64.6	67.9	73.2
18.0–24.9	1463	50.5	11.4	34.5	37.4	39.6	42.6	49.2	56.7	61.7	65.0	71.6
25.0–29.9	1069	53.8	11.7	36.7	40.0	42.4	45.8	52.8	61.2	65.8	68.5	73.5
30.0–34.9	793	55.2	11.4	38.1	40.9	43.4	47.3	54.3	62.6	67.2	70.3	74.8
35.0–39.9	732	56.3	11.9	39.7	43.0	44.9	47.8	54.7	63.3	68.8	71.7	76.7
40.0–44.9	722	56.3	11.2	39.0	42.2	45.3	48.7	55.6	63.8	67.6	70.3	74.4
45.0–49.9	745	55.6	12.0	37.3	41.2	43.6	47.8	55.1	62.6	67.7	71.3	75.5
50.0–54.9	764	54.3	11.6	36.0	40.0	42.7	46.5	53.4	62.0	65.5	68.9	75.3
55.0–59.9	694	54.2	11.4	36.3	40.8	42.7	46.4	53.8	61.6	65.1	68.1	73.3
60.0–64.9	1120	52.6	11.6	34.5	38.7	41.1	44.5	51.8	59.7	64.4	67.2	71.4
65.0–69.9	1488	49.3	11.1	31.3	35.6	38.3	42.1	48.9	56.7	60.4	63.0	67.5
70.0–74.9	1050	47.4	11.1	29.7	33.8	35.9	40.1	46.8	54.3	58.5	61.7	66.1
Females													
1.0–1.9	470	12.4	2.2	8.9	9.7	10.1	10.8	12.3	13.8	14.6	15.3	16.1
2.0–2.9	482	13.3	2.2	10.1	10.6	11.0	11.8	13.2	14.7	15.5	16.2	17.1
3.0–3.9	509	14.3	2.5	10.6	11.3	11.8	12.6	14.3	15.7	16.7	17.5	18.7
4.0–4.9	521	15.3	2.9	11.2	12.2	12.7	13.6	15.1	16.9	17.8	18.5	19.7
5.0–5.9	503	16.6	3.0	12.5	13.2	13.8	14.7	16.3	18.4	19.4	20.6	21.3
6.0–6.9	218	17.6	3.3	13.5	14.1	14.4	15.4	17.3	19.1	20.4	21.8	24.0
7.0–7.9	244	19.2	4.2	14.2	15.1	15.6	16.5	18.8	21.1	22.5	23.9	24.7
8.0–8.9	220	21.1	5.0	15.2	15.8	16.7	18.1	20.6	23.3	24.7	26.5	28.1
9.0–9.9	247	23.0	4.8	17.0	17.7	18.6	19.8	22.2	25.6	27.6	29.2	31.4
10.0–10.9	266	23.9	5.3	17.5	18.3	19.1	20.7	23.4	26.8	28.5	29.8	32.9
11.0–11.9	229	27.3	6.7	19.1	20.2	21.3	22.9	26.1	30.0	33.5	36.8	38.8
12.0–12.9	247	29.5	5.8	21.0	22.4	23.8	25.8	29.0	32.5	35.1	37.2	39.1
13.0–13.9	275	31.9	7.9	22.7	24.3	25.2	26.9	30.5	34.9	38.2	40.4	44.2
14.0–14.9	287	33.7	7.4	24.3	26.4	27.1	29.0	32.8	36.9	39.8	42.0	47.1
15.0–15.9	234	33.4	6.8	24.3	25.4	27.0	29.1	32.6	36.6	39.1	41.1	43.2
16.0–16.9	284	34.3	7.6	24.7	26.5	28.1	29.7	33.5	37.6	39.8	42.7	46.6
17.0–17.9	223	35.6	8.7	25.9	27.4	28.6	30.5	33.9	39.5	43.2	44.4	49.5
18.0–24.9	2058	29.3	8.0	19.2	21.4	22.5	24.3	28.0	32.7	35.7	38.0	42.2
25.0–29.9	1608	30.5	8.7	20.2	21.7	22.9	24.8	29.1	34.2	37.6	40.4	45.8
30.0–34.9	1362	32.1	10.1	21.0	22.8	24.0	25.9	30.1	35.8	39.9	42.9	49.5
35.0–39.9	1194	33.0	10.6	21.0	23.1	24.4	26.8	31.1	37.1	41.6	44.6	50.9
40.0–44.9	1135	33.9	11.7	21.2	23.1	25.1	27.1	31.5	38.2	43.2	47.4	52.8
45.0–49.9	825	34.0	10.8	21.3	22.8	24.4	27.0	32.0	38.4	44.2	47.5	54.0
50.0–54.9	857	34.7	10.4	21.8	24.4	25.5	27.8	32.9	39.1	43.1	47.9	54.1
55.0–59.9	753	36.0	11.9	22.4	24.7	26.1	28.4	33.9	41.4	46.1	50.8	58.0
60.0–64.9	1223	35.8	11.1	22.3	24.5	26.1	29.1	34.0	40.6	44.8	48.3	53.0
65.0–69.9	1644	35.7	11.1	21.9	24.4	26.0	28.5	33.9	40.5	45.2	48.5	55.8
70.0–74.9	1260	35.8	10.7	22.1	24.4	25.9	28.7	34.1	41.1	45.9	48.7	54.6

Note: Values for males and females aged 18 years and older have been adjusted for bone area by subtracting 10.0 cm² and 6.5 cm² respectively from the calculated mid upper arm muscle area.

Appendix B: Table 13.

Means, standard deviations, and percentiles of upper arm muscle area
(cm^2) by height (cm) for White Boys and Girls of 2 to 17 years

Height (cm)	N	Mean	SD	Percentiles								
				5	10	15	25	50	75	85	90	95
Boys: 2 to 11 years												
87–092	54	12.5	2.1	9.1	9.7	10.4	10.9	12.6	14.1	14.6	15.0	16.5
93–098	281	13.5	2.3	10.1	10.8	11.1	11.9	13.4	15.2	15.8	16.5	16.9
99–104	454	14.6	3.3	10.9	11.7	12.3	13.0	14.4	15.9	16.6	17.3	18.4
105–110	476	15.6	3.2	12.0	12.8	13.2	14.0	15.4	16.9	17.7	18.5	19.8
111–116	462	16.7	3.0	12.6	13.5	14.1	15.0	16.6	18.1	18.8	19.5	20.6
117–122	381	18.0	3.6	14.1	14.5	14.9	15.9	17.6	19.6	20.6	21.4	23.0
123–128	285	19.5	3.8	15.0	15.5	16.3	17.4	19.1	21.2	22.3	23.2	24.1
129–134	271	21.2	3.8	16.1	17.2	18.1	19.0	21.0	23.0	24.4	24.9	26.6
135–140	279	22.9	4.5	16.4	18.0	18.6	20.0	22.5	24.9	26.3	28.4	31.7
141–146	264	25.1	5.4	19.3	20.1	20.8	21.8	23.8	27.2	29.0	31.3	34.4
147–152	210	27.6	5.1	21.4	22.4	23.2	24.6	26.7	29.6	32.0	33.2	35.3
153–158	110	29.1	6.4	22.7	23.2	23.8	25.4	28.3	31.5	33.3	35.7	38.7
159–164	44	33.0	7.0	23.6	24.9	25.7	27.5	32.2	35.6	41.0	42.5	45.5
Boys: 12 to 17 years												
141–146	21	26.5	5.0	20.7	20.7	21.4	24.1	25.1	30.3	30.3	32.8	36.3
147–152	70	28.0	4.2	22.2	22.6	23.6	25.1	27.7	29.9	32.2	34.2	36.1
153–158	146	31.6	6.6	22.7	24.8	26.1	27.5	31.1	34.6	36.9	38.9	41.5
159–164	166	34.3	6.8	23.7	26.6	27.4	29.8	33.9	38.3	40.7	42.3	46.4
165–170	253	39.9	8.3	27.4	29.6	31.2	34.1	39.5	44.8	47.8	50.8	55.5
171–176	329	46.2	9.7	32.8	35.4	36.6	39.3	45.6	52.2	55.5	59.1	65.6
177–182	352	49.9	9.3	35.2	38.0	40.5	43.3	49.3	56.2	59.3	62.4	64.6
183–188	223	53.2	11.3	38.7	41.3	42.6	45.7	52.4	57.3	63.0	67.5	74.8
189–194	81	55.5	9.7	41.9	44.9	45.9	48.9	54.7	60.4	65.6	68.5	73.2
Girls: 2 to 10 years												
87–092	119	12.8	2.1	9.1	10.3	10.5	11.1	13.0	14.3	14.8	15.5	16.2
93–098	311	13.1	2.1	10.0	10.6	10.9	11.5	12.8	14.4	15.3	15.7	16.6
99–104	425	14.0	2.4	10.4	11.2	11.7	12.4	14.0	15.5	16.4	16.9	17.9
105–110	429	15.0	2.4	11.7	12.2	12.6	13.4	14.7	16.4	17.3	17.9	19.2
111–116	426	15.9	3.0	12.3	13.0	13.5	14.2	15.6	17.4	18.4	19.1	20.3
117–122	344	16.9	2.8	12.8	13.8	14.4	15.1	16.7	18.6	19.6	20.4	21.4
123–128	268	18.1	2.7	14.4	14.9	15.5	16.2	17.8	19.6	20.8	21.6	22.3
129–134	241	19.9	4.7	15.1	16.0	16.6	17.6	19.5	21.7	22.5	23.5	24.9
135–140	240	21.8	4.3	15.9	17.3	17.9	19.1	21.3	24.0	24.8	26.5	27.9
141–146	206	23.3	4.2	17.6	18.4	19.2	20.3	22.8	25.9	28.0	29.1	30.7
147–152	121	25.4	5.5	17.8	19.8	20.7	22.0	24.9	27.8	30.0	31.2	33.4
153–158	49	26.2	5.7	19.5	21.0	22.6	23.4	25.4	28.8	31.4	34.0	37.2
Girls: 11 to 17 years												
141–146	41	23.2	4.0	17.1	19.5	20.3	21.0	23.3	24.8	25.5	26.5	27.9
147–152	89	25.5	4.7	19.1	19.7	20.9	22.0	24.7	28.4	29.8	30.7	34.4
153–158	233	28.8	6.3	20.3	21.7	22.7	24.3	28.3	32.5	34.4	36.3	38.8
159–164	448	31.9	6.7	23.5	25.0	25.9	27.7	31.0	35.5	38.0	40.0	43.5
165–170	559	33.8	7.3	24.9	26.5	27.7	29.3	33.1	37.1	39.7	42.1	45.6
171–176	285	34.6	8.1	25.7	26.8	27.7	29.8	33.4	37.7	40.1	42.2	47.6
177–182	95	37.0	7.7	28.6	29.3	30.1	31.5	35.1	40.8	43.4	46.5	55.9

Means, standard deviations, and percentiles of upper arm fat area (cm^2)
by age (yrs) for White males and females of 1 to 74 years

Age (yrs)	N	Mean	SD	Percentiles								
				5	10	15	25	50	75	85	90	95
Males												
1.0–1.9	508	7.6	2.2	4.6	4.9	5.3	6.0	7.4	8.9	9.7	10.4	11.8
2.0–2.9	508	7.5	2.3	4.3	4.9	5.2	5.9	7.4	8.8	9.7	10.6	11.6
3.0–3.9	539	7.8	2.4	4.7	5.3	5.6	6.1	7.4	9.0	10.0	10.7	11.9
4.0–4.9	547	7.6	2.5	4.5	5.0	5.4	6.0	7.2	8.7	9.6	10.2	11.6
5.0–5.9	534	7.6	3.0	4.4	4.9	5.2	5.8	7.0	8.6	10.0	11.1	12.8
6.0–6.9	231	8.0	4.0	4.0	4.5	4.8	5.5	7.0	9.0	10.7	11.6	15.6
7.0–7.9	240	8.6	4.1	4.2	4.7	5.1	5.8	7.6	10.0	11.8	13.5	16.2
8.0–8.9	240	9.3	5.0	4.4	5.0	5.3	6.1	7.8	10.7	12.9	15.6	18.5
9.0–9.9	242	11.0	6.5	4.8	5.3	5.8	6.6	9.0	12.8	16.9	18.9	24.5
10.0–10.9	268	12.5	7.2	5.2	5.5	6.3	7.5	10.6	15.5	18.9	22.8	27.6
11.0–11.9	248	14.5	9.7	5.2	6.0	6.4	7.7	11.6	18.2	22.9	26.8	36.5
12.0–12.9	272	14.5	9.1	5.5	6.2	7.0	8.4	11.8	17.0	21.9	29.0	35.5
13.0–13.9	268	14.1	9.7	5.5	6.2	7.0	8.3	11.0	16.3	23.1	26.7	33.2
14.0–14.9	286	14.3	10.9	4.9	6.0	6.8	7.9	11.0	17.0	20.7	26.4	33.5
15.0–15.9	286	12.9	8.8	5.5	6.2	6.7	7.4	9.6	14.8	21.5	24.5	31.0
16.0–16.9	279	14.5	9.8	5.7	6.4	7.1	8.5	11.3	17.4	22.3	26.7	36.6
17.0–17.9	266	13.3	8.6	5.7	6.6	7.1	7.8	10.5	16.2	20.5	23.7	27.9
18.0–24.9	1463	17.3	10.5	6.2	7.2	8.1	9.7	14.5	22.5	27.2	31.0	37.5
25.0–29.9	1069	19.2	11.1	6.6	7.8	9.0	10.8	16.9	24.3	29.8	33.1	39.9
30.0–34.9	793	20.8	11.0	6.8	8.9	10.2	12.6	18.7	26.1	32.2	34.9	41.9
35.0–39.9	732	20.4	10.0	6.8	8.5	10.2	13.5	19.0	25.4	30.1	33.6	39.4
40.0–44.9	722	20.6	11.0	7.7	9.2	10.3	13.0	18.3	25.6	30.4	35.5	42.1
45.0–49.9	745	20.4	10.7	7.9	9.4	10.6	12.8	18.4	25.0	29.9	33.6	39.6
50.0–54.9	764	19.6	10.1	7.4	9.3	10.8	12.6	17.6	23.9	29.2	32.2	39.7
55.0–59.9	694	19.3	9.6	7.1	8.7	10.3	12.7	17.8	23.7	28.1	32.2	38.4
60.0–64.9	1120	19.2	10.0	7.0	9.1	10.2	12.4	17.2	23.7	27.9	31.7	37.6
65.0–69.9	1488	18.4	9.5	5.9	7.6	9.3	11.5	16.9	23.2	27.5	31.1	35.9
70.0–74.9	1050	18.1	9.3	6.4	8.3	9.6	11.6	16.3	22.6	26.2	29.8	35.4
Females												
1.0–1.9	470	7.4	2.4	4.1	4.7	5.1	5.7	7.2	8.6	9.8	10.6	11.8
2.0–2.9	482	7.8	2.4	4.5	5.0	5.5	6.2	7.5	9.2	10.2	11.0	12.1
3.0–3.9	509	8.0	2.4	4.6	5.2	5.7	6.4	8.0	9.4	10.3	11.0	12.2
4.0–4.9	521	8.1	2.4	4.6	5.2	5.7	6.5	7.9	9.4	10.5	11.3	12.6
5.0–5.9	503	8.7	3.2	4.9	5.4	5.9	6.6	8.0	9.9	11.4	12.5	14.4
6.0–6.9	218	9.1	3.7	4.7	5.3	5.7	6.8	8.6	10.3	11.6	13.8	16.4
7.0–7.9	244	10.0	4.4	5.1	5.7	6.4	7.2	9.2	11.3	13.3	15.2	19.3
8.0–8.9	220	11.7	6.8	5.3	6.1	6.8	7.7	10.2	13.7	16.1	18.5	24.4
9.0–9.9	247	13.9	7.4	6.3	6.8	7.6	9.3	12.3	15.8	19.1	22.9	28.3
10.0–10.9	266	14.2	7.4	6.2	7.1	7.4	8.7	12.3	17.8	21.1	24.9	29.9
11.0–11.9	229	16.6	9.2	7.1	8.1	8.9	10.6	13.7	20.5	24.4	28.2	36.9
12.0–12.9	247	16.8	8.3	7.6	8.5	9.5	11.0	15.1	20.7	23.9	27.2	32.7
13.0–13.9	275	19.1	10.8	6.7	7.9	9.8	11.7	16.4	23.4	28.9	32.6	40.8
14.0–14.9	287	20.9	10.5	9.0	10.2	11.3	13.4	18.8	25.5	29.5	35.4	41.2
15.0–15.9	234	20.9	10.5	9.4	10.7	12.1	13.8	18.9	24.6	28.7	32.7	42.0
16.0–16.9	284	23.5	10.5	11.5	13.0	14.2	16.9	20.4	27.7	32.7	35.5	44.4
17.0–17.9	223	24.9	13.1	10.4	12.6	13.6	15.1	22.5	30.1	33.5	38.6	51.6
18.0–24.9	2058	25.3	13.0	10.7	12.5	14.0	16.4	22.2	30.5	36.6	41.4	50.6
25.0–29.9	1608	27.6	14.1	11.1	13.4	15.2	17.6	24.1	33.9	41.0	46.4	55.8
30.0–34.9	1362	30.9	15.4	12.6	15.1	17.4	20.4	27.8	37.6	44.6	50.5	62.1
35.0–39.9	1194	32.5	16.0	13.2	15.7	18.1	21.5	28.9	40.4	47.0	53.8	63.2
40.0–44.9	1135	33.3	15.4	14.0	16.7	19.2	22.7	30.3	40.9	48.1	54.3	63.8
45.0–49.9	825	35.4	15.9	14.6	17.4	20.0	24.3	32.9	43.8	51.1	55.8	65.9
50.0–54.9	857	35.7	15.0	14.5	18.4	21.6	25.5	33.4	43.5	51.0	56.2	63.4
55.0–59.9	753	36.5	16.0	14.0	18.4	20.7	25.6	34.2	44.6	52.9	57.2	66.6
60.0–64.9	1223	36.8	15.7	15.7	19.2	21.9	26.0	34.7	45.2	51.0	56.8	66.5
65.0–69.9	1644	34.4	14.8	14.7	17.7	19.9	24.0	32.3	42.1	48.3	52.8	59.9
70.0–74.9	1260	32.8	14.5	13.1	16.5	18.9	22.8	31.1	40.7	45.8	51.1	57.7

Means, standard deviations, and percentiles of arm fat index (arm fat area / total
arm area x 100) by age (yrs) for White males and females of 1 to 74 years

Age (yrs)	N	Mean	SD	Percentiles								
				5	10	15	25	50	75	85	90	95
Males												
1.0–1.9	508	36.4	7.8	24.5	26.4	28.1	30.6	36.4	41.6	45.0	46.5	49.2
2.0–2.9	508	34.7	7.8	23.0	24.6	26.5	28.8	34.4	40.1	42.7	45.2	49.0
3.0–3.9	539	33.7	7.1	23.4	25.5	26.7	28.6	33.1	37.9	41.7	43.7	46.7
4.0–4.9	547	31.5	6.9	21.7	23.0	24.5	26.4	30.9	35.6	38.1	40.8	44.5
5.0–5.9	534	29.8	7.1	20.1	21.7	22.7	25.0	28.8	34.3	36.9	38.7	42.5
6.0–6.9	231	28.6	7.6	18.5	20.2	21.4	23.0	27.4	34.1	36.6	38.3	40.4
7.0–7.9	240	28.4	8.6	16.7	19.3	20.4	22.0	27.5	32.7	37.4	39.8	45.2
8.0–8.9	240	28.3	8.3	16.9	18.7	19.7	22.4	27.6	32.5	36.3	39.8	44.0
9.0–9.9	242	29.3	9.2	17.1	19.3	20.6	22.1	27.7	34.8	38.7	41.1	47.1
10.0–10.9	268	30.3	9.7	16.3	18.8	20.4	22.7	28.7	36.2	41.0	44.6	49.4
11.0–11.9	248	31.2	11.1	16.4	18.5	20.5	23.0	29.4	37.9	43.8	46.7	51.4
12.0–12.9	272	29.6	10.8	14.2	17.3	18.7	21.5	28.3	35.0	41.8	46.4	51.3
13.0–13.9	268	26.3	11.0	12.9	14.4	15.7	18.2	23.5	31.6	37.9	42.5	47.6
14.0–14.9	286	23.6	10.2	10.8	12.6	13.6	16.4	21.1	28.9	34.6	38.3	43.8
15.0–15.9	286	20.8	9.9	10.8	11.9	12.8	14.0	17.9	24.0	30.2	34.4	41.8
16.0–16.9	279	20.7	8.9	9.9	11.2	12.3	14.4	18.2	25.2	29.6	33.4	39.7
17.0–17.9	266	18.5	7.7	10.0	10.6	11.8	13.2	16.4	22.3	26.1	28.9	33.8
18.0–24.9	1463	21.2	9.1	9.7	11.0	12.2	13.9	19.6	26.7	30.8	33.9	38.8
25.0–29.9	1069	22.1	9.2	9.6	11.4	12.8	15.0	20.7	28.1	31.9	34.7	39.5
30.0–34.9	793	23.3	9.2	9.7	12.2	13.6	16.4	22.3	28.8	33.1	35.6	40.5
35.0–39.9	732	22.8	8.7	10.1	11.9	13.9	16.4	22.2	27.9	31.1	33.9	38.9
40.0–44.9	722	22.9	9.0	10.7	12.4	13.8	16.2	21.5	28.0	32.1	35.2	40.1
45.0–49.9	745	22.9	8.7	11.1	13.0	14.2	16.6	21.6	27.9	32.3	34.8	39.0
50.0–54.9	764	22.6	8.5	11.4	13.1	14.4	16.4	21.3	27.3	31.5	34.9	39.2
55.0–59.9	694	22.4	8.2	10.4	12.5	13.7	16.5	21.5	27.0	30.6	33.4	38.9
60.0–64.9	1120	22.7	8.3	11.1	13.1	14.4	16.5	21.5	27.8	31.1	33.8	38.1
65.0–69.9	1488	22.8	8.5	10.4	12.6	13.9	16.3	21.9	28.0	31.4	34.0	38.5
70.0–74.9	1050	23.1	8.4	11.2	13.4	14.8	17.1	22.1	28.0	31.5	33.6	38.1
Females												
1.0–1.9	470	37.1	8.5	24.3	26.2	28.3	30.4	36.8	42.1	46.0	49.0	51.9
2.0–2.9	482	36.8	7.7	24.3	27.1	28.8	31.3	36.7	41.6	44.8	46.6	50.0
3.0–3.9	509	35.7	7.2	24.9	26.7	28.3	30.4	35.8	40.3	42.6	44.5	47.8
4.0–4.9	521	34.5	7.7	23.1	25.2	26.8	29.3	34.3	39.4	42.1	43.8	46.0
5.0–5.9	503	33.6	7.3	22.4	25.0	26.1	28.7	33.0	38.1	40.6	42.8	45.7
6.0–6.9	218	33.2	7.5	21.5	24.2	25.7	27.8	33.4	37.9	40.0	42.0	45.8
7.0–7.9	244	33.5	8.0	21.5	23.9	25.5	28.1	33.1	37.4	41.6	44.7	47.2
8.0–8.9	220	34.2	9.3	20.2	22.6	24.6	27.7	33.9	38.9	43.8	46.0	49.5
9.0–9.9	247	36.0	9.3	21.9	24.1	25.9	29.4	35.3	41.8	46.2	48.8	52.6
10.0–10.9	266	35.7	9.7	22.1	24.1	25.2	28.4	34.5	42.1	47.2	49.6	52.8
11.0–11.9	229	36.1	9.5	22.1	24.4	26.1	29.6	35.1	41.8	46.6	48.7	52.7
12.0–12.9	247	34.8	8.6	21.9	24.6	25.9	28.7	33.7	40.2	44.5	47.5	49.7
13.0–13.9	275	35.5	9.9	20.1	22.4	24.8	28.4	35.3	42.4	46.3	48.2	52.0
14.0–14.9	287	36.8	9.8	22.1	24.3	26.3	29.7	36.4	43.8	46.5	50.0	53.0
15.0–15.9	234	37.1	9.2	23.1	25.5	27.2	29.7	37.6	42.8	46.5	48.7	53.5
16.0–16.9	284	39.4	9.0	25.5	27.5	29.5	33.2	39.4	45.0	48.3	51.9	54.4
17.0–17.9	223	39.5	10.0	24.6	26.8	28.7	31.6	40.0	45.8	49.5	52.7	56.0
18.0–24.9	2058	39.6	9.9	23.6	26.8	28.9	32.8	39.4	46.4	50.3	53.1	56.2
25.0–29.9	1608	40.9	10.1	24.6	27.8	29.9	33.7	40.7	48.2	52.4	54.4	57.2
30.0–34.9	1362	42.8	10.0	25.7	29.5	32.5	36.0	43.1	49.9	53.5	55.3	58.9
35.0–39.9	1194	43.5	10.0	26.1	30.2	33.0	36.9	43.7	50.6	53.7	56.5	59.2
40.0–44.9	1135	43.8	9.8	27.7	30.3	33.3	37.5	44.7	50.5	53.5	55.6	59.1
45.0–49.9	825	45.1	9.6	28.8	32.1	34.8	39.0	45.5	52.1	55.4	57.2	59.1
50.0–54.9	857	45.1	9.4	27.9	32.3	35.5	39.8	45.6	51.5	54.8	56.8	59.4
55.0–59.9	753	44.8	9.5	27.3	32.5	34.7	39.0	45.3	51.6	54.8	56.0	58.6
60.0–64.9	1223	45.2	9.2	28.8	32.7	35.4	39.6	45.7	51.6	54.5	56.5	58.7
65.0–69.9	1644	43.6	9.2	27.9	31.0	34.0	37.5	44.0	50.2	53.0	54.7	57.5
70.0–74.9	1260	42.3	9.5	25.5	29.6	32.2	36.2	43.1	49.0	51.8	53.5	56.9

Means, standard deviations, and percentiles of triceps skinfold thickness
(mm) by age (yrs) for White males and females of 1 to 74 years

Age (yrs)	N	Mean	SD	Percentiles								
				5	10	15	25	50	75	85	90	95
Males												
1.0–1.9	508	10.5	2.8	6.5	7.0	7.5	8.5	10.0	12.0	13.5	14.0	15.5
2.0–2.9	513	10.1	2.8	6.0	7.0	7.0	8.0	10.0	12.0	13.0	14.0	15.0
3.0–3.9	541	10.1	2.7	6.5	7.0	7.5	8.0	10.0	12.0	13.0	14.0	15.0
4.0–4.9	547	9.6	2.7	6.0	7.0	7.0	8.0	9.0	11.0	12.0	13.0	14.5
5.0–5.9	535	9.3	3.0	5.5	6.5	6.5	7.0	8.5	10.5	12.0	13.0	14.5
6.0–6.9	231	9.3	3.6	5.0	6.0	6.0	6.5	8.5	10.5	12.0	13.0	16.0
7.0–7.9	240	9.6	4.0	5.0	6.0	6.0	7.0	9.0	11.0	13.0	15.0	17.5
8.0–8.9	240	9.9	4.3	5.0	6.0	6.0	7.0	9.0	11.5	13.0	16.0	18.5
9.0–9.9	242	11.1	5.3	5.5	6.0	6.5	7.0	10.0	13.0	16.5	17.0	21.0
10.0–10.9	269	12.0	5.7	5.5	6.0	7.0	8.0	10.5	14.5	18.0	20.0	24.0
11.0–11.9	248	13.2	7.1	5.5	6.0	7.0	8.0	11.5	16.0	20.0	24.0	30.0
12.0–12.9	272	12.8	6.7	5.5	6.0	7.0	8.0	11.0	14.5	20.0	23.0	28.5
13.0–13.9	268	11.9	7.0	5.0	5.5	6.5	7.0	10.0	14.0	18.5	22.0	26.0
14.0–14.9	286	11.1	6.9	4.5	5.0	6.0	6.6	9.0	14.0	16.0	20.0	24.0
15.0–15.9	286	10.0	6.5	5.0	5.0	5.0	6.0	7.5	11.5	15.0	18.0	22.0
16.0–16.9	279	10.4	6.1	4.0	5.0	5.5	6.5	8.5	12.5	15.5	18.5	24.0
17.0–17.9	266	9.3	5.2	4.5	5.0	5.5	6.0	7.5	11.5	14.0	16.0	19.0
18.0–24.9	1463	11.6	6.3	4.5	5.0	6.0	7.0	10.0	15.0	18.0	20.0	24.0
25.0–29.9	1070	12.5	6.5	5.0	5.5	6.0	7.5	11.0	16.0	19.0	21.0	25.0
30.0–34.9	794	13.4	6.5	5.0	6.0	7.0	8.5	12.0	16.5	20.0	22.0	25.5
35.0–39.9	732	13.1	6.0	5.0	6.0	7.0	8.5	12.0	16.0	19.0	21.0	24.5
40.0–44.9	722	13.2	6.4	5.0	6.0	7.0	8.5	12.0	16.0	19.0	22.0	26.0
45.0–49.9	745	13.1	6.2	5.5	6.5	7.0	9.0	12.0	16.0	19.0	21.0	24.5
50.0–54.9	764	12.8	6.0	5.5	6.5	7.5	8.5	12.0	15.5	19.0	20.5	25.0
55.0–59.9	694	12.6	5.7	5.0	6.0	7.0	8.5	11.5	15.0	18.0	20.5	24.0
60.0–64.9	1120	12.6	5.9	5.0	6.5	7.0	8.5	11.5	15.5	18.0	20.0	23.5
65.0–69.9	1489	12.4	5.8	5.0	6.0	6.5	8.0	11.5	15.0	18.0	20.0	23.0
70.0–74.9	1051	12.4	5.7	5.0	6.0	7.0	8.0	11.5	15.0	18.0	20.0	23.0
Females												
1.0–1.9	470	10.5	3.1	6.0	7.0	7.5	8.0	10.0	12.0	13.5	15.0	16.5
2.0–2.9	482	10.7	2.9	6.5	7.0	8.0	9.0	10.5	12.5	14.0	15.0	16.0
3.0–3.9	509	10.6	2.8	6.5	7.0	8.0	8.5	10.5	12.0	13.0	14.0	16.0
4.0–4.9	522	10.5	2.9	6.0	7.0	7.5	8.5	10.0	12.0	13.0	14.0	15.5
5.0–5.9	504	10.6	3.3	6.0	7.0	8.0	8.5	10.0	12.0	14.0	15.0	16.5
6.0–6.9	218	10.8	3.6	6.0	7.0	7.5	8.0	10.5	12.0	13.5	15.0	17.0
7.0–7.9	244	11.4	4.0	6.0	7.0	8.0	9.0	11.0	13.0	15.0	17.0	19.0
8.0–8.9	221	12.5	5.5	6.5	7.0	8.0	9.0	11.5	15.0	17.0	18.0	22.5
9.0–9.9	248	14.1	5.8	7.0	8.0	8.5	10.0	13.0	16.5	19.5	22.0	25.5
10.0–10.9	266	14.2	5.9	7.0	8.0	8.0	10.0	13.0	17.5	20.0	22.5	27.0
11.0–11.9	229	15.4	6.6	7.0	8.5	9.0	11.0	13.0	18.5	21.5	24.5	29.0
12.0–12.9	247	15.2	5.9	8.0	9.0	9.5	11.0	14.0	18.0	20.5	23.0	27.0
13.0–13.9	275	16.4	7.2	7.0	8.0	9.5	11.0	15.0	20.0	24.0	25.0	30.0
14.0–14.9	287	17.5	7.1	9.0	10.0	10.5	12.0	17.0	21.0	23.5	27.0	31.0
15.0–15.9	234	17.6	6.8	8.5	10.0	11.0	12.5	17.0	20.5	23.0	26.0	32.0
16.0–16.9	284	19.4	6.9	10.5	12.0	13.0	14.5	18.0	22.5	26.0	29.0	32.5
17.0–17.9	223	20.0	8.1	10.0	11.5	12.0	14.0	19.0	24.0	26.5	30.0	35.0
18.0–24.9	2058	20.2	8.1	10.0	11.0	12.0	14.5	19.0	24.5	28.0	31.0	35.5
25.0–29.9	1608	21.5	8.5	10.0	12.0	13.0	15.0	20.0	26.0	30.5	33.5	38.0
30.0–34.9	1362	23.5	8.8	11.0	13.0	15.0	17.0	22.5	29.0	32.5	35.0	40.0
35.0–39.9	1194	24.3	9.0	12.0	13.5	15.5	18.0	23.0	30.0	34.0	36.0	40.5
40.0–44.9	1136	24.7	8.7	12.0	14.0	16.0	18.5	24.0	30.0	34.0	36.5	40.0
45.0–49.9	826	25.9	8.9	12.5	15.0	16.5	20.0	25.5	31.0	35.5	37.5	42.0
50.0–54.9	858	26.1	8.6	12.0	15.5	17.5	20.5	25.5	31.5	35.5	37.5	40.5
55.0–59.9	754	26.3	8.8	12.0	15.0	17.0	20.5	26.0	32.0	35.0	37.5	42.0
60.0–64.9	1223	26.5	8.7	13.0	16.0	17.5	20.5	26.0	32.0	35.5	38.0	42.0
65.0–69.9	1644	25.0	8.3	12.0	15.0	16.0	19.0	24.5	30.0	33.0	35.5	39.0
70.0–74.9	1260	24.0	8.3	11.5	14.0	15.5	18.0	24.0	29.5	32.0	34.5	38.0

Means, standard deviations, and percentiles of subscapular skinfold thickness
(mm) by age (yrs) for White males and females of 1 to 74 years

Age (yrs)	N	Mean	SD	Percentiles								
				5	10	15	25	50	75	85	90	95
Males												
1.0–1.9	508	6.3	1.9	4.0	4.0	4.5	5.0	6.0	7.0	8.0	8.5	10.0
2.0–2.9	513	5.8	2.0	3.5	4.0	4.0	4.5	5.5	6.5	7.5	8.5	9.5
3.0–3.9	540	5.5	1.8	3.5	4.0	4.0	4.5	5.0	6.0	7.0	7.0	9.0
4.0–4.9	546	5.3	2.0	3.0	3.5	4.0	4.0	5.0	6.0	6.5	7.0	8.5
5.0–5.9	535	5.2	2.3	3.0	3.5	4.0	4.0	5.0	5.5	6.5	7.0	8.0
6.0–6.9	231	5.6	3.3	3.0	3.5	3.5	4.0	4.5	6.0	7.0	8.0	13.0
7.0–7.9	240	5.9	3.4	3.0	3.5	4.0	4.0	5.0	6.0	7.0	9.0	12.0
8.0–8.9	240	6.0	3.9	3.0	3.5	4.0	4.0	5.0	6.0	7.5	9.0	12.0
9.0–9.9	242	7.1	5.1	3.5	4.0	4.0	4.0	5.5	7.5	10.5	12.5	15.0
10.0–10.9	269	7.7	5.4	3.5	4.0	4.0	4.5	6.0	8.0	11.0	14.0	19.5
11.0–11.9	248	9.3	8.1	4.0	4.0	4.0	5.0	6.0	10.0	15.0	20.0	27.0
12.0–12.9	273	9.1	7.1	4.0	4.0	4.5	5.0	6.5	10.0	14.0	19.0	24.0
13.0–13.9	268	9.3	7.6	4.0	4.0	5.0	5.0	7.0	10.0	14.0	17.0	26.0
14.0–14.9	286	9.4	6.9	4.0	5.0	5.0	5.5	7.0	10.0	14.0	16.0	23.0
15.0–15.9	286	9.2	6.5	5.0	5.0	5.5	6.0	7.0	10.0	12.0	15.5	22.0
16.0–16.9	278	10.2	6.5	5.0	6.0	6.0	6.5	8.0	11.0	14.0	17.0	23.5
17.0–17.9	267	10.1	5.7	5.0	6.0	6.5	7.0	8.0	11.5	14.0	17.0	20.5
18.0–24.9	1461	13.5	7.5	6.0	7.0	7.0	8.0	11.0	16.0	20.0	24.0	30.0
25.0–29.9	1067	15.6	8.0	7.0	7.5	8.0	10.0	13.5	20.0	24.5	26.5	30.5
30.0–34.9	791	17.3	8.2	7.0	8.0	9.0	11.0	16.0	22.0	25.5	28.0	32.5
35.0–39.9	730	17.4	8.0	7.0	8.0	10.0	11.0	16.0	22.0	25.0	27.5	32.0
40.0–44.9	714	17.3	8.0	7.0	8.0	9.5	11.5	16.0	21.5	25.5	28.0	33.0
45.0–49.9	739	18.2	8.2	7.5	9.0	10.0	12.0	17.0	23.0	26.5	30.0	34.0
50.0–54.9	759	17.7	8.1	7.0	8.0	9.0	12.0	16.0	22.5	26.0	30.0	34.0
55.0–59.9	691	17.6	7.8	7.0	8.5	10.0	11.5	16.5	22.5	25.5	28.0	31.0
60.0–64.9	1112	18.1	8.3	7.0	8.0	10.0	12.0	17.0	23.0	26.0	29.0	33.5
65.0–69.9	1486	16.9	8.0	6.0	8.0	9.0	11.0	15.5	21.5	25.0	28.0	32.0
70.0–74.9	1048	16.4	7.6	6.5	7.5	9.0	11.0	15.0	21.0	25.0	27.5	30.5
Females												
1.0–1.9	470	6.4	2.0	4.0	4.0	4.5	5.0	6.0	7.5	8.5	9.0	10.0
2.0–2.9	483	6.3	2.1	4.0	4.0	4.5	5.0	6.0	7.0	8.0	9.0	10.5
3.0–3.9	509	6.2	2.2	3.5	4.0	4.5	5.0	6.0	7.0	8.0	9.0	10.0
4.0–4.9	522	6.0	2.1	3.5	4.0	4.0	4.5	5.5	7.0	8.0	8.5	10.0
5.0–5.9	503	6.2	2.9	3.5	4.0	4.0	4.5	5.5	7.0	8.0	9.0	12.0
6.0–6.9	218	6.4	3.2	3.5	4.0	4.0	4.5	5.5	7.0	9.0	10.0	11.5
7.0–7.9	244	6.8	3.6	4.0	4.0	4.0	4.5	6.0	7.0	9.5	11.0	13.0
8.0–8.9	221	8.0	6.0	3.5	4.0	4.0	5.0	6.0	8.0	11.5	14.5	21.0
9.0–9.9	248	9.4	6.8	4.0	4.5	5.0	5.0	7.0	10.0	14.0	18.5	24.5
10.0–10.9	266	9.8	6.4	4.0	4.5	5.0	5.5	7.0	11.5	16.0	19.5	24.0
11.0–11.9	227	10.7	7.4	4.5	5.0	5.0	6.0	8.0	12.0	16.0	21.0	28.5
12.0–12.9	247	10.9	6.9	5.0	5.5	6.0	6.0	9.0	12.5	15.5	19.5	29.0
13.0–13.9	275	11.9	7.8	5.0	5.5	6.0	7.0	9.5	15.0	19.0	22.0	26.5
14.0–14.9	287	13.0	7.7	6.0	6.5	7.0	7.5	10.5	16.0	21.0	24.5	30.0
15.0–15.9	234	12.7	7.0	6.0	7.0	7.5	8.0	10.0	15.0	20.0	22.0	27.0
16.0–16.9	284	14.2	8.5	6.5	7.5	8.0	9.0	11.5	16.0	22.5	25.5	32.0
17.0–17.9	223	15.4	9.1	6.0	7.0	7.5	9.0	12.5	19.0	24.5	28.0	34.0
18.0–24.9	2058	15.7	9.1	6.0	7.0	8.0	9.0	13.0	19.5	25.0	28.0	35.0
25.0–29.9	1603	16.8	10.1	6.0	7.0	8.0	9.0	14.0	21.5	27.0	32.0	38.0
30.0–34.9	1359	18.6	11.1	6.5	7.0	8.0	10.0	15.5	25.0	30.5	35.5	41.0
35.0–39.9	1189	19.5	11.2	7.0	8.0	9.0	10.8	16.0	26.0	32.0	35.5	43.0
40.0–44.9	1131	19.6	10.7	6.5	7.5	9.0	11.0	17.0	26.0	32.0	35.0	39.5
45.0–49.9	823	20.9	10.8	7.0	8.5	10.0	12.0	19.0	28.0	33.0	35.5	41.5
50.0–54.9	852	21.8	10.8	7.0	9.0	10.0	13.0	20.5	28.0	34.0	37.0	42.0
55.0–59.9	745	22.2	11.2	7.0	9.0	10.5	13.0	20.5	30.0	34.5	36.5	41.5
60.0–64.9	1213	22.2	11.0	7.5	9.0	10.5	13.5	20.5	30.0	34.0	37.5	42.5
65.0–69.9	1636	20.7	10.3	7.0	8.0	10.0	12.5	19.0	27.0	31.5	35.0	40.0
70.0–74.9	1256	20.2	10.0	6.5	8.5	10.0	12.0	19.0	26.0	31.0	35.0	38.0

Means, standard deviations, and percentiles of sum of triceps and subscapular skinfold thicknesses (mm) by age (yrs) for White males and females of 1 to 74 years

Age (yrs)	N	Mean	SD	Percentiles								
				5	10	15	25	50	75	85	90	95
Males												
1.0–1.9	508	16.8	4.0	11.0	12.0	12.5	14.0	16.5	19.0	21.0	22.5	24.0
2.0–2.9	513	16.0	4.2	10.0	11.5	12.0	13.0	15.5	18.0	20.0	21.5	24.0
3.0–3.9	540	15.6	4.0	11.0	11.5	12.0	13.0	15.0	17.5	19.5	20.5	23.0
4.0–4.9	546	14.9	4.3	10.0	10.5	11.0	12.0	14.0	17.0	18.0	19.0	22.5
5.0–5.9	535	14.5	4.9	9.5	10.0	11.0	11.5	13.5	16.5	18.0	19.2	22.0
6.0–6.9	231	14.8	6.5	8.6	9.5	10.0	11.0	13.0	16.0	19.0	21.0	28.0
7.0–7.9	240	15.5	6.9	8.5	9.5	10.0	11.0	14.0	17.5	20.5	23.0	28.5
8.0–8.9	240	15.9	7.8	9.0	9.5	10.0	11.0	14.0	17.0	21.0	25.0	29.5
9.0–9.9	242	18.2	9.9	9.0	10.0	10.5	12.0	15.0	21.0	27.0	31.0	35.5
10.0–10.9	269	19.7	10.5	9.5	10.0	11.0	13.0	16.5	23.5	28.0	33.5	42.5
11.0–11.9	248	22.6	14.4	9.5	10.5	11.0	13.0	17.5	26.0	36.4	41.5	55.0
12.0–12.9	272	21.8	12.9	9.5	10.5	11.5	13.0	17.5	24.0	34.0	41.0	53.0
13.0–13.9	268	21.2	14.1	10.0	11.0	11.5	13.0	16.0	23.5	31.5	41.0	49.0
14.0–14.9	286	20.5	13.3	9.5	11.0	11.5	13.0	16.0	23.0	28.5	35.0	47.0
15.0–15.9	286	19.2	12.5	10.0	11.0	11.0	12.0	15.0	21.5	29.5	32.5	42.0
16.0–16.9	278	20.5	11.8	10.0	11.5	12.0	13.0	16.5	23.5	29.0	35.5	46.5
17.0–17.9	266	19.4	10.4	10.5	11.5	12.0	13.0	16.0	23.5	28.0	32.0	39.0
18.0–24.9	1460	25.0	12.9	11.0	12.5	13.5	16.0	21.5	30.5	37.0	42.0	50.5
25.0–29.9	1066	28.0	13.4	12.0	13.5	15.0	17.5	25.5	35.5	41.0	46.0	53.0
30.0–34.9	791	30.6	13.6	12.5	15.0	17.0	20.5	28.5	38.5	44.0	48.5	56.5
35.0–39.9	729	30.4	12.7	12.5	15.0	17.5	21.0	29.0	37.0	42.0	47.0	52.0
40.0–44.9	713	30.3	12.9	13.0	15.5	17.5	21.5	28.5	37.0	42.5	47.5	55.0
45.0–49.9	736	31.1	13.0	14.0	16.5	18.0	21.5	29.5	39.0	43.5	47.5	55.0
50.0–54.9	759	30.3	12.7	13.5	16.0	17.5	21.5	28.5	37.5	43.0	48.0	55.5
55.0–59.9	691	30.1	12.1	12.5	16.0	18.0	21.0	29.0	37.0	42.5	47.0	52.5
60.0–64.9	1111	30.6	12.8	13.0	16.0	18.0	21.5	29.0	37.5	42.5	47.0	55.0
65.0–69.9	1486	29.3	12.7	11.5	14.0	16.5	20.0	27.5	36.0	42.0	46.5	53.0
70.0–74.9	1048	28.7	12.1	12.0	15.0	17.0	20.0	27.0	35.0	41.0	44.5	51.0
Females												
1.0–1.9	470	16.9	4.6	10.5	12.0	12.0	14.0	16.5	19.5	21.5	23.0	25.0
2.0–2.9	482	17.0	4.5	11.0	12.0	13.0	14.0	16.5	19.0	22.0	23.5	25.5
3.0–3.9	509	16.8	4.4	10.5	12.0	12.5	14.0	16.5	19.0	20.5	22.0	25.0
4.0–4.9	522	16.4	4.4	10.5	11.5	12.0	13.5	16.0	18.5	20.5	22.0	24.0
5.0–5.9	503	16.9	5.6	10.5	11.5	12.0	13.5	16.0	18.5	21.0	23.5	28.5
6.0–6.9	218	17.2	6.2	10.0	11.0	12.0	13.5	16.5	19.5	22.0	24.0	28.0
7.0–7.9	244	18.2	7.1	10.0	11.5	12.0	14.0	16.5	20.5	24.0	26.0	32.5
8.0–8.9	221	20.5	11.0	10.5	11.5	13.0	14.0	17.5	23.0	28.5	32.0	41.5
9.0–9.9	248	23.4	12.0	11.5	12.5	13.5	16.0	20.0	26.5	30.5	40.0	49.0
10.0–10.9	266	24.0	11.8	12.0	13.0	13.5	15.5	20.5	28.5	34.5	41.0	50.5
11.0–11.9	227	25.9	13.0	13.0	14.0	15.0	17.0	22.0	31.0	37.0	42.5	55.0
12.0–12.9	247	26.1	12.0	13.0	14.5	16.0	18.0	23.0	31.0	36.3	41.0	52.0
13.0–13.9	275	28.3	14.4	12.5	14.0	16.0	18.5	24.5	36.0	42.5	46.0	56.5
14.0–14.9	287	30.5	14.0	15.0	16.5	18.0	20.5	27.0	38.0	44.5	48.5	61.5
15.0–15.9	234	30.3	13.2	15.5	18.0	19.0	21.5	27.0	34.5	42.5	48.0	60.5
16.0–16.9	284	33.6	14.6	17.5	20.0	21.5	24.0	29 5	39.5	46.0	53.5	64.5
17.0–17.9	223	35.4	16.4	17.0	19.0	20.5	23.0	31.5	42.0	50.0	56.5	69.0
18.0–24.9	2057	35.8	16.2	17.0	19.4	21.5	24.5	32.0	43.5	51.0	57.0	69.0
25.0–29.9	1598	38.1	17.5	17.5	20.0	22.0	25.0	34.0	47.0	57.0	63.5	73.0
30.0–34.9	1357	42.0	18.8	18.5	22.0	24.5	28.0	38.0	52.0	62.0	68.5	80.5
35.0–39.9	1187	43.7	18.9	19.0	22.5	25.0	29.5	39.5	54.0	63.5	69.0	81.0
40.0–44.9	1128	44.1	18.0	20.0	23.5	26.0	30.5	41.0	54.5	63.0	70.0	77.5
45.0–49.9	820	46.7	18.4	21.0	24.0	27.5	33.0	44.5	58.0	66.5	71.5	80.0
50.0–54.9	849	47.7	17.8	21.0	25.5	29.5	35.0	46.0	59.0	67.0	73.0	79.5
55.0–59.9	744	48.2	18.5	21.0	26.0	29.0	34.5	46.5	60.0	67.5	72.0	80.0
60.0–64.9	1212	48.6	18.2	22.5	27.0	29.5	35.0	46.5	60.0	67.5	73.0	82.5
65.0–69.9	1633	45.6	17.1	21.0	25.0	28.5	33.5	43.0	56.0	63.5	69.0	76.5
70.0–74.9	1255	44.2	16.8	18.5	23.5	27.0	32.5	42.5	55.0	61.0	66.5	74.5

Appendix B: Table 19.
Means, standard deviations, and percentiles of weight (kg) by age (yrs)
for adult White males of small, medium, and large frames

Age (yrs)	N	Mean	SD	Percentiles 5	10	15	25	50	75	85	90	95
Males with small frames
18.0–24.9	370	70.4	11.1	54.5	57.4	59.8	63.2	69.3	76.4	81.0	83.9	89.6
25.0–29.9	273	74.5	12.2	57.9	60.9	62.1	66.1	73.1	81.6	85.8	88.3	97.9
30.0–34.9	202	76.4	11.5	59.6	63.0	65.1	68.4	75.4	83.3	87.0	91.5	97.6
35.0–39.9	187	76.3	11.4	56.6	61.7	63.3	67.9	76.5	83.9	88.6	91.6	96.0
40.0–44.9	183	79.5	12.0	62.3	64.6	68.8	71.9	77.6	87.4	93.0	96.8	101.3
45.0–49.9	189	76.9	11.5	58.8	62.3	63.8	68.3	76.8	84.1	89.4	92.6	96.4
50.0–54.9	195	75.9	11.7	57.3	62.8	65.2	67.5	75.4	83.0	88.2	90.5	99.4
55.0–59.9	176	74.7	12.2	54.0	58.2	61.8	66.4	75.1	81.5	87.2	90.9	94.7
60.0–64.9	283	74.0	11.9	56.4	60.2	62.5	65.8	73.6	80.8	85.7	88.4	93.3
65.0–69.9	376	71.6	12.0	51.1	56.0	59.0	62.9	71.4	79.9	84.1	86.8	91.8
70.0–74.9	267	70.5	11.7	50.1	54.5	58.7	62.6	70.5	78.1	82.6	84.9	92.2
Males with medium frames
18.0–24.9	733	74.7	12.7	57.9	60.8	62.4	65.9	72.3	81.0	87.0	93.1	100.5
25.0–29.9	535	77.7	13.1	59.5	63.0	65.2	69.3	76.7	84.6	88.9	93.2	100.7
30.0–34.9	399	78.8	13.0	60.0	63.4	66.2	69.7	78.1	85.7	91.6	94.0	99.1
35.0–39.9	367	80.8	12.0	60.9	66.3	69.8	73.7	80.6	87.1	91.5	94.6	101.6
40.0–44.9	361	80.7	12.4	61.2	65.3	68.4	72.5	79.9	88.4	93.4	97.8	102.6
45.0–49.9	375	80.7	12.9	60.1	65.2	67.3	72.1	79.8	88.6	93.3	96.7	101.3
50.0–54.9	383	79.3	13.4	58.6	63.4	66.4	70.9	78.5	86.4	91.7	96.7	102.2
55.0–59.9	347	79.0	11.9	60.2	65.8	67.1	71.2	78.0	85.4	91.1	95.4	100.9
60.0–64.9	561	76.9	11.9	58.4	61.8	65.3	69.2	76.9	84.5	88.6	91.5	97.8
65.0–69.9	743	75.6	11.8	56.7	60.7	63.4	67.9	75.1	83.2	87.0	90.8	96.7
70.0–74.9	527	74.4	11.9	55.2	59.1	62.9	66.6	73.7	81.8	86.6	90.3	93.9
Males with large frames
18.0–24.9	362	77.4	14.5	58.4	61.5	62.7	67.6	75.0	85.4	91.2	95.0	103.3
25.0–29.9	265	83.6	15.9	61.2	66.0	68.3	72.8	82.0	90.9	99.3	102.1	113.5
30.0–34.9	196	86.5	14.5	64.6	69.1	70.9	76.3	86.0	94.0	101.0	104.3	115.5
35.0–39.9	178	84.8	15.0	59.6	67.4	71.4	75.4	83.6	92.6	98.4	104.1	115.3
40.0–44.9	179	84.8	16.3	63.6	67.4	68.7	73.4	81.8	92.2	100.3	107.4	113.8
45.0–49.9	184	85.2	15.7	64.2	67.3	69.4	75.3	83.9	92.5	97.9	103.2	113.2
50.0–54.9	189	84.0	14.7	64.3	66.6	68.8	73.0	82.4	92.5	100.9	102.8	110.2
55.0–59.9	170	85.5	15.0	64.8	68.1	71.5	75.1	84.5	92.8	100.0	102.6	116.3
60.0–64.9	277	82.1	14.3	62.7	66.7	69.5	73.1	80.1	89.4	94.5	98.9	107.3
65.0–69.9	368	79.6	13.5	58.2	62.0	66.3	71.0	78.9	87.5	92.2	95.7	103.9
70.0–74.9	258	77.2	13.2	55.8	61.6	64.8	68.4	76.9	83.2	90.5	94.7	99.6

Means, standard deviations, and percentiles of weight (kg) by age (yrs)
for adult White females of small, medium, and large frames

Age (yrs)	N	Mean	SD	Percentiles								
				5	10	15	25	50	75	85	90	95
Females with small frames												
18.0–24.9	518	56.2	8.3	44.0	46.7	48.5	50.6	54.9	60.9	64.5	66.9	71.5
25.0–29.9	408	56.9	9.5	44.4	47.3	48.5	51.3	55.9	60.9	63.7	66.1	72.6
30.0–34.9	346	58.6	9.4	46.1	48.3	50.0	52.6	57.0	62.5	66.8	68.8	77.1
35.0–39.9	302	60.7	10.7	45.9	48.2	50.8	53.4	59.4	66.2	71.0	74.7	78.4
40.0–44.9	288	60.3	9.1	48.0	50.3	51.8	54.5	58.8	65.2	70.5	73.1	78.1
45.0–49.9	212	60.9	10.5	46.5	48.8	50.9	53.5	60.1	66.3	70.5	73.1	79.7
50.0–54.9	218	61.0	9.8	46.8	49.3	51.5	54.4	60.1	66.7	70.4	72.9	76.5
55.0–59.9	192	60.4	9.6	45.4	49.3	51.6	54.4	59.2	64.9	69.6	72.3	79.1
60.0–64.9	310	61.6	10.5	46.6	48.5	50.6	54.2	60.7	67.9	71.4	73.9	79.8
65.0–69.9	416	60.8	10.4	45.1	48.4	51.1	53.5	60.0	67.3	70.8	73.5	79.0
70.0–74.9	318	60.1	11.4	42.6	45.9	48.5	51.5	59.6	66.4	72.0	74.2	79.3
Females with medium frames												
18.0–24.9	1031	59.3	10.0	46.6	48.8	50.2	52.6	57.9	64.1	68.1	71.9	77.8
25.0–29.9	808	60.5	11.4	46.9	49.1	50.2	52.7	58.1	66.1	72.2	76.0	81.6
30.0–34.9	685	62.6	12.4	47.2	50.0	51.7	54.2	60.1	68.3	73.7	78.6	83.6
35.0–39.9	600	63.1	11.3	49.2	51.7	53.0	55.9	60.8	67.6	72.8	76.7	83.5
40.0–44.9	572	64.2	12.8	49.0	51.0	53.2	56.1	61.6	68.8	75.4	80.1	90.6
45.0–49.9	415	64.9	12.7	47.7	50.9	53.0	55.9	62.8	71.2	76.9	81.9	89.0
50.0–54.9	432	65.8	12.0	48.8	52.4	54.5	57.3	63.6	72.3	78.0	81.6	89.6
55.0–59.9	378	66.2	13.4	48.2	50.6	53.6	57.3	64.5	73.3	78.4	84.1	89.2
60.0–64.9	613	65.5	11.8	49.1	51.7	53.3	57.3	64.2	72.7	77.6	81.1	87.2
65.0–69.9	823	65.7	12.6	48.5	51.3	53.3	56.3	64.4	72.7	78.1	81.1	87.8
70.0–74.9	630	63.9	11.6	47.1	50.6	52.5	56.6	62.5	70.2	75.9	79.1	83.9
Females with large frames												
18.0–24.9	511	66.8	16.5	48.6	50.8	52.7	55.3	62.1	74.3	81.9	86.4	102.1
25.0–29.9	401	70.5	17.6	49.8	52.7	55.1	57.8	66.0	79.7	87.7	96.3	104.0
30.0–34.9	340	74.3	19.1	50.5	53.6	56.8	60.1	69.3	87.2	95.6	101.3	109.4
35.0–39.9	295	75.5	18.7	52.3	55.0	56.7	61.5	71.8	86.1	94.5	98.9	108.9
40.0–44.9	282	76.9	18.6	52.3	56.8	59.9	64.0	73.5	86.8	94.9	100.6	110.8
45.0–49.9	204	78.9	17.6	56.0	60.3	63.2	65.8	76.0	86.1	97.6	102.2	112.5
50.0–54.9	213	75.9	15.9	50.6	58.7	61.2	65.5	73.0	85.5	93.1	98.5	106.7
55.0–59.9	185	78.1	15.6	55.9	59.8	61.9	66.1	76.4	88.2	92.9	99.1	105.6
60.0–64.9	302	76.9	15.8	56.0	58.5	61.3	65.7	75.8	84.7	91.3	98.8	104.2
65.0–69.9	408	75.3	15.6	54.8	58.4	60.8	63.8	73.8	82.5	90.8	97.2	105.7
70.0–74.9	311	74.3	13.2	53.9	57.6	60.7	65.7	74.4	81.9	87.0	90.0	93.9

Appendix B: Table 21.

Means, standard deviations, and percentiles of muscle area (cm^2) by age
(yrs) for adult White males of small, medium, and large frames

Age (yrs)	N	Mean	SD	Percentiles								
				5	10	15	25	50	75	85	90	95
Males with small frames												
18.0–24.9	370	45.5	10.5	31.3	33.7	35.7	38.9	44.4	51.1	55.0	57.5	63.2
25.0–29.9	273	48.4	9.9	33.3	36.8	39.2	42.0	47.8	53.9	58.0	61.3	63.7
30.0–34.9	200	49.5	9.6	35.5	37.9	39.0	41.8	48.6	55.4	58.7	62.4	66.2
35.0–39.9	187	51.4	10.0	36.2	39.5	41.2	44.6	50.7	57.3	61.7	65.1	70.0
40.0–44.9	183	52.0	9.9	35.5	39.0	41.2	45.3	52.0	58.5	61.8	64.7	66.8
45.0–49.9	189	49.1	10.5	32.8	36.2	38.9	42.3	48.7	55.6	59.1	62.5	65.9
50.0–54.9	195	49.1	11.0	33.3	35.0	38.2	41.9	48.6	55.7	60.4	62.9	68.0
55.0–59.9	176	47.3	10.0	29.8	35.3	37.2	41.0	47.4	53.7	57.2	61.1	64.9
60.0–64.9	283	48.5	11.1	32.6	36.6	38.7	41.1	47.6	54.6	58.8	61.6	66.4
65.0–69.9	376	44.6	10.4	26.7	31.3	34.2	37.3	44.3	52.2	56.0	57.9	61.1
70.0–74.9	266	42.8	9.9	27.4	30.8	32.0	35.7	42.7	48.9	52.3	55.4	58.4
Males with medium frames												
18.0–24.9	731	50.6	10.6	35.7	38.2	40.9	43.4	49.5	56.4	60.7	64.0	70.6
25.0–29.9	534	53.9	11.3	37.3	40.1	42.6	46.0	53.0	60.7	65.8	68.0	73.0
30.0–34.9	398	54.5	10.0	38.5	41.5	44.8	47.8	54.1	60.4	64.5	67.5	70.8
35.0–39.9	366	56.4	11.1	41.1	43.4	45.5	48.8	55.6	63.2	68.6	70.8	74.1
40.0–44.9	360	56.4	10.9	39.2	42.4	45.7	48.9	55.7	63.2	67.5	70.4	74.4
45.0–49.9	373	56.6	11.2	39.1	42.8	45.5	49.5	55.9	63.6	69.2	72.6	76.2
50.0–54.9	382	54.5	10.6	37.8	41.8	44.4	47.6	53.6	61.9	64.7	67.0	73.1
55.0–59.9	347	55.0	10.3	39.5	42.5	44.4	48.4	54.7	61.6	65.1	68.0	73.1
60.0–64.9	560	52.3	10.7	34.5	38.9	41.6	44.9	52.1	59.1	63.3	66.2	70.3
65.0–69.9	743	49.6	10.1	33.4	37.3	39.7	42.8	49.4	56.3	59.5	61.9	66.3
70.0–74.9	526	47.7	10.4	30.7	34.7	36.7	40.8	47.5	54.3	58.5	61.6	65.4
Males with large frames												
18.0–24.9	360	55.2	11.7	37.6	40.8	42.6	47.3	54.1	62.1	66.7	70.2	74.6
25.0–29.9	262	59.5	11.3	42.8	45.7	48.0	51.5	58.9	66.5	69.9	73.2	79.3
30.0–34.9	194	62.6	11.9	44.6	47.6	50.2	54.2	63.6	70.3	74.6	77.1	82.0
35.0–39.9	178	61.0	13.2	43.2	46.0	47.7	51.6	59.2	69.0	74.0	78.2	81.9
40.0–44.9	179	60.5	11.6	43.0	46.5	49.3	51.9	59.1	67.9	70.6	75.0	83.2
45.0–49.9	183	60.3	12.2	44.2	46.3	48.0	51.8	59.5	67.0	69.5	73.6	83.2
50.0–54.9	187	59.0	11.8	41.2	45.1	47.4	50.8	58.7	66.8	71.7	74.8	79.2
55.0–59.9	169	59.5	11.4	42.4	45.0	47.9	52.6	58.5	66.4	70.6	73.3	79.1
60.0–64.9	275	57.4	12.0	38.9	43.6	46.1	48.9	56.8	65.6	68.1	71.5	77.3
65.0–69.9	367	53.5	11.7	35.6	39.3	41.5	46.0	53.0	61.4	65.1	67.9	73.4
70.0–74.9	258	51.5	12.0	33.0	38.3	40.3	43.5	50.9	58.6	63.3	66.3	72.2

Note: Values for males aged 18 years and older have been adjusted for bone area by subtracting 10.0 cm² from the calculated mid upper arm muscle area (see text).

Means, standard deviations, and percentiles of muscle area (cm^2) by age
(yrs) for adult White females of small, medium, and large frames

Age (yrs)	N	Mean	SD	Percentiles								
				5	10	15	25	50	75	85	90	95
Females with small frames												
18.0–24.9	517	26.0	6.0	17.9	19.4	20.3	22.2	25.4	29.0	31.2	32.8	36.2
25.0–29.9	407	27.4	7.0	19.4	20.5	21.2	22.9	26.4	30.5	32.5	34.8	36.7
30.0–34.9	346	28.1	7.9	19.1	21.6	22.4	24.2	27.4	30.8	32.7	35.2	37.6
35.0–39.9	301	29.4	10.1	19.4	21.7	23.1	24.5	28.5	32.2	34.7	36.4	40.3
40.0–44.9	285	29.3	6.5	20.5	21.8	22.8	25.3	28.6	32.4	35.5	37.8	41.8
45.0–49.9	209	28.7	6.8	18.3	21.0	22.1	24.0	28.0	32.5	34.9	38.2	39.1
50.0–54.9	218	29.9	6.2	20.8	22.1	23.9	25.6	29.0	33.4	36.4	37.9	40.7
55.0–59.9	192	30.5	7.6	19.8	22.2	23.1	25.5	29.9	34.2	37.1	38.9	43.5
60.0–64.9	310	31.5	8.5	20.5	22.4	23.6	25.8	31.0	35.8	38.4	40.4	44.5
65.0–69.9	416	31.1	7.9	19.5	22.1	23.7	25.7	30.1	35.2	39.0	41.6	45.2
70.0–74.9	317	31.7	9.6	19.2	22.4	23.9	25.8	30.3	35.9	39.6	42.6	47.3
Females with medium frames												
18.0–24.9	1030	28.8	6.6	19.7	21.7	22.9	24.7	27.9	32.2	34.6	36.5	39.8
25.0–29.9	807	29.9	7.4	20.7	22.1	23.1	24.7	28.7	33.6	36.5	38.9	42.8
30.0–34.9	685	31.5	8.8	21.5	22.9	24.0	25.9	30.4	35.2	38.4	40.3	44.6
35.0–39.9	598	31.8	8.1	21.2	23.1	24.4	26.8	30.8	36.0	39.6	42.1	45.2
40.0–44.9	569	32.5	9.1	21.1	23.1	24.2	26.8	30.8	36.1	40.8	44.1	49.0
45.0–49.9	415	33.2	8.7	22.0	23.5	24.9	27.4	31.9	37.2	42.2	44.9	49.3
50.0–54.9	430	34.5	9.7	22.7	24.9	26.0	28.3	33.0	39.1	43.5	46.7	52.8
55.0–59.9	376	35.0	9.5	23.5	25.2	26.5	28.5	33.6	39.3	42.7	45.4	48.7
60.0–64.9	613	34.6	8.8	22.9	25.3	26.4	29.2	34.2	40.2	44.1	48.1	51.9
65.0–69.9	821	35.4	10.0	22.1	24.7	26.4	28.8	33.7	40.2	43.5	46.1	51.2
70.0–74.9	630	35.0	9.5	22.5	24.4	26.1	28.9	33.7	39.2	43.5	46.1	51.2
Females with large frames												
18.0–24.9	511	33.5	10.1	21.7	23.7	25.0	27.2	31.7	37.3	40.9	45.7	53.5
25.0–29.9	394	35.2	10.8	21.4	24.2	26.1	28.1	33.1	39.7	43.5	48.6	56.7
30.0–34.9	331	37.4	12.1	23.1	24.9	26.3	28.8	34.5	44.1	49.2	52.8	60.7
35.0–39.9	295	39.2	12.9	23.4	26.5	27.8	31.1	37.0	44.6	50.4	53.7	63.2
40.0–44.9	281	41.4	16.2	25.8	27.6	29.4	32.0	38.8	47.2	52.0	55.8	65.6
45.0–49.9	201	41.2	14.0	23.7	26.9	28.7	32.0	38.8	47.5	55.1	60.2	64.4
50.0–54.9	209	40.1	12.5	24.0	25.9	29.1	32.0	37.5	47.9	53.5	57.8	63.5
55.0–59.9	184	44.0	15.4	26.5	28.6	31.8	35.7	41.4	50.1	57.8	59.3	63.5
60.0–64.9	298	42.6	14.3	25.8	28.6	30.8	33.2	40.3	48.9	53.0	56.3	67.7
65.0–69.9	406	40.9	13.3	25.6	27.6	29.2	32.2	37.5	46.4	53.6	58.1	66.5
70.0–74.9	311	41.5	11.8	25.6	27.9	30.2	32.7	40.0	48.4	51.1	54.8	60.8

Note: Values for males aged 18 years and older have been adjusted for bone area by subtracting 6.5 cm^2 from the calculated mid upper arm muscle area (see text).

Subject Index